Lippincott's
ANESTHESIA REVIEW:
1,001
QUESTIONS AND ANSWERS

Lippincott's
ANESTHESIA REVIEW:
1,001
QUESTIONS AND ANSWERS

Paul Sikka, MD, PhD

*Department of Anesthesia and
Perioperative Medicine
Signature Healthcare Brockton Hospital,
Brockton, Massachusetts
Affiliate of Beth Israel Deaconess Medical
Center, Boston, Massachusetts (Former
Faculty—Brigham and Women's Hospital,
Harvard Medical School)*

**Edward A. Bittner, MD, PhD,
  FCCP, FCCM**

*Program Director, Critical Care Medicine-
Anesthesiology Fellowship, Associate
Director, Surgical Intensive Care Unit,
Assistant Professor of Anaesthesia,
Harvard Medical School, Massachusetts
General Hospital, Department of
Anesthesia, Critical Care, and Pain
Medicine, Boston, Massachusetts*

**Thomas M. Halaszynski, DMD,
  MD, MBA**

*Associate Professor of Anesthesiology,
Director of Regional Anesthesia/
Acute Pain Medicine, Department of
Anesthesiology, Yale University School of
Medicine, Yale New Haven Hospital, New
Haven, Connecticut*

Thoha M. Pham, MD

*Associate Clinical Professor, University
of California, San Francisco (UCSF),
Department of Anesthesia and
Perioperative Care, San Francisco, California*

**Ashish C. Sinha, MD, PhD,
  DABA**

*Vice Chairman, Anesthesiology &
Critical Care, Drexel University College
of Medicine, Hahnemann University
Hospital, Philadelphia, Pennsylvania*

. Wolters Kluwer

Philadelphia • Baltimore • New York • London
Buenos Aires • Hong Kong • Sydney • Tokyo

Acquisitions Editor: Brian Brown
Product Development Editor: Nicole Dernoski
Editorial Assistant: Lindsay Burgess
Production Project Manager: Bridgett Dougherty
Design Coordinator: Stephen Druding
Manufacturing Coordinator: Beth Welsh
Marketing Manager: Dan Dressler
Prepress Vendor: S4C Publishing Services

9 8 7 6 5 4 3 2 1

Printed in China (or the United States of America)

Library of Congress Cataloging-in-Publication Data

Sikka, Paul, author.
Lippincott's anesthesia review : 1001 questions and answers / Paul Sikka, Edward Bittner, Thomas Halaszynski, Thoha Pham, Ashish Sinha.
    p. ; cm.
  Anesthesia review
   ISBN 978-1-4511-3200-7 (paperback) — ISBN 1-4511-3200-X (paperback)
  I. Bittner, Edward A., 1967- author.   II. Halaszynski, Thomas, author.   III. Pham, Thoha, author.   IV. Sinha, Ashish, author.   V. Title.   VI. Title: Anesthesia review.
  [DNLM: 1. Anesthesia--Examination Questions.   2. Anesthetics—Examination Questions. WO 218.2]
  RD82.3
  617.9'6076—dc23
                                                                                      2014019574

LWW.com

"Dedicated to our Parents and Teachers"
who selflessly pass on their values and knowledge to us

Mian Ahmad, MD
Department of Anesthesiology and Perioperative
    Medicine, Drexel University College of Medicine,
    Philadelphia, Pennsylvania

Sheri M. Berg, MD
Instructor, Department of Anesthesia,
    Critical Care, and Pain Medicine,
    Massachusetts General Hospital,
    Boston, Massachusetts

Edward A. Bittner, MD, PhD, FCCP, FCCM
Program Director, Critical Care
    Medicine-Anesthesiology Fellowship,
    Associate Director, Surgical Intensive Care Unit,
    Assistant Professor of Anaesthesia,
    Harvard Medical School,
    Massachusetts General Hospital,
    Department of Anesthesia, Critical Care,
    and Pain Medicine,
    Boston, Massachusetts

Yuriy S. Bronshteyn, MD
Surgical Critical Care Fellow, Massachusetts
    General Hospital, Department of Anesthesia,
    Critical Care, and Pain Medicine,
    Boston, Massachusetts

Thomas M. Halaszynski, DMD, MD, MBA
Associate Professor of Anesthesiology, Director
    of Regional Anesthesia/Acute Pain Medicine,
    Department of Anesthesiology,
    Yale University School of Medicine,
    Yale New Haven Hospital,
    New Haven, Connecticut

Darrin J. Hyatt, MD
Anesthesia Chief Resident, Department of
    Anesthesia, Critical Care, and Pain Medicine,
    Massachusetts General Hospital,
    Boston, Massachusetts

Daniel W. Johnson, MD
Assistant Professor, Fellowship Director, Critical Care
    Anesthesiology, Department of Anesthesiology,
    University of Nebraska Medical Center,
    Omaha, Nebraska

Rebecca Kalman, MD
Clinical Instructor in Anesthesia,
    Massachusetts General Hospital,
    Boston, Massachusetts

Jean Kwo, MD
Anesthesiologist, Department of Anesthesia,
    Critical Care, and Pain Medicine,
    Massachusetts General Hospital,
    Assistant Professor of Anaesthesia,
    Harvard Medical School,
    Boston, Massachusetts

Jinlei Li, MD
Assistant Professor of Anesthesiology,
    Yale University School of Medicine,
    Yale New Haven Hospital,
    New Haven, Connecticut

Dipty Mangla, MD
Staff Anesthesiologist,
    Cumberland Pain Management,
    Cumberland, Maryland

Ala Nozari, MD
Assistant Professor, Department of Anesthesia,
    Critical Care, and Pain Medicine,
    Massachusetts General Hospital,
    Boston, Massachusetts

Thoha M. Pham, MD
Associate Clinical Professor,
    University of California, San Francisco (UCSF),
    Department of Anesthesia
    and Perioperative Care,
    San Francisco, California

Manish Purohit, MD
Department of Anesthesiology and Perioperative
    Medicine, Drexel University College of Medicine,
    Philadelphia, Pennsylvania

Paul Sikka, MD, PhD
Department of Anesthesia and Perioperative
    Medicine, Signature Healthcare Brockton
    Hospital, Brockton, Massachusetts,
    Affiliate of Beth Israel Deaconess Medical Center,
    Boston, Massachusetts
    (Former Faculty—Brigham and Women's
    Hospital, Harvard Medical School)

Ashish C. Sinha, MD, PhD, DABA
Vice Chairman, Anesthesiology & Critical Care,
    Drexel University College of Medicine,
    Hahnemann University Hospital,
    Philadelphia, Pennsylvania

Preet Mohinder Singh, MD
Department of Anesthesia,
    All India Institute of Medical Sciences,
    New Delhi, India

David L. Stahl, MD
Clinical Fellow, Department of Anesthesia,
    Critical Care and Pain Medicine,
    Massachusetts General Hospital,
    Boston, Massachusetts

Deppu Ushakumari, MD
Department of Anesthesiology and Perioperative
    Medicine, Drexel University College of Medicine,
    Philadelphia, Pennsylvania

The practice of anesthesiology requires a solid foundation of knowledge. It is with extreme pleasure that we introduce *Lippincott's Anesthesia Review: 1,001 Questions and Answers.* The book is designed to rapidly review anesthesiology to help residents pass the written examinations taken during and after residency. The book is broadly divided into 21 chapters to cover almost all relevant topics tested. Each question is followed by four possible answers, among which one is the best or most likely answer.

The editors acknowledge the work of all who have given their valuable time and effort to complete this book. These include all authors, proofreaders (including Shilpa Shah, MD), and the team at Lippincott Williams & Wilkins. We would also like to thank our families for their support while we prepared this manuscript.

We hope that this review book proves to be a valuable educational resource for anesthesia residents and young practitioners to help them pass the boards. For any constructive suggestions, please contact us by email: Anes1001@outlook.com.

The Editors

CONTENTS

Contributors vii
Preface ix

1. Perioperative Evaluation and Management 1
PREET SINGH, MANISH PUROHIT, ASHISH SINHA, AND PAUL SIKKA

2. Airway Management 25
YURIY BRONSHTEYN AND EDWARD BITTNER

3. Anesthesia Machine 39
PAUL SIKKA

4. Patient Monitoring 47
DARREN HYATT, ALA NOZARI, AND EDWARD BITTNER

5. Fluid Management and Blood Transfusion 61
REBECCA KALMAN AND EDWARD BITTNER

6. Anesthetic Pharmacology 71
MIAN AHMAD AND ASHISH SINHA

7. Spinal and Epidural Anesthesia 103
THOMAS HALASZYNSKI

8. Peripheral Nerve Blocks 113
THOMAS HALASZYNSKI

9. Pain Management 127
THOMAS HALASZYNSKI

10. Orthopedic Anesthesia 137
THOMAS HALASZYNSKI

11. Cardiovascular Anesthesia 145
DEPPU USHAKUMARI AND ASHISH SINHA

12. Thoracic Anesthesia 173
DEPPU USHAKUMARI AND ASHISH SINHA

13. Neuroanesthesia 191
DIPTY MANGLA AND ASHISH SINHA

14. Gastrointestinal, Liver, and Renal Diseases 205
THOHA PHAM

15. Endocrine Diseases 223
JEAN KWO AND EDWARD BITTNER

16. Ophthalmic, Ear, Nose, and Throat Surgery 231
THOHA PHAM

17. Obstetric Anesthesia 247
THOHA PHAM

18. Pediatric Anesthesia 267
DIPTY MANGLA AND ASHISH SINHA

19. Critical Care 283
DAVID STAHL, DANIEL JOHNSON, AND EDWARD BITTNER

20. Postoperative Anesthesia Care 299
SHERI BERG AND EDWARD BITTNER

21. Miscellaneous Topics 313
PAUL SIKKA AND THOMAS HALASZYNSKI

Perioperative Evaluation and Management

Preet Singh, Manish Purohit, Ashish Sinha, and Paul Sikka

1. Preoperative application of scopolamine patch to prevent postoperative nausea and vomiting should be avoided in

   A. Female, 35 years old
   B. Smoker, 20 years old
   C. Patient with a blood pressure of 160/96 mm Hg
   D. Male, 70 years old

2. Which of the following drugs is least likely to be effective for prophylaxis for postoperative nausea and vomiting?

   A. Ondansetron
   B. Scopolamine patch
   C. Aprepitant
   D. Metoclopramide

3. Famotidine, when used for stress ulcer prophylaxis, must be avoided preoperatively in which of the following patients?

   A. Patients with replaced mitral valve on warfarin
   B. Patients with idiopathic thrombocytopenic purpura (ITP) for splenectomy
   C. Patients with achalasia cardia for esophageal myotomy
   D. Patients with a history of coronary stenting on aspirin

4. Which of the following drugs antagonizes substance P in the central nervous system and is used as premedication to prevent postoperative nausea and vomiting?

   A. Palonosetron
   B. Aprepitant
   C. Metoclopramide
   D. Prochlorperazine

5. Which of the following predictors is likely to be associated with lower incidence of perioperative nausea and vomiting?

   A. Female gender
   B. Use of fentanyl for pain relief
   C. Patients with a history of smoking
   D. Patients undergoing laparoscopic surgery

6. All of the following have an antiemetic action, except
   A. Promethazine
   B. Propofol
   C. Etomidate
   D. Haloperidol

7. Cefazolin, as a component of perioperative antimicrobial prophylaxis for surgery, must begin within what time before incision?
   A. Simultaneously with incision
   B. Within 30 minutes prior to incision
   C. Within 60 minutes prior to incision
   D. Within 120 minutes prior to incision

8. Vancomycin, as a component of perioperative antimicrobial prophylaxis for surgery, must begin within what time before incision?
   A. Simultaneously with incision
   B. Within 30 minutes prior to incision
   C. Within 60 minutes prior to incision
   D. Within 120 minutes prior to incision

9. A 65-year-old male with a history of hypertension and diabetes presents to emergency department with altered sensation with a likely subdural hematoma. To assess his cardiorespiratory status, he is asked about his level of physical activity. If he is capable of performing at least which of the following activities independently, he is less likely to have significant cardiopulmonary ailment during surgery?
   A. Walk to washroom on level floor
   B. Play the accordion
   C. Walk one block
   D. Climb a flight of stairs

10. In preoperative assessment of patients, physical activity is graded in terms of metabolic equivalents (METs). The value that corresponds to oxygen consumption of 1 MET in an adult is
    A. 2 mL/kg/min
    B. 7 mL/kg/min
    C. 3.5 mL/kg/min
    D. 5.5 mL/kg/min

11. As per American Society of Regional Anesthesia (ASRA) guidelines, intravenous infusion of unfractionated heparin should be stopped how long prior to a planned epidural?
    A. 1 to 1.5 hours
    B. 2 to 4 hours
    C. at least 12 hours
    D. at least 24 hours

12. For emergent surgery, anticoagulation produced by warfarin can be reversed by using
    A. Fresh-frozen plasma (FFP)
    B. Injectable vitamin K
    C. Prothrombin complex concentrate
    D. Factor VIII concentrate

13. Neuraxial block is not contraindicated for patients on which of the following drugs?

    A. Warfarin
    B. Low-molecular-weight heparin
    C. Aspirin
    D. Clopidogrel

14. All of the following are risk factors for obstructive sleep apnea, except

    A. Obesity
    B. Short neck
    C. Enlarged tonsils
    D. Female gender

15. A 70-year-old male, who is diabetic for the last 20 years, is scheduled for an elective surgery. Which of the following is *not* a sign of autonomic diabetic neuropathy?

    A. History of recurrent diarrhea
    B. History of postural hypotension
    C. History of recurrent constipation
    D. History of urinary retention

16. Which of the following perioperative factors in patients undergoing dialysis prior to surgery predicts the possibility of hypotension (due to increased volume removed)?

    A. Change in serum sodium
    B. Change in body weight
    C. Change in serum potassium
    D. Change in pH after dialysis

17. A patient with a history of severe asthma is scheduled for an appendectomy. Which of the following induction agents will cause the least respiratory depression?

    A. Ketamine
    B. Propofol
    C. Etomidate
    D. Thiopental

18. Which of the following drugs can significantly prolong the QT interval on the ECG?

    A. Dexamethasone
    B. Dropcridol
    C. Aprepitant
    D. Glycopyrrolate

19. Which of the following tests is used to confirm coagulation after stopping low-molecular-weight heparin (LMWH)?

    A. PT
    B. aPTT
    C. ACT
    D. None of the above

20. Effect of combined administration of midazolam and fentanyl is

    A. Additive
    B. Synergistic
    C. Competitively antagonistic
    D. Noncompetitively antagonistic

21. Preoperative anesthetic evaluation is likely to bring down the incidence of all the following, except

    A. Case cancellations
    B. Patient morbidity
    C. Preoperative anxiety
    D. Direct procedural costs

22. For elective procedures, an anesthesia provider must obtain informed and preferably written consent

    A. Just prior to transferring the patient to the operating room for surgery
    B. During preoperative anesthetic evaluation
    C. At the same time that a surgeon obtains consent for the surgical procedure
    D. Just prior to induction of anesthesia in the operating room

23. An optimal preoperative evaluation is designed

    A. To screen for and properly manage comorbid conditions
    B. To assess the risk of anesthesia and surgery and lower it
    C. To identify patients who may require special anesthetic techniques or postoperative care
    D. All the above

24. ASA classification for risk stratification is validated for predicting preoperative morbidity associated with the following, except

    A. General or regional anesthesia
    B. Conscious sedation
    C. Monitored anesthesia care
    D. Surgical procedure

25. A healthy pregnant patient in labor has which of the following ASA classifications?

    A. I
    B. II
    C. III
    D. IV

26. Sedatives, as premedication, must be avoided in which of the following patients?

    A. Uncontrolled hypertensive
    B. Toddler for tonsillectomy
    C. Brain tumor patients
    D. Patients with alcohol abuse

27. As per the American Society of Regional Anesthesia (ASRA) guidelines, which of the following drugs can be continued preoperatively in patients planned for neuraxial blockade for an elective procedure?

    A. Aspirin
    B. Clopidogrel
    C. Warfarin
    D. Low-molecular-weight heparin

28. As per ASA classification, a controlled hypertensive patient with no target end-organ damage scheduled for elective surgery will be classified as

    A. ASA I
    B. ASA II
    C. ASA III
    D. ASA VI

29. A brain-dead organ donor undergoing laparotomy for "kidney harvesting" will be classified as an

    A. ASA III
    B. ASA IV
    C. ASA V
    D. ASA VI

30. A moribund patient who is not expected to survive without the operation is categorized as an

    A. ASA III
    B. ASA IV
    C. ASA V
    D. ASA VI

31. A patient with a history of uncontrolled hypertension, diabetes, and angina, who is to undergo a laparoscopic cholecystectomy, will be classified as an

    A. ASA II
    B. ASA III
    C. ASA IV
    D. ASA V

32. A 65-year-old male with a history of mitral valve replacement 2 years back presents for a knee replacement. He is on warfarin since the time of valve replacement. As per ASRA guidelines, the ideal time to stop his warfarin prior to surgery would be

    A. 12 hours
    B. 3 days
    C. 5 days
    D. 10 days

33. A 26-year-old female, with a history of rheumatic mitral stenosis, is scheduled for an elective cesarean section at 38 weeks of gestation. Just prior to surgery, she is diagnosed to have atrial fibrillation (AF) with no hemodynamic instability. The first step in preparation for surgery is

    A. Perform an echocardiogram to rule out left-atrial clot
    B. Synchronized DC cardioversion under sedation
    C. Antiarrhythmic medication
    D. Plan for therapy postdelivery

34. A 72-year-old patient with a history of hypertension and angina at moderate activity is to undergo a laparoscopic cholecystectomy. Due to decreased effort tolerance and a significant blockade of left anterior descending coronary artery onstress thallium, a preprocedure coronary intervention is planned. Which of the following procedures performed prior to the elective surgery is least likely to delay the laparoscopic surgery?

    A. Coronary artery bypass graft (CABG)
    B. Percutaneous coronary stenting—bare-metallic stent
    C. Percutaneous coronary stenting—drug-eluting stent
    D. Percutaneous balloon dilatation

35. Which of the following is *not* seen as a result of primary renal disease in patients with chronic renal failure?

    A. Hypocoagulable state
    B. Hypercoagulable state
    C. Hyperproteinemia
    D. Anemia

36. A 2-year-old child is to undergo a tonsillectomy. The child had formula milk 2 hours ago. As per ASA guidelines, optimal NPO status would be to wait another _____ before proceeding to surgery:

    A. No waiting, since it is a child
    B. 2 hours
    C. 4 hours
    D. 6 hours

37. A 45-year-old patient is scheduled for an abdominal hysterectomy. She states that her aunt had a severe reaction to anesthesia and was in the ICU for 1 week. You would avoid which of the following drugs for her general anesthesia?

    A. Droperidol
    B. Ketamine
    C. Sevoflurane
    D. Etomidate

38. Elective surgery should be postponed after a myocardial infarction for at least

    A. 30 days
    B. 6 weeks
    C. 3 months
    D. 6 months

39. The most significant risk factor for developing pulmonary complications is

    A. Site of surgery (abdominal/thoracic)
    B. Presence of respiratory infection
    C. Presence of obstructive sleep apnea
    D. Smoking

40. Maximum international normalized ratio (INR) before proceeding for elective surgery should be

    A. 1.0
    B. 1.2
    C. 1.4
    D. 1.6

41. A 73-year-old patient has residual weakness on the right arm and leg following a stroke 5 years ago. He is now scheduled for laparoscopic cholecystectomy under general anesthesia. Which of the following sites should be preferably used to monitor the train of four muscle twitches for estimating neuromuscular blockade?

    A. Right ulnar nerve–innervated muscles
    B. Right posterior tibial nerve–innervated muscles
    C. Left ulnar nerve–innervated muscles
    D. Left facial nerve

42. A 32-year-old patient after being involved in a road traffic accident due to alcohol intoxication is taken to the operating room for open fracture reduction of an ankle fracture. His blood alcohol level is above the legal limit. Compared to a patient who is not intoxicated with alcohol, you would expect the minimum alveolar concentration (MAC) of sevoflurane to be

    A. Higher
    B. Lower
    C. Equal
    D. Unpredictable due to pharmacodynamic variations

43. A 55-year-old patient with a history of asthma and heart failure is to undergo a hernia repair. On physical examination, you notice that the patient is wheezing. Following treatment with albuterol, the patient should be monitored for which electrolyte?

    A. Potassium
    B. Calcium
    C. Sodium
    D. Chloride

44. Smoking cessation for 24 hours before a scheduled surgery will lead to

    A. Improvement of ciliary function
    B. Decrease in mucous production
    C. Decrease in airway irritability
    D. Decrease in level of carboxyhemoglobin

45. Which of the following tests is likely to detect clinically relevant bleeding tendency most efficiently?

    A. Activated partial thromboplastin time
    B. Prothrombin time
    C. Activated clotting time
    D. Thromboelastogram (TEG)

46. As per AHA guidelines, which of the following is not a major clinical risk predictor in a patient with cardiac disease scheduled for noncardiac surgery?

    A. Recent myocardial infarction
    B. Symptomatic mitral stenosis
    C. Presence of congestive cardiac failure
    D. Uncontrolled systolic hypertension

47. Glycopyrrolate, when given preoperatively, can cause all of the following, except

    A. Skin flushing
    B. Dry mouth
    C. Bronchoconstriction
    D. Tachycardia

48. Which of the following is true about metoclopramide?

    A. Decreases lower esophageal sphincter tone
    B. Delays gastric emptying
    C. Can cause extrapyramidal side effects
    D. Useful in preventing postoperative nausea

49. Which of the following occurs during the preoxygenation of a patient?

    A. Increase in functional residual capacity
    B. Denitrogenation
    C. Increase in CO_2 clearance from lungs
    D. Increase in closing capacity of lungs

50. Which of the following agents is associated with the highest incidence of hepatitis postoperatively?

    A. Halothane
    B. Isoflurane
    C. Desflurane
    D. Sevoflurane

51. The inhalation agent of choice in a 2-year-old child for ophthalmologic surgery is
    A. Halothane
    B. Desflurane
    C. Sevoflurane
    D. Nitrous oxide

52. Which of the following is true of nitrous oxide?
    A. Acts on central nervous system GABA receptors
    B. Lowers pulmonary vascular resistance
    C. Suppresses EEG pattern in the cerebral cortex
    D. Precipitates vitamin B_{12} deficiency anemia

53. The antiemetic effect of propofol is thought to occur due to
    A. Depressant effect on the chemoreceptor trigger zone
    B. Inhibition of dopamine activity
    C. Inhibition of glutamate release
    D. All of the above

54. Which of the following is the preferred intravenous agent of induction of anesthesia for maintaining spontaneous breathing and airway tone?
    A. Midazolam
    B. Propofol
    C. Ketamine
    D. Diazepam

55. Succinylcholine is contraindicated in a patient with
    A. Chronic renal failure
    B. Duchene muscular dystrophy
    C. Myasthenia gravis
    D. Patient with full stomach

56. A 75-year-old patient with a history of hypertension is to undergo laparoscopic colectomy for carcinoma colon. Continuing of which of the following antihypertensive drugs, preoperatively, in the geriatric age group, can be associated with profound hypotension on induction of general anesthesia?
    A. Metoprolol
    B. Angiotensin-converting-enzyme (ACE) inhibitors
    C. Hydrochlorothiazide
    D. Furosemide

57. Which of the following findings in the preoperative evaluation cannot be attributed to obesity with obstructive sleep apnea (OSA) in a patient planned for bariatric surgery?
    A. Pulmonary artery hypertension
    B. Congestive heart failure
    C. Peripheral neuropathy
    D. Dementia

58. All of the following medications can be administered via an epidural anesthesia, except
    A. Fentanyl
    B. Sufentanil
    C. Alfentanil
    D. Remifentanil

59. Ondansetron causes its antiemetic effect by acting as an

   A. Agonist at 5-HT$_2$ receptors
   B. Antagonist at 5-HT$_2$ receptors
   C. Agonist at 5-HT$_3$ receptors
   D. Antagonist at 5-HT$_3$ receptors

60. Which of the following statements is false regarding scopolamine patch applied preoperatively?

   A. May produce sedation
   B. Decreases the risk of nausea
   C. Adds to the analgesia
   D. Inhibits muscarinic receptors

61. Overdose with dexmedetomidine results in

   A. Hypertension
   B. Bradycardia
   C. Hypertension and bradycardia
   D. Hypotension and bradycardia

62. Abrupt withdrawal of steroids can lead to

   A. Malignant hypertension
   B. Sickle cell crisis
   C. Addisonian crisis
   D. Psychosis

63. Promethazine primarily inhibits which of the following receptors?

   A. Serotonin
   B. Dopamine
   C. Muscarinic
   D. Acetylcholine

64. All of the following surgeries are associated with an increased risk of postoperative nausea and vomiting, except

   A. Shoulder arthroscopy
   B. Laparoscopic surgery
   C. Strabismus repair
   D. Tympanoplasty

65. Abrupt stoppage of total parenteral nutrition (TPN) would most likely cause

   A. Hypoglycemia
   B. Hyperglycemia
   C. Hyperphosphatemia
   D. Hypophosphatemia

66. Glycopyrrolate causes all of the following, except

   A. Sedation
   B. Tachycardia
   C. Antisialagogue effect
   D. Lowers lower esophageal sphincter tone

67. In general, herbal medications should be stopped before surgery for at least _____ days:

A. 3
B. 7
C. 10
D. 14

68. Which of the following antibiotics can prolong the action of neuromuscular-blocking drugs?

A. Gentamicin
B. Penicillin
C. Levofloxacin
D. Cephalexin

69. Estrogen in birth control pills increases the perioperative risk of

A. Diarrhea
B. Thromboembolism
C. Stroke
D. Myocardial infarction

70. A 42-year-old patient is scheduled for a hernia repair under general anesthesia. His medications include fluoxetine, alprazolam, and lithium for bipolar disorder. In the preoperative area, he appears confused, has tremors, and is ataxic. Your next step would be to

A. Cancel the case
B. Proceed with the case
C. Order a lithium blood level
D. Consult a psychiatrist

71. A 34-year-old patient is to undergo an appendectomy under general anesthesia. He is taking a monoamine oxidase inhibitor (MAOI) for depression. Intraoperatively, his blood pressure drops to 72/36 mm Hg and a medication is administered. His blood pressure suddenly increases to 220/120 mm Hg. The most likely medicine that was administered is

A. Ephedrine
B. Meperidine
C. Phenylephrine
D. Norepinephrine

72. All of the following are true about diabetic patients, except

A. Patients should take half or one-third of their insulin dose the morning of the surgery
B. Patients should continue their oral hypoglycemic agents the morning of the surgery
C. Finger-stick blood glucose should be tested before taking the patient to the operating room
D. Patient with an insulin pump should continue the insulin at their basal rate

73. Digoxin toxicity is most likely exacerbated by

A. Hyperkalemia
B. Hypokalemia
C. Hypercalcemia
D. Hypocalcemia

74. The most common complication of inserting a central venous catheter is

A. Carotid artery puncture
B. Thrombosis
C. Cardiac arrhythmias
D. Air embolism

75. A patient is administered cephalexin preoperatively. Within 5 minutes of starting the antibiotic, the patient starts to wheeze and develops tachycardia, and the blood pressure drops to 78/42 mm Hg. Your next step would be to administer

   A. Ephedrine
   B. Phenylephrine
   C. Epinephrine
   D. Oxygen

76. All of the following may occur with an interscalene block, except

   A. Subarachnoid injection
   B. Radial nerve blockade
   C. Median nerve blockade
   D. Ulnar nerve blockade

77. An axillary nerve block would not produce loss of sensation of the

   A. Lateral aspect of the forearm
   B. Medial aspect of the forearm
   C. The entire forearm
   D. None of the above

78. The femoral nerve lies

   A. Medial to the femoral artery
   B. Anterior to the femoral artery
   C. Posterior to the femoral artery
   D. Lateral to the femoral artery

79. All of the following nerves are blocked by an ankle block, except

   A. Sural
   B. Superficial peroneal
   C. Deep peroneal
   D. Anterior tibial

80. Sore throat is

   A. More common after using an endotracheal tube
   B. More common after using a laryngeal mask airway
   C. Similar incidence with either endotracheal tube or a laryngeal mask airway
   D. More common after using an oral airway

81. A patient with hypertrophic obstructive cardiomyopathy (HOCM) presents with dyspnea and angina on exertion. Which of the following is the best agent to treat these symptoms?

   A. Hydrochlorothiazide
   B. Metoprolol
   C. Morphine
   D. Nitroglycerin

82. St. John wort (*Hypericum perforatum*) potentiates the effects of

   A. Heparin
   B. Warfarin
   C. Aspirin
   D. Clopidogrel

83. The most powerful predictor of atrial fibrillation post–cardiac surgery is

    A. History of diabetes
    B. History of hypertension
    C. Age
    D. Time on bypass

84. A patient with Parkinson disease undergoes a general anesthetic. Your plan to treat his nausea would include all of the following, except

    A. Dexamethasone
    B. Scopolamine patch
    C. Metoclopramide
    D. Ondansetron

85. A 65-year-old patient is being treated for congestive cardiac failure. He is able to take a shower but gets dyspneic on mowing the lawn. His New York Heart Association classification is

    A. Class 1
    B. Class 2
    C. Class 3a
    D. Class 3b

86. The percentage of postdural puncture headaches that would resolve spontaneously by 1 week is approximately

    A. 30%
    B. 50%
    C. 50%
    D. 70%

87. A 46-year-old lady is seen at the preoperative assessment clinic. She is taking 180 mg/day methadone. The most likely change to be found in her preoperative ECG is

    A. Prolonged PR interval
    B. Prolonged QTc
    C. U wave
    D. Tented T-waves

88. You are about to anesthetize a 55-year-old man who is undergoing liver resection for removal of metastatic carcinoid tumor. The drug of choice to treat intraoperative hypotension is

    A. Octreotide
    B. Dobutamine
    C. Milrinone
    D. Vasopressin

89. You are performing an interscalene brachial plexus block on an awake 40-year-old patient who is healthy with no significant medical history. Soon after injecting 20 mL of 0.25% bupivacaine the patient becomes agitated, has a seizure, and loses consciousness. Your first step in management is

    A. Administer intralipid
    B. Administer midazolam or propofol to control the seizure
    C. Establish airway and give 100% O_2 via a face mask
    D. Administer epinephrine

90. Patients with dilated cardiomyopathy exhibit all of the following, except

    A. Decreased myocardial contractility
    B. Afterload should be maximized
    C. Increased preload
    D. Left ventricular hypertrophy

91. A septic patient has a central venous pressure of 10 mm Hg, a blood pressure of 80/40 mm Hg, and a pulse rate of 96 beats/min. The best agent to treat the hypotension is

    A. Dopamine
    B. Dobutamine
    C. Noradrenaline
    D. Epinephrine

92. Which of the following organs is least tolerant of ischemia for removal for transplantation?

    A. Cornea
    B. Heart
    D. Kidney
    E. Pancreas

93. You have administered a patient 1.2 mg/kg of rocuronium to do an intubation. You are unable to intubate or ventilate the patient and decide to reverse the patient's paralysis with sugammadex. The dosage you would use is

    A. 2 mg/kg
    B. 4 mg/kg
    C. 8 mg/kg
    D. 16 mg/kg

94. A young female patient with anorexia nervosa has just started eating again. After 4 days, she develops dyspnea and is found to have cardiac failure. Which of the following is most important to correct?

    A. Potassium
    B. Phosphate
    C. Glucose
    D. Sodium

95. A pregnant lady is to undergo general anesthesia for acute appendicitis. At what gestational age should you monitor fetal heart rate?

    A. 16 weeks
    B. 18 weeks
    C. 24 weeks
    D. 28 weeks

96. Which of the following is the best predictor of a difficult intubation in a morbidly obese patient?

    A. Pretracheal tissue volume
    B. Body mass index
    C. Mallampati score
    D. Thyromental distance

97. A patient with a history of chronic obstructive pulmonary disease presents for lung volume–reduction surgery. Which of the following is a contraindication for surgery?

    A. Age >60 years
    B. Chronic asthma
    C. FEV <25%
    D. Evidence of bullous disease

98. All of the following help increase the excretion of calcium, except

    A. Bisphosphonates
    B. Calcitonin
    C. Furosemide
    D. IV crystalloids

99. Which of the following is contraindicated to use during pregnancy?

    A. Aspirin
    B. Enalapril
    C. Metoprolol
    D. Hydralazine

100. During scoliosis surgery, monitoring of somatosensory-evoked potentials indicates monitoring of

    A. Anterior horn
    B. Anterior corticospinal tract
    C. Dorsal column
    D. Spinothalamic tract

101. The desflurane vaporizer is heated because of desflurane's

    A. High vapor pressure
    B. High boiling point
    C. High minimum alveolar concentration
    D. High volatility

102. Which of the following is the most effective way to reduce renal failure in a patient having an abdominal aortic aneurysm repair?

    A. Fluid bolus prior to aortic clamping
    B. Fluid bolus after aortic clamp release
    C. Administration of mannitol
    D. Minimization of cross-clamp time

CHAPTER 1 ANSWERS

1. **D.** Scopolamine, an anticholinergic drug, is often applied as a transdermal patch preoperatively for the prevention of postoperative nausea and vomiting. However, like atropine, and unlike glycopyrrolate, scopolamine passes through the blood–brain barrier and can cause confusion, especially in the elderly. Hence, application of scopolamine patch should be avoided in the elderly. Treatment of scopolamine-induced confusion may require administration of physostigmine.

2. **D.** Metoclopramide is a prokinetic agent and helps to increase gastric motility. The ASA does not recommend preoperative administration of metoclopramide for prevention of postoperative nausea and vomiting. All the other agents have proven benefit in preventing postoperative nausea and vomiting.

3. **B.** Famotidine is known to cause thrombocytopenia (both quantitative and qualitative platelet dysfunction). Patients with ITP already have low platelets; thus, such premedication should be avoided. Warfarin does not affect platelet function or number, thus has no relation to perioperative bleeding due to platelet pathology; however, it is an independent risk factor for bleeding.

4. **B.** Aprepitant is an NK_1 receptor antagonist that antagonizes the action of substance P in the central nervous system to prevent nausea and vomiting. Palonosetron is a $5\text{-}HT_3$ antagonist, metoclopramide is an antidopaminergic agent, and prochlorperazine is a dopamine (D_2) receptor antagonist (antipsychotic drug) with additional antiemetic activity.

5. **C.** The Apfel score can be used to predict patients with a high risk for perioperative nausea and vomiting (PONV). It includes four factors: female gender, nonsmoking, postoperative use of opioids, and previous PONV or motion sickness in the patients' history. Surgeries like laparoscopy, middle-ear surgery, and strabismus surgery are associated with a higher risk of PONV.

6. **C.** Etomidate administration can cause an increase in the incidence of perioperative nausea and vomiting (PONV). Promethazine, haloperidol, and propofol all are used in the treatment of PONV. The latter two are usually used for the treatment of refractory PONV.

7. **C.** β-Lactam antibiotics must be given within 60 minutes prior to incision. Vancomycin and fluoroquinolones require administration within 120 minutes prior to incision.

8. **D.** Vancomycin and fluoroquinolones require administration within 120 minutes prior to incision. β-Lactam antibiotics must be given within 60 minutes prior to incision.

9. **D.** Effort tolerance of around 4 METs (metabolic equivalent of tasks) or more is suggested to be a good predictor for postoperative cardiopulmonary outcome. These activities are classified as per physical strain involved.

10. **C.** One metabolic equivalent is defined as the amount of oxygen consumed at rest, and is equal to 3.5 mL O_2/kg/min. The energy cost of any activity can be determined by multiplying 3.5 to the oxygen consumption (mL O_2/kg/min). METs can be assessed as follows:
    - 1 MET—can take care of self (eating, dressing, toilet)
    - 4 METs—can walk up a flight of steps or a hill
    - 4 to 10 METs—can do heavy household work (scrubbing floors, lifting heavy furniture)
    - >10 METs—can participate in strenuous sports (swimming, tennis, basketball, skiing)

11. **B.** As per ASRA guidelines 2010, heparin infusion should be stopped at least 2 to 4 hours before placing an epidural. This is to prevent the potential formation of an epidural hematoma.

12. **A.**   As per the AHA/ACC Scientific Statement, reversal of warfarin can be achieved by using all, except choice D. However, for emergent surgery the fastest method is the administration of fresh-frozen plasma. Peak action of injectable vitamin K takes up to 6 to 12 hours.

13. **C.**   As per ASRA guidelines (2010), aspirin intake by the patient is no more considered as a contraindication to performing a neuraxial block.

14. **D.**   The assessment of preoperative predictability for obstructive sleep apnea can be done by using the "STOP-BANG" questionnaire. In this scoring, male gender, and not female gender, is classified as a risk factor (S, snoring; T, tired during daytime; O, observed for apnea during sleep; P, high blood pressure; B, BMI >35 kg/m²; A, age >50 years; N, neck circumference >40 cm; G, male gender). In addition to the questionnaire, upper airway anatomical abnormalities that increase the likelihood of obstruction are tonsillar hypertrophy, tumors of the upper airway, or facio maxillary abnormalities.

15. **D.**   All, except choice D, are signs of diabetic autonomic neuropathy. Urinary retention at this age is more likely due to prostate hypertrophy.

16. **B.**   Weight loss due to dialysis is attributed to actual volume (ultrafiltrate) removed from the body. Thus, a high weight loss can predict higher circulatory volume lost, which can lead to poor compensation of hypotension in patients undergoing surgery.

17. **A.**   Ketamine causes the least respiratory depression among the intravenous induction agents. Therefore, it may be beneficial as an induction agent in patients with severe asthma. However, ketamine causes an increase in secretions, and may produce emergence delirium (vivid dreams). Pretreatment with glycopyrrolate and midazolam alleviates these effects of ketamine. The other induction agents cause dose-dependent respiratory depression.

18. **B.**   Droperidol can cause a significant prolongation of the QT interval on the ECG. Patients should have a preoperative ECG, and ECG monitoring should be continued postoperatively for at least 2 hours, before discharging the patient.

19. **D.**   At present, no conventional test (PT, PTT) can be used to quantify the clinical effects of LMWH on the coagulation system. Anti–Factor Xa estimation may be used in specific patients to monitor the coagulative effects of LMWH.

20. **B.**   As these drugs act on different receptors, their effects are generally considered to be synergistic. Patients receiving both these drugs may be prone to greater sedation and respiratory depression than when receiving the drug alone.

21. **D.**   Preoperative evaluation in fact includes a battery of tests and adds additional costs to the total perioperative costs. However, preoperative evaluation is vital, as it recognizes patient comorbidities, which can worsen perioperatively and cause increased patient morbidity. Preoperative evaluation eventually lowers indirect costs that may be incurred to treat the worsening aliment, postoperatively. During preoperative interaction, patient anxiety is usually lowered as the risks and procedure are explained to the patient.

22. **B.**   An anesthesia consent should be obtained during preanesthetic evaluation, whenever possible. This is one of the prime aims that need to be fulfilled as a component of preoperative anesthetic evaluation.

23. **D.**   The goals of preanesthetic evaluation include all those listed in the question. In addition, other targets of preanesthetic evaluation include education of patients and families about anesthesia and the anesthesiologist's role, obtaining informed consent, motivation of patients to stop smoking and lose weight, or commit to other preventive care.

24. **D.** ASA classification does not include the nature of procedure in predicting perioperative morbidity and mortality. It only includes patient-based morbidity rather than type of surgery.

25. **B.** Healthy pregnant patients in labor are classified as an ASA II. Patients with controlled diabetes or essential hypertension are still classified as an ASA II. Presence of preeclampsia will step up the classification to an ASA III.

26. **C.** Sedatives typically alleviate anxiety in hypertensive patients (preventing blood pressure elevations due to surgery-related anxiety), in patients with chronic alcohol abuse, and in children to maintain cooperation for induction of anesthesia. In neurosurgical patients, sedatives can lead to depression of respiratory drive, which can cause hypercarbia and an increase in intracranial pressure.

27. **A.** As per ASRA guidelines, warfarin must be stopped at least 5 days prior and clopidogrel 7 to 10 days prior to elective surgery. Low-molecular-weight heparin in therapeutic doses must be stopped at least 24 hours prior, and when being used in prophylactic doses, it must be stopped at least 12 hours prior to an elective surgery requiring central neuraxial blockade. Aspirin use is no more considered as a contraindication to performing a neuraxial block.

28. **B.** ASA classifies any medical comorbidity without functional limitation (i.e., hypertensive without coronary artery disease or angina) as an ASA II. Once the patient's activity is limited due to the disease, the patient is then categorized as an ASA III.

29. **D.** By definition, such patients are categorized as ASA Class VI.

30. **C.** By definition, these patients require surgery despite being really sick. Most often, the surgical correction of the underlying pathology (that may have led to multiorgan involvement) may be the only option of improving their chances of survival. A hemodynamically unstable patient secondary to perforation peritonitis, with an acute kidney injury, would be an example. Although the patient may be extremely sick, until the perforation peritonitis is surgically treated, the chances of survival may not improve.

31. **B.** ASA III is a patient with severe systemic disease that is a constant threat to life (functionality incapacitated).

32. **C.** Warfarin should be stopped at least 5 days prior to surgery. On the day of the surgery, the prothrombin time (international normalized ratio or INR) is checked. An INR of 1.4 or less is desirable to perform the surgery.

33. **A.** Before any rate/rhythm control in patients likely to have AF for more than 48 hours, left-atrial clots must be ruled out. An undiagnosed clot can lead to catastrophic embolic consequences.

34. **D.** For a drug-eluting stent, it is advised to avoid elective surgery for a year (to continue dual antiplatelet medication), and for a bare-metallic stent, it is advised to avoid elective surgery for about 4 weeks. Performing laparoscopic surgery post–CABG surgery is highly risky. So when surgery needs to be planned in the near future, the patient should be advised to undergo balloon dilatation and then delay the elective procedure for 2 to 3 weeks thereafter.

35. **C.** Renal failure can induce platelet dysfunction, and therefore, central neuraxial blockade is still debated in these patients. They also have coagulation factor abnormalities that may predispose them to deep vein thrombosis. Anemia is a result of decreased erythropoietin production and is often labeled as "anemia of chronic disease."

36. **C.** As per ASA guidelines, it is recommended to wait at least 6 hours after ingestion of non-human milk before performing an elective operation in a child.

37. **C.**   Volatile inhalation agents and succinylcholine are considered triggers for malignant hyperthermia (MH) reaction. MH has a genetic component, and runs in families. Since her aunt had a severe reaction to anesthesia, further details should be obtained from the history. If any doubt about the history, the patient should be assumed to be prone to developing MH. Volatile agents and succinylcholine should be avoided in this patient.

38. **B.**   Elective surgery should be postponed for at least 6 weeks after a myocardial infarction. Risk of reinfarction is approximately 5.5% for surgeries between 0 and 3 months, 2.5% between 3 and 6 months, and 2% after 6 months of a myocardial infarction.

39. **A.**   The most significant risk factor for developing pulmonary complications is the upper abdominal or thoracic site of surgery. As such, all patients undergoing such surgeries should be optimally prepared for the surgery. This includes pulmonary toilet: chest physiotherapy/exercises, and postural drainage of mucus and secretions.

40. **C.**   There is no specific value of INR before a patient is taken to the OR for elective surgery. However, it is recommended that an INR value of 1.4 or less should be aimed for before taking the patient to the OR for elective surgery. In case of emergency, the INR can be normalized by infusing fresh-frozen plasma.

41. **C.**   The paralyzed muscles due to central denervation eventually develop atrophy. Extrajunctional receptors are then synthesized at the muscle sites, which remain resistant to the effects of neuromuscular blockade for varying degrees. Thus, these paralyzed muscles give an exaggerated response on direct stimulation with a nerve stimulator. Therefore, muscle twitch monitoring should be done on the nonaffected sites to correctly monitor the degree of neuromuscular blockade.

42. **B.**   MAC typically is found to be lower for patients on sedatives, anxiolytics, alcohol intoxication, hypothermia, extremes of age, moribund/sick patients, and patients with obtunded consciousness. Chronic alcohol abuse, however, increases MAC.

43. **A.**   All β_2 agonists are known to cause internalization of potassium (from plasma to cell), thus causing hypokalemia. This principle is sometimes used in the treatment of patients with hyperkalemia.

44. **D.**   Smoking cessation for 24 hours before surgery reduces carboxyhemoglobin (COHb) levels. Reduced levels of COHb increases levels of oxygenated Hb, which decreases the risk of myocardial ischemia and perioperative cardiac morbidity. Delayed benefits (cessation more than 8 weeks) are known to improve airway immunologic and ciliary function.

45. **D.**   Among all these tests, TEG has the highest positive predictive value for diagnosing a bleeding tendency. Deranged values from other tests listed have not shown to always correlate well with bleeding tendency. For example, the other tests will be deranged in a patient with sepsis but may not show a clinically relevant bleeding tendency.

46. **D.**   All the other choices need evaluation/optimization prior to elective noncardiac surgery. Uncontrolled systolic hypertension without target end-organ damage is a minor predictor/risk factor. It can be usually controlled with intraoperative antihypertensive medications without evidence of significant adverse outcomes.

47. **C.**   Glycopyrrolate is a synthetic quaternary amine with antimuscarinic properties and no central side effects like sedation. All the other choices are as a result of direct consequence of cholinergic blockade.

48. **C.**   Metoclopramide is a prokinetic agent that enhances gastric clearance and increases lower esophageal sphincter tone, preventing vomiting, but may not actually work for nausea

(vomiting rather than nausea is prevented). It blocks the dopaminergic receptors to cause parkinsonism-like extrapyramidal side effects.

49. **B.**   Preoxygenation of lungs primarily acts to increase safe apnea time by denitrogenating functional residual capacity (FRC) and increasing dissolved oxygen content in the blood. It does not alter any physical measurements of lungs; that is, it has no effect on FRC or on closing volume/capacity.

50. **A.**   Halothane, especially on repeated administration, can cause two subtypes of hepatitis (type 1 is immunogenic—mild—and type 2 is due to direct effect of halothane on liver cells). The incidence of halothane hepatitis is around 1 in 10,000 to 1 in 35,000 halothane anesthetics.

51. **C.**   Both halothane and sevoflurane have been used for inhalation induction in the pediatric population. Sevoflurane has largely replaced halothane due to a better safety profile, and has emerged as the induction agent of choice in pediatric population.

52. **D.**   Nitrous oxide is known to inhibit the enzyme "methionine synthase," inhibiting DNA synthesis and precipitating B_{12} deficiency, causing pernicious megaloblastic anemia. Nitrous oxide is also known to act on NMDA receptors and also increase pulmonary vascular resistance.

53. **D.**   All the mechanisms have been proposed for propofol in preventing nausea and vomiting in the postoperative period (PONV). Propofol, when used, is used in refractory cases of PONV and in low doses.

54. **C.**   Ketamine preserves spontaneous respiration and airway tone without causing apnea at induction doses. Propofol and benzodiazepines are associated with respiratory depression at induction doses and cause apnea.

55. **B.**   Succinylcholine should not be used in patients with a history of muscular dystrophy or patients with a history of malignant hyperthermia. Myasthenia gravis patients may show resistance to Phase I block of succinylcholine. In patients with full stomach, succinylcholine is used in "rapid sequence intubation" to prevent aspiration.

56. **B.**   Multiple studies have shown propensity of ACE inhibitors to precipitate profound hypotension at induction of general anesthesia, especially in the geriatric age group. Hence, ACE inhibitors should be with held on the day of the surgery, especially in the elderly and for major surgeries.

57. **D.**   Morbidly obese patients with OSA are often subject to persistent hypoxia, which leads to increased pulmonary vascular resistance, eventually leading to pulmonary artery hypertension. Obese patients are also known to have a higher incidence of cardiac problems, including a dilated heart and heart failure. Compression neuropathies are also common in this subpopulation. Dementia is a central-nervous-system–related complication not associated directly with obesity.

58. **D.**   Remifentanil preparations available in the market have glycine as the preservative, which can cause direct neurotoxicity. Thus, it is recommended that remifentanil preparations be not used for central neuraxial blockade.

59. **D.**   Ondansetron exerts its antiemetic effect by acting as an antagonist on the 5-HT$_3$ receptors. Drugs in the same category include palonosetron and granisetron. Rarely reported side effects of these agents include QT prolongation, hypotension, and headache.

60. **C.**   Scopolamine is an antimuscarinic drug that can cross the blood–brain barrier and cause sedation and confusion, especially in the elderly. It does not produce analgesia.

61. D.   Dexmedetomidine is an α_2 receptor agonist, with about eight times greater affinity for the receptor than clonidine. Continuous infusion is more likely to result in hypotension and bradycardia.

62. C.   Addisonian crisis or acute adrenal insufficiency during the perioperative period occurs in patients with known adrenal insufficiency or in those receiving chronic steroid therapy. The latter causes hypothalamic–pituitary axis suppression. Patients with adrenal insufficiency may present with refractory shock with electrolyte and glucose abnormalities. Treatment consists of administration of hydrocortisone and correction of associated derangements.

63. B.   Promethazine is commonly used as an antiemetic. It has antidopaminergic activity, and in addition also has antihistaminic and anti–α-adrenergic activity.

64. A.   Factors that are associated with an increased risk of postoperative nausea and vomiting include previous history of postoperative nausea and vomiting, female gender, obesity, nonsmoking, pain, eye or ear surgery, laparoscopic surgery, anesthetic drugs, and gastric distention.

65. A.   Abrupt withdrawal of TPN will most commonly result in hypoglycemia due to the high circulating insulin levels.

66. A.   Glycopyrrolate is an anticholinergic drug with a quaternary ammonium structure, which prevents it from crossing the blood–brain barrier. Therefore, it has no central nervous system effects (sedation). Glycopyrrolate increases the heart rate, causes dryness of secretions, and lowers the lower esophageal sphincter tone. The latter may predispose a patient to pulmonary aspiration of gastric contents.

67. B.   Patients taking herbal medications for their alleged benefits are often unaware of their potential side effects (bleeding tendency, platelet dysfunction, etc.). Most medications must be stopped for at least 7 days prior to surgery.

68. A.   Gentamicin is an aminoglycoside antibiotic that blocks acetylcholine release from the presynaptic terminals and reduces postsynaptic responsiveness. This may prolong neuromuscular blockade associated with nondepolarizing muscle relaxants.

69. B.   Estrogen intake can lead to a hypercoagulable state, predisposing women to thromboembolic events. Other risk factors for thromboembolism include major surgery, multiple trauma (hip fracture), lower extremity paralysis, increasing age, cardiac or respiratory failure, prolonged immobility, presence of central venous lines, and a wide variety of hematologic conditions (inherited or acquired).

70. C.   Because of its narrow therapeutic index, lithium dosing requires constant surveillance with monitoring of levels and dosage adjustment. Three types of lithium intoxication can occur—acute, acute or chronic, and chronic. Chronic lithium intoxication occurs in those patients on long-term lithium therapy.

- Mild toxicity: manifests as lethargy, drowsiness, coarse hand tremor, muscle weakness, nausea, vomiting, and diarrhea
- Moderate toxicity: manifests as confusion, dysarthria, nystagmus, ataxia, myoclonic twitches, and flat or inverted T-waves on ECG
- Severe toxicity: may be life-threatening. It may present with grossly impaired consciousness, increased deep tendon reflexes, seizures, syncope, renal insufficiency, coma, and death.

71. A.   Patients under treatment with MAOIs have an increased availability of endogenous norepinephrine. Therefore, treatment with an indirect-acting drug such as ephedrine can lead to an exaggerated response. Hypotension in these patients is better managed with a direct-acting drug such as phenylephrine.

72. **B.** Patients taking oral hypoglycemic agents may experience delayed hypoglycemia in the absence of caloric intake in the intraoperative and postoperative periods. Hence, patients should be advised not to take oral hypoglycemic agents the morning of the surgery. In addition, metformin should be stopped at least 48 hours before surgery as it may precipitate the development of lactic acidosis during surgery. Patients on an insulin pump should continue the insulin at the basal rate.

73. **B.** Digoxin is an inotrope that blocks the Na^+/K^+ ATPase pump on the myocardial cell. It causes calcium ions to enter the cells, but causes a net K^+ loss from the cell. Thus, hypokalemia, more so than hypercalcemia, will exacerbate digitalis toxicity. Signs and symptoms of digoxin toxicity include drowsiness or confusion, nausea/vomiting, loss of appetite, diarrhea, disturbed color vision (yellow or green halos around objects), agitation, and cardiac dysrhythmias. Characteristic EKG changes include bradycardia, a prolonged PR interval, or an accelerated junctional rhythm.

74. **C.** During central line insertion, the guide wire or the tip of the catheter enters the right atrium and may result in an arrhythmia, which returns to sinus rhythm when the guide wire/catheter tip is withdrawn out of the heart.

75. **C.** Antibiotic allergies may result in an anaphylactic or anaphylactoid reaction. Based on the patient's presentation, anaphylactic shock is the most consistent diagnosis and needs to be treated with epinephrine first, which reverses most of the manifestations of anaphylaxis.

76. **D.** The ulnar nerve is frequently spared with an interscalene block. Complications of an interscalene block include stellate ganglion block, phrenic nerve block, recurrent laryngeal nerve block, Horner syndrome, vertebral artery injection, epidural/subarachnoid/subdural injection, and pneumothorax.

77. **A.** An axillary nerve block produces blockade of the median, ulnar, and the radial nerves. Sensation to the lateral aspect of the forearm is provided by the musculocutaneous nerve, which must be blocked separately (deep injection into the coracobrachialis muscle).

78. **D.** The femoral nerve lies lateral to the femoral artery, which is lateral to the femoral vein (VAN—vein, artery, nerve; medial to lateral).

79. **D.** The ankle block blocks the deep peroneal nerve, the saphenous nerve, the posterior tibial nerve, the sural nerve, and the superficial peroneal nerve.

80. **A.** Laryngopharyngitis is more common after an endotracheal intubation than when using a laryngeal mask airway. The incidence of sore throat can vary from 15% to 40%, and depends on operator experience (less trauma). Use of smaller endotracheal tubes, smaller cuff sizes (less area of contact with tracheal mucosa), and low pressure in the tracheal cuff decrease the incidence of postoperative sore throat. Using lidocaine jelly to lubricate the endotracheal tube (rather than lubricating jelly) increases the incidence of sore throat. Most cases of sore throat resolve spontaneously.

81. **B.** In HOCM, obstruction of the ventricular outflow tract can occur from systolic anterior motion of the mitral valve against the hypertrophied septum. In patients with a severe HOCM, myocardial depression is beneficial, which can be obtained by using β-blockers (metoprolol) or calcium channel blockers.

82. **D.** St. John wort is a commonly used herbal medication that is a CYP2C19- and CYP3A4 inducer. As clopidogrel is activated by the cytochrome P450 system, St. John wort may be used to increase the effect of clopidogrel in hyporesponders. It reduces the effect of warfarin and heparin, with little effect on aspirin.

83. C.   Advanced age is the most important predictor of atrial fibrillation not only in patients following cardiac surgery but also in the general population.

84. C.   Parkinson disease is characterized by a loss of dopamine in the nigrostriatum, resulting in bradykinesia, rigidity, postural instability, and pill-rolling resting tremor. Metoclopramide (and droperidol) has significant antidopaminergic properties and should be avoided in these patients in the treatment of nausea and vomiting.

85. B.   The New York Heart Association classification for heart failure is based on both a functional and objective assessment of the patient's capabilities and symptoms. This patient is asymptomatic at rest and can go about his activities of daily living without issues. However, with more strenuous activity, he becomes dyspneic. His classification would, therefore, be 2 (Tables 1-1 and 1-2).

Table 1-1 Functional capacity: How a patient with cardiac disease feels during physical activity

Class I: Patients with cardiac disease but resulting in no limitation of physical activity.	Ordinary physical activity does not cause undue fatigue, palpitation, dyspnea, or anginal pain.
Class II: Patients with cardiac disease resulting in slight limitation of physical activity.	They are comfortable at rest. Ordinary physical activity results in fatigue, palpitation, dyspnea, or anginal pain.
Class III: Patients with cardiac disease resulting in marked limitation of physical activity.	They are comfortable at rest. Less-than-ordinary activity causes fatigue, palpitation, dyspnea, or anginal pain.
Class IV: Patients with cardiac disease resulting in inability to carry on any physical activity without discomfort.	Symptoms of heart failure or the anginal syndrome may be present even at rest. If any physical activity is undertaken, discomfort increases.

Table 1-2 Objective assessment

Class A: No objective evidence of cardiovascular disease.	No symptoms and no limitation in ordinary physical activity.
Class B: Objective evidence of minimal cardiovascular disease.	Mild symptoms and slight limitation during ordinary activity. Comfortable at rest.
Class C: Objective evidence of moderately severe cardiovascular disease.	Marked limitation in activity due to symptoms, even during less-than-ordinary activity. Comfortable only at rest.
Class D: Objective evidence of severe cardiovascular disease.	Severe limitations. Experiences symptoms even while at rest.

86. D.   In the event of a postdural puncture headache (PDPH), 53% of headaches resolve in 4 days, 72% in 7 days, and 85% within 6 weeks. Mild–moderate PDPH is usually treated conservatively (fluids, caffeine drinks, analgesics). Severe PDPH may require an epidural blood patch.

87. B.   Following a rash of sudden deaths in patients taking methadone, the FDA in 2006 issued a black box warning for all practitioners, specifically detailing the high risk of prolonged QT syndrome and sudden death in patients prescribed this medication.

88. A.   Surgery for carcinoid tumor debulking or resection may precipitate a carcinoid crisis in the patient consisting of flushing, hypotension, bronchospasm, acidosis, and ventricular tachycardia. Patients who received octreotide experienced no significant intraoperative complications.

89. **C.**   Injection of large amount of local anesthetic into the vertebral artery or into the sub-arachnoid or subdural space resulting in a seizure is a well-known complication of the inter-scalene block. Treatment for this patient is to first establish an airway (ABCs) and then treat the seizure.

90. **B.**   Patients with dilated cardiomyopathy are extremely sensitive to changes in afterload. Therefore, afterload should be minimized to maintain stroke volume.

91. **C.**   In septic shock, both dopamine and norepinephrine can be used to treat persistent hypotension. However, dopamine may promote further tissue acidosis in the splanchnic circulation, whereas norepinephrine does not, thus making it the drug of choice for this scenario.

92. **B.**   The heart, because of its high oxygen requirements, is the least tolerant of ischemia. Hyperkalemic crystalloid cardioplegia at 4°C for a maximum of 4 hours is used to preserve the heart. Thus, reducing the ischemic time of donor hearts will decrease morbidity and costs of cardiac transplantations.

93. **D.**   Sugammadex reverses neuromuscular blockade by nondepolarizing muscle relaxants by directly binding to rocuronium, vecuronium, and pancuronium, without any side effects. Reversal of neuromuscular blockade is achieved in a dose-dependent manner and can be used in the event of failed intubation. For normal reversal, that is, with two twitches, the dose is 2 mg/kg. When the blockade is deeper, the dose must be increased. When reversing following a failed intubation, a dose of 8 mg/kg of sugammadex will effectively reverse rocuronium given at 0.6 mg/kg. If the dose of rocuronium given is 1.2 mg/kg, reversal with sugammadex requires a dose of 16 mg/kg.

94. **B.**   With prolonged periods of starvation followed by reintroduction of enteral or parenteral nutrition, the increased release of pancreatic insulin leads to an anabolic state and an intracellular shift of phosphate, magnesium, and potassium. Of these derangements, hypophosphatemia leads to the most severe conditions, including cardiac failure.

95. **C.**   Fetal heart rate and uterine monitoring should be performed during induction, emergence, recovery, and, if possible, during the surgery in any pregnancy of more than 24 weeks' gestation. The fetus becomes viable at this gestation age.

96. **A.**   Airway management in obese patients begins first with an adequate physical exam as these patients are more likely to be both more difficult to ventilate and to intubate. The best predictor of difficulty is a short, thick neck (pretracheal tissue volume) and a history of obstructive sleep apnea.

97. **C.**   In pulmonary resections, preoperative impairment is directly related to operative risk. Using routine pulmonary function tests, criteria have been established for high-risk patients.
    - $PaCO_2$ >45 mm Hg or PaO_2 <50 mm Hg on room air
    - FEV <25%
    - FEV_1 <2 L preoperatively or <0.8 L or <40% of predicted postoperatively
    - FEV_1/FVC <50% predicted
    - Maximum breathing capacity <50% of predicted
    - Maximum VO_2 <10 mL/kg/min

98. **A.**   Bisphosphonates are used in the treatment of osteoporosis as they inhibit osteoclastic resorption of bone. Biphosphonates do not affect the excretion of calcium.

99. B. Enalapril exposure during the first trimester of pregnancy has been associated with multiple fetal defects, affecting the cardiac, pulmonary, renal, and musculoskeletal systems.

100. C. Somatosensory-evoked potentials are usually monitored on the posterior tibial nerves of the legs during spinal surgery and are used to assess the integrity of the dorsal columns of the spinal cord.

101. A. The main issue with desflurane is that it has a high saturated vapor pressure at room temperature (669 mm Hg at 20°C). It boils at just 22.8°C compared with sevoflurane at 58.5°C or isoflurane at 48.5°C. Therefore, the desflurane vaporizer is heated to 39°C and pressurized at 2 atm.

102. D. The incidence of renal failure after abdominal aortic aneurysm surgery is 5.4%, of which 0.6% requires hemodialysis. Loop diuretics (furosemide), dopamine, mannitol, fenoldopam, and *N*-acetylcysteine are proposed renal protective agents; however, there is no concrete evidence to support their use. The mainstay of renal preservation is by reducing aortic cross-clamping time, adequate fluid resuscitation, and avoidance of nephrotoxins (nonsteroidal anti-inflammatory drugs, angiotensin-converting-enzyme inhibitors, aminoglycoside antibiotics).

2

Airway Management

Yuriy Bronshteyn and Edward Bittner

1. A major difference between the adult and neonatal airway is that the

   A. Neonate's larynx is located more superiorly in the neck
   B. Neonate's epiglottis is angled more superiorly
   C. Narrowest segment of a neonate's upper airway occurs at the level of the vocal cords
   D. Neonate is at lower risk of postextubation stridor compared to the adult

2. The narrowest segment of a 14-day-old child's upper airway is located at the

   A. Hyoid bone
   B. Thyroid cartilage
   C. Vocal cords
   D. Subglottic region

3. Airway obstruction in Pierre Robin syndrome most likely occurs

   A. Between the tongue and pharyngeal wall
   B. At the level of the glottis
   C. In the subglottic trachea
   D. At the bronchial level

4. Airway management in Klippel–Feil syndrome is most likely to be challenging because of

   A. Micrognathia
   B. Macroglossia
   C. Subglottic stenosis
   D. Cervical spine fusion

5. One of the following statements regarding airway management in patients with congenital syndromes is most accurate:

   A. Laryngoscopy is often challenging in Turner syndrome because of a high frequency of laryngeal distortion
   B. Airway management in Treacher Collins syndrome is complicated by a high incidence of cervical spine instability
   C. Intubation in patients with Goldenhar syndrome is often challenging due to a high rate of subglottic stenosis
   D. Airway management of patients with trisomy 21 is complicated by a high incidence of cervical spine instability

6. A healthy 2-year-old male is scheduled to undergo a laparoscopic inguinal hernia repair. His airway was managed uneventfully with mask ventilation followed by direct laryngoscopy and intubation with a 4.5-mm uncuffed endotracheal tube (ETT). Manual ventilation produces an air leak in the oropharynx beginning at a peak pressure of 20 cm H_2O. The best next step in the anesthetic management is to

   A. Continue current management
   B. Replace the ETT with a smaller-sized uncuffed tube
   C. Replace the ETT with a larger-sized uncuffed tube
   D. Replace the ETT with a 4.0-mm cuffed ETT

7. A 4-year-old patient scheduled for laparoscopic gastrostomy tube placement undergoes induction of general anesthesia and endotracheal intubation with a 4.5-mm cuffed endotracheal tube. The tube is taped 14 cm at the gumline, and the patient is placed on volume-control ventilation. The most likely first sign of a right main stem intubation is

   A. Arterial desaturation
   B. Hypercapnia
   C. Increased peak inspiratory pressures
   D. Hypotension

8. A 6-year-old patient scheduled for laparoscopic bilateral inguinal hernia repair undergoes inhalational induction and intubation with a 5.0-mm cuffed endotracheal tube. The tube is secured with the 15-cm mark at the patient's gumline. Auscultation reveals equal breath sounds bilaterally. Inflation of the pilot balloon results in palpation of the inflated tube cuff just above the cricoid cartilage. A leak test reveals leak of air into the oropharynx at a positive pressure of 20 cm H_2O. The next best step in management is

   A. No change in anesthetic care is indicated
   B. The tube cuff should be deflated until a leak is present starting at 15 cm H_2O of positive pressure
   C. The tube cuff should be deflated and the tube advanced until the cuff, when inflated, is palpable below the cricoid cartilage
   D. The tube cuff should be deflated and the tube withdrawn until ventilator peak pressures decrease

9. A 4-year-old boy with autism and failure-to-thrive undergoes a gastrostomy tube placement. At the completion of the operation, the patient remains unresponsive but is breathing spontaneously and has a mild gag response to oral suctioning. The anesthesiologist extubates the patient and immediately shuts off the volatile agent. The anesthesiologist then inserts an appropriately sized oropharyngeal airway and places a face mask connected to the ventilator circuit over the patient's face, allowing the patient to breathe 100% oxygen. Despite providing a chin lift, jaw thrust, and positive-pressure breaths, the anesthesiologist notes that the ventilator shows no end-tidal carbon dioxide. Auscultation over the sternal notch reveals no air movement. The pulse oximeter reading then rapidly drops to 70% from 100%. The next best step in management is

   A. Administration of albuterol
   B. Insertion of a nasal trumpet
   C. Endotracheal reintubation
   D. Administration of succinylcholine

10. In the scenario above, if the patient's postextubation condition is left untreated, the patient will most likely experience

   A. Aspiration
   B. Bronchospasm
   C. Pulmonary edema
   D. Croup

11. A 2-year-old child weighing 13 kg is scheduled for inguinal hernia repair. She is at the 55th percentile for height for her age. An appropriately-sized cuffed endotracheal tube for this patient will have an internal diameter of

   A. 3.0 mm
   B. 4.0 mm
   C. 5.0 mm
   D. 6.0 mm

12. The superior surface of the epiglottis is innervated by the

   A. Hypoglossal nerve
   B. Recurrent laryngeal nerve
   C. Internal branch of the superior laryngeal nerve
   D. External branch of the superior laryngeal nerve

13. Tactile sensation from the anterior third of the tongue is carried by fibers of the

   A. Trigeminal nerve
   B. Facial nerve
   C. Glossopharyngeal nerve
   D. Hypoglossal nerve

14. A 48-year-old female patient with temporomandibular joint dysfunction and associated limited mouth opening is scheduled for a thyroidectomy for goiter. Due to concern for challenging laryngoscopy, the anesthesiologist elects to perform an awake fiberoptic intubation. In order to anesthetize the posterior third of the tongue, the anesthesiologist should perform a nerve block of the

   A. Cranial nerve V
   B. Cranial nerve VII
   C. Cranial nerve IX
   D. Cranial nerve XII

15. A patient who suffers acute, bilateral denervation of the external branch of the superior laryngeal nerve will most likely present with

   A. No symptoms
   B. Hoarseness
   C. Stridor
   D. Aspiration

16. To anesthetize the supraglottic laryngeal mucosa, the local anesthetic should be injected into one of the following areas:

   A. The base of the anterior tonsillar pillar
   B. Medial to the lesser cornu of the hyoid bone
   C. Superior to the superior cornu of the thyroid cartilage
   D. Through the cricothyroid membrane

17. The efferent limb of the glottic closure reflex, which is involved in laryngospasm, primarily involves the

   A. Internal branch of the superior laryngeal nerve
   B. Hypoglossal nerve
   C. Recurrent laryngeal nerve
   D. Glossopharyngeal nerve

18. A 65-year-old woman undergoes a thyroidectomy for papillary thyroid cancer. Immediately after emergence and extubation, she is aphonic and has minimal chest movement, despite spontaneously moving her limbs and head. Auscultation reveals lack of breath sounds over the chest. There is no evidence of a surgical site hematoma. The anesthesiologist provides a jaw thrust and positive-pressure breaths, which slightly improve the patient's oxygenation and ventilation. The surgeon suggests a bilateral block of both the internal and external branches of the patient's superior laryngeal nerve. If performed this block would likely result in

A. Worsening of the patient's respiratory distress and no change in her aphonia
B. Improvement of the patient's respiratory distress and no change in her aphonia
C. No change in the patient's respiratory distress and improvement of her aphonia
D. No change in the patient's respiratory distress and no change in her aphonia

19. A 48-year-old woman with temporomandibular joint dysfunction and limited mouth opening is scheduled for thyroidectomy for goiter. Due to concern for a difficult laryngoscopy, the anesthesiologist elects to perform an awake oral fiberoptic intubation. To reliably blunt the afferent limb of the cough reflex, the anesthesiologist should perform a bilateral block of the

A. Superior laryngeal nerve and the recurrent laryngeal nerve
B. Glossopharyngeal nerve and internal branch of the superior laryngeal nerve
C. Glossopharyngeal nerve and external branch of the superior laryngeal nerve
D. Internal and external branches of the superior laryngeal nerve

20. If an adult patient were to suffer an acute, bilateral transection of cranial nerve X, awake laryngoscopy would most likely reveal

A. Fully adducted vocal cords
B. Fully abducted vocal cords
C. Vocal cords in a partially adducted position with 2 to 3 mm of space between them
D. Vocal cords oscillating between adducted and abducted position

21. Several hours after undergoing repair of an ascending aortic dissection, a 65-year-old male patient is extubated in the intensive care unit. All of the arch vessels were preserved during the operation. After extubation, the patient's voice is noted to be hoarse. Awake fiberoptic laryngoscopy would most likely show the following during inspiration:

A. Vocal cords in a fully abducted position
B. Vocal cords in a fully adducted position
C. Left vocal cord in an adducted position and right vocal cord fully abducted
D. Left vocal cord in an abducted position and right vocal cord fully adducted

22. An awake tracheostomy would be facilitated by a regional block of the

A. Trigeminal nerve
B. Glossopharyngeal nerve
C. Superior laryngeal nerve
D. Recurrent laryngeal nerve

23. One of the following statements regarding the innervation of airway structures is most correct:

A. The afferent limb of the gag reflex is primarily carried by fibers of the recurrent laryngeal nerve
B. Trigeminal nerve block would facilitate awake nasotracheal intubation
C. The superior surface of the epiglottis is primarily innervated by the glossopharyngeal nerve
D. Tactile sensation from the posterior one-third of the tongue is carried by the hypoglossal nerve

24. A nasal trumpet would be most appropriate for management of anesthetic-induced upper airway obstruction in one of the following patients:

    A. A 25-year-old passenger ejected out of a motorcycle now with Glasgow Coma Scale of 13 and some periorbital bruising

    B. A 32-year-old term parturient, otherwise healthy except for gestational thrombocytopenia, who requires emergent cesarean section under general anesthesia

    C. A 45-year-old female with temporomandibular joint syndrome and breast cancer scheduled for bilateral mastectomy

    D. A 65-year-old male with a mechanical mitral valve on therapeutic anticoagulation undergoing emergent coronary catheterization for unstable angina

25. A 55-year-old woman with severe anxiety and rheumatoid arthritis is scheduled for thyroidectomy for medullary thyroid cancer. Her airway exam in the upright position is notable for a nonvisible uvula with the tongue protruded, a 2 fingerbreadth mouth opening, a thyromental distance of 2.5 fingerbreadths, and neck range-of-motion at the atlanto-occipital joint of about 70 degrees. Examination of her neck reveals an enlarged, fixed, and nonmobile mass that appears to be contiguous with the thyroid gland when the patient swallows. The trachea cannot be palpated. The patient is highly anxious and tells you that under no circumstance will she let you insert a "breathing tube inside my airway while I'm awake." The next best step in anesthetic management is

    A. Induction of general anesthesia followed by fiberoptic bronchoscopy

    B. Induction of general anesthesia followed by rigid bronchoscopy

    C. Induction of general anesthesia followed by laryngeal mask airway placement

    D. Cancel the case

26. After rapid sequence induction of general anesthesia, a patient is unable to be intubated. Subsequent attempts at ventilation by face mask and a supraglottic airway device are also unsuccessful. One of the following statements regarding transtracheal jet ventilation and surgical cricothyrotomy in this situation is most correct:

    A. Transtracheal jet ventilation does not require a patent natural airway

    B. Ventilation through a surgical cricothyrotomy allows both inhalation and exhalation to occur

    C. The development of laryngospasm during ventilation through a cricothyrotomy would rapidly cause pulmonary overinflation and barotrauma

    D. Transtracheal jet ventilation can be continued for a longer period of time than can ventilation via a cricothyrotomy

27. Use of a laryngeal mask airway would be most appropriate for airway management in the following patient:

    A. An obese patient with acute appendicitis who, after rapid sequence induction, cannot be intubated

    B. An elderly patient with restrictive lung disease scheduled for inguinal hernia repair

    C. An obese male patient with a hiatal hernia and GERD scheduled for umbilical hernia repair

    D. A full-term parturient brought to the OR for emergent cesarean section because of fetal bradycardia

28. After undergoing an uneventful operation, one of the following patients would be the best candidate for "deep extubation":

    A. A 23-year-old woman with asthma who has just undergone an exploratory laparotomy for small bowel obstruction

    B. A 65-year-old man with gastroesophageal reflux who has just undergone an inguinal hernia repair

C. An 18-year-old patient with scoliosis who has just undergone a 6-hour posterior thoraco-lumbar spinal instrumentation and fusion

D. A 64-year-old female with coronary artery disease who has just undergone a total hip arthroplasty under general anesthesia

29. One of the following is a primary risk factor for difficult mask ventilation:

A. Limited mouth opening

B. Thyromental distance less than 3 fingerbreadths

C. High arched palate

D. Inability to bring mandibular incisors anterior to the maxillary incisors

30. An otherwise healthy patient with a history of daytime sleepiness and snoring from laryngeal papillomatosis undergoes polysomnography and spirometry, which shows dynamic inspiratory obstruction. The flow–volume loop that would be most consistent with this patient's condition is

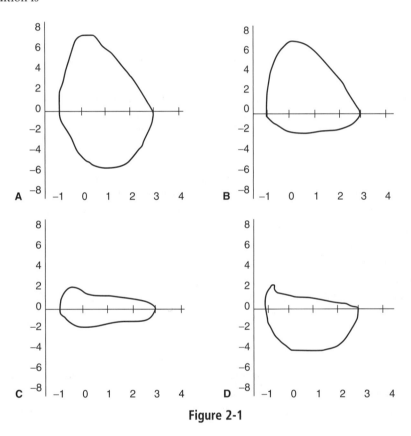

Figure 2-1

A. Figure 2-1A

B. Figure 2-1B

C. Figure 2-1C

D. Figure 2-1D

CHAPTER 2 ANSWERS

1. **A.** The neonate's larynx is located more superiorly in the neck than the adult's. The location of the adult's larynx is at C4–C5 level of the spine, while the neonate's is at C3–C4 level. The neonate's epiglottis is relatively longer, stiffer, and angled more *posteriorly* compared to the adult's, which is one of the reasons why straight blades are more popular among pediatric anesthesiologists. The narrowest part of the upper airway is at the level of the cricoid cartilage in neonates, and at the level of the vocal cords in adults. The child's airway takes on adult characteristics between the ages of 5 and 10 years. The neonate is at greater risk of postextubation stridor compared to the adult. Resistance through a cylindrical tube (such as the trachea) is inversely proportional to the radius raised to the fourth power (Poiseuille law). Thus, a 1-mm reduction in tracheal diameter due to edema results in a marked rise in airway resistance in small children, which may be inconsequential in adults.

2. **D.** According to classical teaching, the narrowest portion of a child's upper airway is at the level of the cricoid cartilage, whereas the narrowest portion of an adult's upper airway is at the level of the vocal cords. However, a more recent bronchoscopic study of airway dimensions in children found that between the ages of 6 months and 13 years, the glottis, not the cricoid cartilage, is the narrowest portion of the child's airway. This study did not measure airway dimensions in children younger than 6 months.

3. **A.** Pierre Robin is a congenital syndrome associated with enlarged tongue, small mouth, and mandibular anomalies typically manifested as micrognathia. All of these limit the oropharyngeal space, contributing to airway obstruction between the tongue and posterior pharyngeal wall. When you see Pierre Robin, think PR: Posterior Restriction behind the tongue.

4. **D.** Klippel–Feil is a congenital syndrome associated with the phenotypical triad of short neck, low posterior hair line, and congenital spinal fusion causing limited neck mobility. Fused segments of the cervical spine in patients with this syndrome promote hypermobility at unfused spine segments, increasing the risk of neurologic compromise during neck manipulation. When you see Klippel–Feil, think KF: Cervical Fusion.

5. **D.** Airway management of patients with trisomy 21 (Down syndrome) is complicated by several factors. These patients tend to have small mouths and large tongue, resulting in limited oropharyngeal space. They are prone to laryngospasm. They also have a high incidence of subglottic stenosis, such that endotracheal tubes should be downsized by 0.5 mm from the caliber expected for a patient of the same size without Down syndrome. Finally, they have a high incidence of cervical spine instability. The other three syndromes share a common feature of micrognathia (small jaw), which renders these patients a challenge for direct laryngoscopy. Turner syndrome occurs in females who lack a complete second X chromosome (monosomy). These women tend to have short necks and small jaws. Laryngeal distortion (choice A) has not been described in this population. Treacher Collins is a rare syndrome characterized by abnormal development of facial bones (e.g., maxillary and mandibular). A high incidence of cervical spine instability (choice B) has not been described in this population. Goldenhar syndrome is manifested by dysplastic growth of the face (especially the ears, eyes, and mouth) and vertebral anomalies (e.g., scoliosis). A high incidence of subglottic stenosis (choice D), although a common finding in patients with trisomy 21, has not been described in the Goldenhar population.

6. **A.** A positive-pressure leak test provides information about the tightness of the seal formed between an ETT and its surrounding mucosa. A leak at pressures below 25 cm H_2O places the tracheal mucosa at a very low risk of ischemic injury. Pressures above 30 cm H_2O, the arteriolar-capillary perfusion pressure, can cause mucosal ischemia, with resulting inflammation, ulceration, stridor, and later scarring and stenosis.

7. **C.**   When an endotracheal tube migrates from an intratracheal to an endobronchial position while on volume-control ventilation, the first sign of migration is generally an increase
in peak inspiratory pressures. Peak inspiratory pressure results from the resistance to flow of
the large airways and the static compliance of the lung. A fixed volume of air moving out of
an endobronchial tube would encounter significantly more large airway resistance compared
to the same volume moving out of an endotracheal tube (remember: resistance is inversely
proportional to radius raised to the fourth power). Thus, the first sign of an endobronchial
intubation would be an elevation in peak inspiratory pressures. Because the nonventilated
lung has some reserve of oxygen, passive oxygenation would delay onset of hypoxemia briefly
(choice A). Hypercapnia (choice B) would eventually develop in an endobronchially intubated patient on controlled ventilation if the minute ventilation were kept constant. Hypotension (choice D) might occur if the right lung is allowed to hyperinflate, restricting venous
return. However, this would not be as immediate as a rise in peak inspiratory pressures.

8. **C.**   Palpation of the endotracheal tube cuff palpable above the cricoid cartilage implies that the
cuff's position is intralaryngeal. This is problematic for two reasons: (1) an inflated cuff in the
larynx may cause laryngeal injury and postoperative respiratory compromise, and (2) such a high
tube position may increase the risk of inadvertent extubation. The cuff should be deflated and
the tube advanced until the cuff (when inflated) is palpable below the cricoid cartilage. Choice B
is incorrect: a cuff inflated to enable air leak at 20 to 25 cm H_2O of positive pressure should not
cause airway injury and edema in routine circumstances. Choice D would likely result in the tip
of the endotracheal tube moving from an intralaryngeal to a supralaryngeal position.

9. **D.**   The scenario describes extubation of a child during a "light" plane of anesthesia when
laryngeal reflexes are hypersensitive. Return of a gag reflex is a characteristic of this lighter,
hyperexcitable stage. If a patient is extubated while lightly anesthetized, there is an increased
risk of laryngospasm. Stimulation of the laryngeal mucosa by secretions or a foreign body
(e.g., the endotracheal tube or an oral airway) can result in laryngospasm during the excitation stage of anesthesia or sometimes even during awake states.

    Laryngospasm and other causes of upper airway obstruction (e.g., tongue collapsed against
the posterior pharyngeal wall) may not be immediately distinguishable. However, the initial
treatment is identical: anterior displacement of the mandible using a chin lift or jaw thrust
combined with positive-pressure ventilation. If these measures fail to relieve the laryngospasm
and hypoxemia develops, pharmacologic therapy should be initiated emergently. In a patient
with no contraindications, a small dose of succinylcholine (0.25–0.5 mg/kg) or deepening of the
anesthetic (e.g., with propofol or another general anesthetic) should break the laryngospasm.

10. **C.**   Left untreated, upper airway obstruction in a spontaneously breathing patient can result in
the development of negative-pressure pulmonary edema (also called postobstructive pulmonary
edema). Forceful inspiration against a closed upper airway generates a large negative intrathoracic pressure which can result in pulmonary edema by increasing capillary transmural pressure
and/or by acutely elevating left ventricular end-diastolic pressure. Aspiration (choice A) would
be impossible during laryngospasm. Bronchospasm (choice B) would not be expected as a direct
consequence of prolonged laryngospasm. Croup or laryngotracheal bronchitis (choice D) is a
form of upper airway obstruction that typically occurs in response to a viral or bacterial upper
respiratory tract infection in children between the ages of 6 months and 6 years. This clinical
scenario is not suggestive of an infectious etiology for the upper airway obstruction.

11. **B.**   A commonly used formula for estimating the internal diameter of an *uncuffed* endotracheal tube in children is

$$\text{Internal diameter (in mm)} = (\text{Age} + 16)/4$$

The resulting value should be reduced by 0.5 mm when using a *cuffed* endotracheal tube to
allow space in the tracheal lumen for cuff inflation. Since this child appears to have a height
and weight appropriate for her age, the formula would be reasonable to use. For the patient
in this question, the internal diameter is (2 + 16)/4 = 4.5 mm for an uncuffed tube, which is
reduced to 4.0 mm for a cuffed tube.

12. C.   The vagus nerve provides sensory innervation to the structures of the airway beginning with the epiglottis and moving caudally. It has two major branches that innervate distinct parts of the airway: the superior laryngeal nerve (SLN) and recurrent laryngeal nerve (RLN). Above the vocal cords, the sensory innervation of the larynx is via the SLN. Below the vocal folds, sensory innervation of the airway is provided by branches of the recurrent RLN. The vocal cords themselves receive dual innervation from both nerves. The SLN has two branches: internal and external. The internal SLN branch (choice C) is exclusively a sensory nerve that innervates both the superior and inferior surfaces of the epiglottis. The external branch of the SLN is a motor nerve that innervates the cricothyroid muscle (Fig. 2-2). The RLN (choice B) is a mixed motor and sensory nerve. The motor branch innervates all of the laryngeal muscles, except the cricothyroid muscle, while the sensory branch innervates the subglottic mucosa of the airway. The hypoglossal nerve (choice A) is a purely motor nerve that innervates the muscles of the tongue.

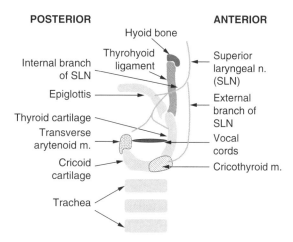

Figure 2-2. Subdivisions of the superior laryngeal nerve in the sagittal view.

13. A.   The tongue has innervation for both gustatory (aka "taste") and tactile (general sensory) input. Gustatory (taste) sensation for the anterior two-thirds of the tongue is provided by the facial nerve (CN VII), and for the posterior third of the tongue by the glossopharyngeal nerve (CN IX). Tactile sensation for the anterior two-thirds of the tongue is provided by the trigeminal nerve (CN V), and for the posterior one-third of the tongue by the glossopharyngeal nerve (CN IX). In addition, a small portion of sensory innervation of the posterior tongue is provided by fibers of the superior laryngeal nerve's internal branch ("spillover fibers" from that nerve's innervation of the epiglottis) (Fig. 2-3). The hypoglossal nerve (choice D) is a purely motor nerve that innervates the muscles of the tongue.

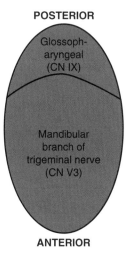

Figure 2-3. General sensory innervation of tongue.

14. C.   The glossopharyngeal nerve (CN IX) is a mixed motor and sensory nerve. Its sensory fibers carry information about general sensation and taste from the posterior third of the tongue (Fig. 2-3). Of note, the glossopharyngeal nerve does not provide sensory innervation to the epiglottis; it is provided by the superior laryngeal nerve. The trigeminal nerve (CN V) (choice A) carries general sensory information from the anterior two-thirds of the tongue. The facial nerve (CN VII) (choice B) is a mixed motor and sensory nerve. It carries taste sensation from the anterior two-thirds of the tongue and oral cavity. The hypoglossal nerve (CN XII) (choice D) is a purely motor nerve that innervates the muscles of the tongue.

15. B.   The superior laryngeal nerve (SLN) is a mixed motor and sensory nerve that receives sensory information from the supraglottic larynx and provides motor innervation to the cricothyroid muscle. The cricothyroid muscle tenses and adducts the vocal cords. This action raises the pitch of speech and enables singing. Acute, bilateral denervation of the external branch of the SLN may cause hoarseness and other subtle voice findings. However, the ability to adduct and abduct the vocal cords would remain intact.

16. C.   Sensory innervation of the larynx above the vocal cords is carried by fibers of the superior laryngeal nerve (SLN). The internal branch of the SLN provides sensory innervation to the supraglottic portion of the larynx, including all of the epiglottis and the supraglottic mucosa. The external branch of the SLN is primarily a motor nerve that innervates the cricothyroid muscle. The SLN can be blocked as it descends between the greater cornu of the hyoid bone and the superior cornu of the thyroid cartilage. As shown in Figure 2-4, "SLN block" is likely to block the internal branch of the SLN, but not the external "motor" branch. Choice A describes a glossopharyngeal block. Choice B does not describe a clinically relevant procedure (i.e., the injection would be too medial to reliably block the SLN). Choice D describes a transtracheal topicalization of RLN fibers.

17. C.   The efferent limb of the glottic closure reflex involved in laryngospasm is primarily mediated by the recurrent laryngeal nerve (RLN), while the afferent limb is mediated by the superior laryngeal nerve (SLN). The RLN innervates all of the muscles of the larynx except the cricothyroid muscle. The external branch of the SLN (not one of the listed options) is a motor nerve that innervates the cricothyroid muscle. The cricothyroid muscle contributes to laryngospasm by lengthening, and thus tensing the vocal cords.

18. B.   The presentation of acute aphonia and respiratory distress immediately after thyroidectomy are suggestive of bilateral injury to the recurrent laryngeal nerve (RLN), a recognized complication of this surgery. Bilateral RLN injury leaves the vocal cords tensed and closed due to the unopposed action of the cricothyroid muscles. The cricothyroid muscle is innervated by the external (motor) branch of the superior laryngeal nerve (SLN). Blockade of the motor branch of the SLN should improve the patient's respiratory distress by relaxing the vocal cords but would have no impact on the aphonia. Practically speaking, a typical "SLN block" (i.e., injection of ~2 mL of local anesthetic between the greater cornu of the hyoid cartilage and the superior cornu of the thyroid cartilage) is likely to only block the internal (sensory) branch of this nerve as opposed to the motor branch (Fig. 2-4).

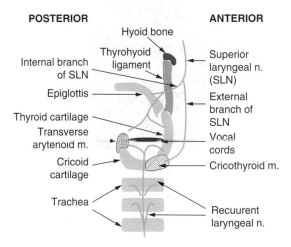

Figure 2-4. Gross anatomic distribution of the SLN and RLN.

19. **A.**   A cough occurs through the stimulation of a complex reflex arc. This is initiated by the irritation of cough receptors, which are found in the pharynx, larynx, trachea, carina, branching points of large airways, and more distal smaller airways. When triggered, impulses travel via the internal branch of the superior laryngeal nerve and the recurrent laryngeal nerve, which stem from the vagus nerve, to the medulla of the brain. This is the afferent neural pathway. The efferent neural pathway then follows, with relevant signals transmitted back from the cerebral cortex and medulla via the vagus and superior laryngeal nerves to the glottis, external intercostals, diaphragm, and other major inspiratory and expiratory muscles.

20. **B.**   Acute, bilateral injury to the vagus nerve (CN X) terminates all of the motor innervation to the larynx. This leaves the vocal cords in a fully open or abducted position. In contrast, bilateral injury to the recurrent laryngeal nerve (a branch of the vagus) would leave the cords paralyzed in a partially adducted position because of unopposed action of the cricothyroid muscle. This adducted position may cause stridor and respiratory distress, especially if the patient has any concurrent laryngeal edema. Choice A would be observed during laryngospasm. Choice D would be observed in a patient with a normal larynx who is alternating between breathing and phonating.

21. **C.**   Postoperative hoarseness can result from injury to the motor nerves which innervate the larynx. The left recurrent laryngeal nerve (RLN) is particularly vulnerable to injury during cardiothoracic surgeries and many neck surgeries due to its anatomic location. After branching off the left vagus nerve in the chest, the left RLN passes between the left pulmonary artery and the arch of the aorta above before ascending alongside the trachea to the larynx. The right RLN, in contrast, branches off the right vagus nerve in the lower neck where it passes under the root of the right subclavian artery before ascending alongside the trachea to the larynx. An aortic arch repair that spares the arch vessels would be more likely to damage the left RLN than the right RLN.

      Acute injury to the left RLN would leave the left vocal cord subject to the unopposed action of the cricothyroid muscle (the only laryngeal muscle NOT innervated by the RLN). This muscle stretches and tenses the vocal cords, an action that shifts the vocal cords toward midline (adduction). During inspiration, both vocal cords normally abduct, maximizing the glottic opening for air movement. During inspiration, a patient with acute left RLN palsy would be expected to have an adducted left vocal cord and an abducted right vocal cord.

22. **D.**   Above the vocal cords, the sensory innervation of the larynx is via the superior laryngeal nerve. Below the vocal cords, sensory innervation is via branches of the recurrent laryngeal nerve (RLN). The vocal cords themselves receive dual innervation from both nerves. The trigeminal nerve (choice A) provides tactile sensation, among other things, to the anterior two-thirds of the tongue and the nasal passages. The glossopharyngeal nerve (choice B) provides tactile and gustatory sensation to the posterior one-third of the tongue. None of the choices except for the RLN would be stimulated during an awake tracheostomy.

23. **B.**   The ophthalmic (V1) and maxillary (V2) divisions of the trigeminal nerve (CN V) convey sensory information from the nasal mucosa. Blockade of these nerves would facilitate awake nasotracheal intubation. The gag reflex is elicited primarily by tactile stimulation of the posterior one-third of the tongue. The afferent limb of this reflex is carried by the glossopharyngeal nerve (CN IX), not the recurrent laryngeal nerve (choice A) or the hypoglossal nerve (choice D). The superior surface of the epiglottis is innervated by the superior laryngeal nerve (SLN), not the glossopharyngeal (choice C). In general, the SLN provides sensory innervation to all structures of the larynx above the vocal cords, including the epiglottis.

24. **C.**   Both nasotracheal intubation and nasal trumpet insertion are contraindicated in patients with facial or skull injuries (choice A), with coagulopathy (choice B), and those on anticoagulation (choice D). In choice A, the patient's mechanism of injury and findings of periorbital bruising suggest an underlying skull fracture. In addition to periorbital ecchymoses, other classic signs of a basilar skull fracture include leakage of blood or cerebrospinal fluid from the nares, ecchymoses on the skin overlying the mastoid process, and hemotympanum or

bleeding from the ears. For a patient with temporomandibular joint dysfunction who has none of the above contraindications (choice C), the nasal trumpet would be a reasonable way to bypass the patient's limited mouth opening and relieve upper airway obstruction.

25. **D.**   This patient has multiple risk factors for difficult intubation, including Mallampati class > 2, thyromental distance < 3 fingerbreadths, mouth opening < 3 fingerbreadths, and total atlanto-occipital range-of-motion < 80 degrees. Patients with inflammatory rheumatoid arthritis (RA) have an increased incidence of temporomandibular joint disease (and associated limited mouth opening) and immobile cervical vertebra (associated with limited neck range-of-motion). Additionally, patients with RA can have occult airway abnormalities not apparent on physical exam, such as laryngeal rotation, cricoarytenoid arthritis, and cervical spine instability. The patient's thyroid malignancy may result in other airway abnormalities including tracheal deviation and/or compression. Were such a patient to be induced and mask ventilation turn out to unsuccessful, there would be no reliable backup method of airway management. The safest way to secure this patient's airway would be an awake fiberoptic intubation. Since the patient has refused this option and the case is not urgent, the anesthesiologist should cancel the operation and discuss the options for airway management with the patient so that a mutually acceptable plan can be reached.

26. **B.**   The "cannot intubate, cannot ventilate" scenario is an emergency and necessitates immediate invasive airway access to prevent anoxic injury. Two options include transtracheal jet ventilation and surgical cricothyrotomy. Transtracheal jet ventilation requires that the airway be cannulated in some way. In emergent circumstances, this may be accomplished by cannulating the cricothyroid membrane with an intravenous catheter (e.g., 14/16G) and then attaching the end of the catheter to a jet ventilator. Jet ventilation requires a pathway for expired air to egress out of the lungs. Thus, when using transtracheal ventilation, laryngospasm (choice C), or another cause of upper airway obstruction (choice A), would rapidly cause pulmonary overinflation and barotrauma. In contrast, a surgical cricothyrotomy permits both inhalation and exhalation through the lumen of inserted tube (choice B) and so is not dependent on upper airway patency in order to function safely. Transtracheal jet ventilation is a temporary way to provide oxygenation until a definitive airway can be established. With prolonged jet ventilation, the delivered high pressures can expel the catheter out of the trachea. When the catheter migrates into the anterior cervical soft tissues, catastrophic subcutaneous emphysema can rapidly develop rendering other attempts at invasive airway access impossible. Surgical cricothyrotomy, on the other hand, *is* a definitive method of securing the airway that can be used for up to 72 hours.

27. **A.**   The ASA Difficult Airway Algorithm recommends use of supraglottic devices such as the laryngeal mask airway (LMA) as rescue tools when laryngoscopy and mask ventilation are unsuccessful. Although the patient in choice A ideally would be treated with "full stomach" precautions, if a rapid sequence induction and intubation are unsuccessful, an LMA may be a life-saving tool to oxygenate and ventilate the patient. Aside from its use as a rescue device, the LMA can be used as a supraglottic airway for elective surgery. Relative contraindications to the elective use of the LMA include low airway compliance (choices B and C), incompetence of the gastroesophageal sphincter (choice C), and in patients with a full stomach (choice D).

28. **D.**   "Deep extubation" refers to the technique of removing the endotracheal tube in a patient breathing spontaneously who remains anesthetized such that his or her protective airway reflexes are still abolished. This technique decreases the chance of a patient coughing during emergence in response to the presence of an endotracheal tube. Deep extubation may be performed because of potential benefit related to a patient's medical comorbidities or for surgical reasons. For example, a patient with coronary artery disease or heart failure may benefit from deep extubation to avoid the sympathetic surge associated with awake extubation and a patient undergoing abdominal hernia repair may benefit from deep extubation to avoid the increased intra-abdominal pressure associated with coughing. However, deep extubation should not be

attempted in patients with contraindications to this technique. These include patients with a full stomach (choices A and B) and in patients who may be challenging to mask ventilate or reintubate. Choice C would fall into this latter category because of the potential for airway edema from prolonged prone positioning.

29. **D.** Mask ventilation can be made difficult by anything that prevents the face mask from forming an adequate seal with the patient's face (e.g., a beard) or increases the resistance to airflow between the mouth and larynx. Edentulousness, a history of snoring, history of neck radiation, multiple attempts at laryngoscopy, male gender, obesity, and Mallampati status ≥ 3 are all factors associated with difficult mask ventilation. Choices A, B, and C represent risk factors for difficult intubation. In general, factors that make it difficult to align the oral axis with the laryngeal axis result in difficult intubation. These factors include prominent maxillary teeth, a highly arched or very narrow palate, and an acute angle between the mouth and larynx.

30. **B.** Flow–volume loops can help differentiate fixed vs. dynamic causes of airway obstruction. They can also help to distinguish extrathoracic vs. intrathoracic sources of the obstruction. During the inspiratory phase of spontaneous ventilation, an extrathoracic obstruction is drawn into the pathway of air movement by subatmospheric intraluminal pressures. In contrast, an intrathoracic obstruction is stented open during inspiration by the negative extraluminal intrathoracic pressure. During expiration in a spontaneously breathing patient, an extrathoracic obstruction is stented open by supra-atmospheric intraluminal pressure. In contrast, an intrathoracic obstruction is exacerbated during expiration, since the extraluminal intrathoracic pressure exceeds the intraluminal pressure. Choice A represents a normal flow–volume loop. Choice C represents a fixed obstruction, that is, one present during both inspiration and expiration. Choice D represents a dynamic intrathoracic obstruction, which would be expected in a patient with asthma or chronic obstructive pulmonary disease.

Anesthesia Machine

Paul Sikka

1. Pipeline gases are supplied at pressures of about _____ psi:

   A. 25
   B. 40
   C. 50
   D. 75

2. Which of the following prevents delivery of hypoxic gas mixture once the oxygen pressure falls below 25 psi?

   A. Diameter index safety system
   B. Pin index safety system
   C. Inspiratory check valve
   D. Fail-safe valve

3. The oxygen-flush valve provides which of the following oxygen flows (L/min) to the common gas outlet?

   A. 10
   B. 25
   C. 50
   D. 90

4. Gas flowmeters

   A. Are gas-specific
   B. Have a gas flow rate which depends on viscosity at high turbulent flows
   C. Have a gas flow rate which depends on density at low laminar flows
   D. Are cylindrical in shape

5. Which of the following flowmeters is situated nearest to the gas outlet?

   A. Nitrous oxide
   B. Oxygen
   C. Air
   D. None of the above

6. Modern vaporizers are

   A. Agent-specific
   B. Temperature-compensated
   C. Pressure-compensated
   D. Both A and B

7. The Tec 6 desflurane vaporizer

    A. Is electrically heated to 39°C
    B. Is pressurized to 3 atm
    C. Is pressure-compensated
    D. All of the above

8. Variable bypass vaporizers should be located

    A. Between the common gas outlet (upstream) and the flowmeters (downstream)
    B. Between the flowmeters (upstream) and the common gas outlet (downstream)
    C. Between the gas pipeline and the flowmeters
    D. Inside the circle system

9. A standing or ascending bellow is preferred for anesthesia ventilators, as disconnection is indicated by

    A. Collapse
    B. Filling by gravity
    C. Disconnection alarm
    D. Stoppage of flowmeter gas

10. The National Institute for Occupational Safety and Health (NIOSH) recommends limiting operating-room concentration of nitrous oxide to _____ ppm:

    A. 10
    B. 25
    C. 50
    D. 100

11. The National Institute for Occupational Safety and Health (NIOSH) recommends limiting operating-room concentration of volatile inhalational agents to _____ ppm:

    A. 0.2
    B. 0.5
    C. 1
    D. 2

12. Capacity of an oxygen "E" cylinder is approximately _____ L:

    A. 500
    B. 600
    C. 650
    D. 750

13. If pressure in a full nitrous oxide "E" cylinder is 745 psi at 20°C, the pressure in a half-full cylinder will be about _____ psi:

    A. 186
    B. 248
    C. 372
    D. 745

14. Which of the following system prevents the wrong gas cylinder being attached to the anesthesia machine?

    A. Diameter index safety system
    B. Pin index safety system
    C. Hanger yoke assembly system
    D. Gauge-safety system

15. A line-isolation monitor

    A. Warns that an electrical shock is imminent
    B. Warns of a fault between the power line and the ground
    C. Warns of the presence of two faults
    D. Trips the ground leakage circuit breaker

16. The highest content of soda lime is

    A. Calcium hydroxide
    B. Potassium hydroxide
    C. Sodium hydroxide
    D. Silica

17. End products of the reaction in a soda lime CO_2 canister are

    A. Carbonates, water, heat
    B. Carbonates, heat, sodium hydroxide
    C. Sodium hydroxide, water, heat
    D. Carbonates, sodium hydroxide, water, heat

    1. $CO_2 + H_2O \rightarrow H_2CO_3$
    2. $H_2CO_3 + 2\,NaOH$ (or KOH) $\rightarrow Na_2CO_3$ (or K_2CO_3) $+ 2\,H_2O$ + Energy
    3. Na_2CO_3 (or K_2CO_3) $+ Ca(OH)_2 \rightarrow CaCO_3 + 2\,NaOH$ (or KOH)

18. If you notice that the CO_2 absorbent is exhausted during the surgical procedure, which of the following minimal fresh gas flows (L/min) will make the CO_2 absorbent unnecessary?

    A. 3
    B. 5
    C. 7
    D. 10

19. Compared to the Mapleson A system, the circle system

    A. Is less bulky
    B. Has a decreased risk of disconnection
    C. Has decreased resistance to patient breathing
    D. Better conserves humidity

20. Incorrect statement regarding the mechanisms of an Ambu bag is

    A. It contains a nonrebreathing valve, same as the circle system
    B. It is capable of delivery of nearly a 100% O_2 concentration
    C. It allows for positive-pressure ventilation
    D. Patient valve has low resistance to both inspiration and expiration

21. You are preparing to set up for anesthesia in an off-floor location in the interventional radiology suite. The radiography equipment is consuming the limited space that is available in the suite, and therefore, the decision is made to double the extension tube length from the ventilator to the patient table. What is the impact on the dead-space ventilation that would have occurred secondary to doubling the extension tubing length?

    A. It would double as well
    B. It has been decreased to half the original volume
    C. It would have increased by 4-fold
    D. It would have not changed

22. Malfunction of which of the following valves within a circle system may cause rebreathing of carbon dioxide and could potentially result in hypercapnia?

    A. Inspiratory valve
    B. Expiratory valve
    C. Both A and B
    D. None of the above

23. Since fresh gas flow equal to minute ventilation is sufficient to prevent rebreathing, which of the following Mapleson circuit breathing/ventilation systems is the most efficient for spontaneous ventilation of the patient?

    A. Mapleson A
    B. Mapleson B
    C. Mapleson C
    D. Mapleson D

24. Different semi closed anesthetic ventilation/breathing systems (classically referred to as Mapleson systems and designated A to F) are pictured below. While setting up for anesthesia delivery in an "off-floor" location and planning for controlled ventilation of an asthmatic patient, which of the Mapleson systems provides for the best efficacy?

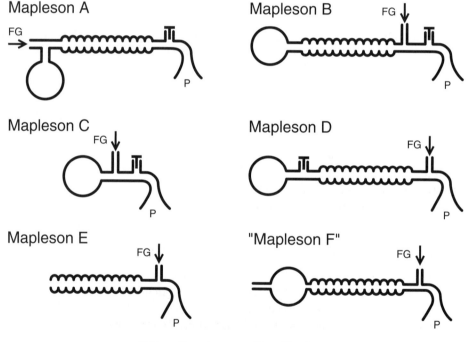

FG = Fresh gas   P = Patient

Figure 3-1.

    A. $D > B > C > A$
    B. $A > B > C > D$
    C. $D > C > B > A$
    D. $C > A > D > B$

25. Degradation of sevoflurane by soda lime results in the production of

    A. Compound A
    B. Compound B
    C. Compound C
    D. Compound D

26. In a CO_2-absorbent canister, the greatest amount of carbon monoxide is produced by which of the following volatile agents?

    A. Sevoflurane
    B. Halothane
    C. Isoflurane
    D. Desflurane

CHAPTER 3 ANSWERS

1. **C.**   Pipeline gases are supplied at pressures between 45 and 55 psi. This is in contrast to cylinder gas pressures, which are much higher, and are reduced by pressure regulators to less than 50 psi.

2. **D.**   The fail-safe valve automatically closes nitrous oxide (and other gases) to prevent delivery of hypoxic gas mixture to the patient. The fail-safe valve is designed to be activated when oxygen pressure falls below 25 psi.

3. **C.**   The oxygen-flush valve provides gas flow at pipeline pressures of about 45 to 55 psi at 35 to 75 L/min. The high flow of oxygen is provided directly to the common gas outlet, bypassing the flowmeters and vaporizers. One should be careful when using the oxygen-flush valve, as high gas flows at high pressures can cause lung barotrauma in the patient.

4. **A.**   Gas flowmeters are calibrated for a particular gas. Gas flow rate depends on its viscosity at low laminar flows, and its density at high turbulent flows. Flowmeters are tapered in shape, with the diameter the smallest near the bottom of the tube.

5. **B.**   The oxygen flowmeter is situated nearest to the gas outlet. This is because, if a leak develops in the flowmeter tubes, a hypoxic gas mixture can be delivered to the patient. To minimize this, the oxygen flowmeter is positioned downstream and nearest to the gas outlet.

6. **D.**   Modern vaporizers are agent-specific and temperature-compensated. Also, specific fillers are available for each volatile agent, which prevent filling on the wrong agent. A constant concentration of agent is delivered, unaffected by temperature or flow rates. Temperature compensation is achieved by a metallic strip composed of two different metals, which expands/contracts to deliver a constant concentration of vapor.

7. **A.**   The Tec 6 desflurane vaporizer is electrically heated to 39°C and pressurized to 2 atm. This is done because desflurane boils at room temperature at sea level (1 atm). The heating and pressurization optimizes the delivery of desflurane.

8. **B.**   Vaporizers are located between the flowmeters (upstream) and the common gas outlet (downstream). In other words, vaporizers are located outside the circle system. This decreases the likelihood of delivery of high vapor concentrations when using the oxygen-flush valve.

9. **A.**   An ascending bellow collapses when disconnection occurs. A descending bellow, however, continues to fill by gravity when disconnection occurs. Therefore, ascending bellows are preferred for anesthesia ventilators.

10. **B.**   NIOSH recommends limiting operating-room concentration of nitrous oxide to 25 ppm. Minimizing operating-room pollution is important to prevent health-related effects in healthcare providers. Waste-scavenging systems are utilized to decrease operating-room pollution.

11. **D.**   NIOSH recommends limiting operating-room concentration of volatile agents to 2 ppm. Minimizing operating-room pollution is important to prevent health-related effects in healthcare providers. Waste-scavenging systems are utilized to decrease operating-room pollution.

12. **C.**   The capacity of an "E" cylinder of oxygen is about 625 to 700 L. The pressure in a full cylinder is about 1,800 psi at 20°C. Cylinders are color-coded, with oxygen being green, nitrous oxide being blue, and air being yellow.

13. D.   Pressure in a half-full "E" cylinder of nitrous oxide will still be 745 psi. Nitrous oxide is present in the cylinder as a liquid, and therefore, the volume remaining in the cylinder does not reflect the pressure in the cylinder. Capacity of an "E cylinder" of nitrous is about 1590 L. It is not until three-fourth of the gas is consumed (about 400 L remaining) that the pressure in the cylinder begins to fall. Therefore, the reliable way to determine the remaining nitrous oxide in the cylinder is to weigh the cylinder. The empty weight of the cylinder is stamped on the cylinder.

14. B.   Cylinder manufactures have adopted the pin index safety system, which prevents attachment of wrong gas cylinder to the anesthesia machine. The diameter index safety system prevents attachment of the wrong gas hose from the wall supply. Hanger yoke assembly is the method of attachment of gas cylinders to the anesthesia machine.

15. B.   A line-isolation monitor, when alarming, indicates that a single fault has occurred between the power line and the ground. As soon as the alarm is triggered, the equipment should be checked, especially the last equipment that was plugged in. A single fault does not cause an electrical shock, as two faults are required to produce a shock.

16. A.   The highest content of soda lime is calcium hydroxide (75%). Other constituents include sodium (3%) and potassium hydroxide (1%), water (20%), and silica, which is added to produce hardness. An indicator dye, such as ethyl violet, is added to indicate the degree of exhaustion.

17. D.   End products of the reaction occurring in a soda lime CO_2 canister are carbonates, sodium hydroxide (regeneration), water, and heat. Following are the reactions:

18. B.   Advantages of a circle system include the use of low fresh gas flow rates because of the presence of a CO_2-absorbent canister. However, if the CO_2 absorbent is exhausted during a surgical procedure, the fresh gas flow rate has to be increased. A minimum fresh gas flow rate of 5 L/min will make the use of the absorbent unnecessary. Newer anesthesia machines allow changing the CO_2-absorbent canister during the surgical procedure, if necessary.

19. D.   Advantages of the circle system include economy (low fresh gas flow rates, decreased use of volatile agents), conservation of heat and humidity, and decreased operating-room pollution. Disadvantages of circle system include greater size, decreased portability, increased risk of disconnection, and increased resistance to patient breathing.

20. A.   While resuscitation devices such as Ambu bags or bag-mask units have nonrebreathing valves, neither the Mapleson (only has adjustable pressure-limiting valve) nor the circle system (only has unidirectional valves and does allow rebreathing) has this component. Ambu resuscitation bags do allow for positive-pressure ventilation as the intake valve closes during bag compression. The patient valve has low resistance, but can become obstructed by exhaled moisture. Ambu bags have a reservoir system to prevent room air entrapment and are able to deliver nearly 100% oxygen.

21. D.   One advantage of the circle system ventilation when compared to the Mapleson system is the presence of unidirectional valves (inspiratory and expiratory valves). With the use of such valves, the volume of dead-space ventilation is limited *only* to that volume distal to Y-piece (including the endotracheal tube), where inspiratory and expiratory gases mix and converge, regardless of the length of tubing proximal to the Y-piece (to the anesthesia machine).

22. C.   Malfunction in either of the unidirectional valves within a circle system could result in the accumulation and eventual CO_2 rebreathing that may result in hypercapnia.

23. **A.** During spontaneous ventilation/breathing of the patient, the Mapleson circuit providing for the most efficacy ranges from A > D > C > B (in the order of decreasing efficiency).

24. **A.** The efficiency of Mapleson systems drops from D > B > C > A for controlled ventilation. The Mapleson D circuit is most efficient during controlled ventilation, as its fresh gas flow drives expired air away from the patient and toward the expiratory/exhaust valve.

25. **A.** Sevoflurane is degraded by soda lime, resulting in the production of a potentially nephrotoxic compound A. Compound A production is increased by using low fresh gas flow rates, using high concentrations of sevoflurane, and for long hours (>6 hours).

26. **D.** Desflurane produces the highest amount of carbon monoxide in the CO_2-absorbent canister, which can increase carboxyhemoglobin blood concentration. Production of carbon monoxide is increased by using low fresh gas flow rates, high concentrations of volatile agent, and a dry absorbent.

Patient Monitoring

Darren Hyatt, Ala Nozari, and Edward Bittner

1. To help encourage universal quality and safety practices, the ASA has adopted and mandates the use of all the following monitors during general anesthesia, except

   A. An oxygen analyzer
   B. Capnography
   C. Continuous visual display of an ECG
   D. A peripheral nerve stimulator

2. Current ASA standards require that during anesthesia, systemic blood pressure and heart rate be evaluated at least every

   A. 3 minutes
   B. 5 minutes
   C. 7 minutes
   D. 10 minutes

3. Lead II of an ECG is represented by placing the

   A. Positive electrode on the right arm and the negative electrode on the left leg
   B. Negative electrode on the right arm and the positive electrode on the left leg
   C. Positive electrode on the right arm and the negative electrode on the left arm
   D. Negative electrode on the right arm and the positive electrode on the left arm

4. During the course of a complicated cardiac case, the surgeon informs you that he is worried about damage to the right coronary artery in a patient with a right-dominant coronary system. During reperfusion, you are looking for signs of ischemia, and are most interested in leads

   A. V1–V3
   B. V4–V6
   C. II, III, and AvF
   D. I and AvL

5. Use of lead V5 alone on ECG results in the detection of _____ (%) of ischemic episodes:

   A. 35
   B. 55
   C. 75
   D. 95

6. You are taking over a case from another anesthesia provider with a patient in the beach chair position and a history of moderate carotid artery disease. You are told during pass-off that the patient's blood pressures have consistently been 90/50 mm Hg. You notice the blood pressure cuff on the left arm is one or two sizes small and barely stays on the patient. A blood pressure cuff that is too small will

   A. Incorrectly underestimate the true blood pressure
   B. Incorrectly overestimate the true blood pressure
   C. Randomly both over- and underestimate the true blood pressure
   D. Not give an incorrect blood pressure, but will be uncomfortable in an awake patient

7. When performing the oscillometric method to measure blood pressure, for example, when you do not have a stethoscope or automated blood pressure cuff, it is important to remember that you will not be able to measure the

   A. Systolic blood pressure
   B. Diastolic blood pressure
   C. Mean arterial pressure
   D. Diastolic or mean arterial blood pressure

8. The diastolic blood pressure recorded with an automated blood pressure cuff using the oscillometric method will be

   A. Approximately 10 mm Hg higher when compared to direct arterial measurement
   B. Approximately 10 mm Hg lower when compared to direct arterial measurement
   C. Equal to direct arterial measurement
   D. Random and unreliable

9. When measuring blood pressure manually and listening for Korotkoff sounds, the diastolic blood pressure is measured at the onset of

   A. Phase 1
   B. Phase 2
   C. Phase 3
   D. Phase 5

10. You are preparing for an emergent mitral valve repair that will need to be done on cardiopulmonary bypass (CPB). While on CPB

    A. A pulse oximeter can be used to monitor oxygen saturation
    B. A noninvasive blood pressure cuff can be used to monitor perfusion pressures
    C. An arterial line can be used to measure perfusion pressures
    D. None of the above

11. The incidence of distal ischemia resulting from arterial cannulation is less than

    A. 10%
    B. 1%
    C. 0.1%
    D. 0.01%

12. When considering the advantages and disadvantages of different sites for arterial cannulation such as radial, ulnar, femoral, brachial, and dorsalis pedis, the

    A. Radial artery provides the principal source of blood to the hand
    B. Cannulation of ulnar artery is commonly associated with damage to the median nerve
    C. Dorsalis pedis artery is commonly used during emergencies and low-flow states
    D. Cannulation of the femoral artery risks local and retroperitoneal hematoma

13. Systolic blood pressures are generally higher and diastolic blood pressures are generally lower in which of the following conditions?

    A. The further you are from the heart when using a direct arterial measurement
    B. The closer you are to the heart when using a direct arterial measurement
    C. When using an automated noninvasive blood pressure cuff compared to a direct arterial measurement
    D. When recording from an over dampened arterial tracing

14. While taking care of a patient, you notice that the arterial monitor transducer has slipped off its stand and is hanging approximately 30 cm lower than where it was originally leveled. This would correspond to a blood pressure reading that is

    A. 30 mm Hg lower than the actual pressure
    B. 30 mm Hg higher than the actual pressure
    C. 22 mm Hg lower than the actual pressure
    D. 22 mm Hg higher than the actual pressure

15. An important consideration in using the subclavian approach for central venous access includes the

    A. Ease of compressibility if a hematoma or laceration develops
    B. Lower risk of pneumothorax when compared to internal jugular approach
    C. Ability of the vessel to remain patent in the setting of hypovolemia
    D. Increased risk of damaging the brachial plexus when compared to internal jugular approach

16. When interpreting a CVP waveform, the end of systole best coincides with the

    A. A wave
    B. C wave
    C. V wave
    D. X decent

17. When interpreting a CVP waveform, the beginning of systole is best represented by the

    A. A wave
    B. C wave
    C. V wave
    D. X decent

18. After placing a central line in an unstable patient in the ICU, you notice the initial CVP tracing shows very prominent C–V waves. If an echocardiogram was then obtained, you might expect to find

    A. Cardiac tamponade
    B. Significant tricuspid regurgitation
    C. Atrial fibrillation
    D. AV dissociation

19. You receive a patient from the emergency department with multiple stab wounds to the upper abdomen. The patient is unstable, and needs to emergently come to the operating room with minimal to no time for fluid resuscitation. After placing a central line, you notice loss of the Y descent on the CVP tracing, as well as universally elevated filling pressures. If you were to then do an echocardiogram, you might expect to find which of the following?

    A. Cardiac tamponade
    B. Significant tricuspid regurgitation
    C. Descending thoracic aortic dissection
    D. AV dissociation

20. The risk of complication from pulmonary artery catheter placement is less than

    A. 0.05%
    B. 0.5%
    C. 5%
    D. 15%

21. Insertion of a pulmonary artery catheter can be beneficial in the management of all of the following cases, except

    A. Helping to determine cardiogenic versus noncardiogenic pulmonary edema
    B. Following cardiac output in an unstable patient with acute-onset tricuspid regurgitation
    C. Following the response to therapy in a patient with severe pulmonary hypertension
    D. Following response to therapy in an unstable septic patient using mixed venous oxygen tension

22. During placement of a pulmonary artery catheter, you are watching the pressure tracing, as shown. At the point indicated by the arrow, the catheter tip is located in the

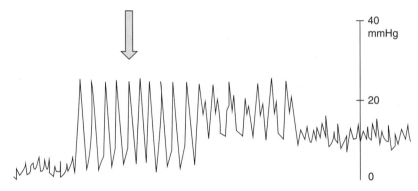

Figure 4-1.

    A. Right atrium
    B. Right ventricle
    C. Pulmonary artery
    D. Wedge position

23. The tip of a pulmonary artery catheter typically enters the pulmonary artery at approximately

    A. 15 to 25 cm
    B. 25 to 35 cm
    C. 35 to 45 cm
    D. 45 to 55 cm

24. Typical mixed venous oxygen tension in a healthy adult is

    A. 25 mm Hg
    B. 40 mm Hg
    C. 55 mm Hg
    D. 75 mm Hg

25. A pulmonary artery catheter is placed to help guide management of hypotension. Cardiac output is found to be markedly decreased with low central venous, pulmonary artery, and pulmonary artery occlusion pressures. Systemic vascular resistance is moderately elevated. Of the options listed below, the most beneficial intervention at this time would be to

    A. Administer volume
    B. Begin diuresis
    C. Start an infusion of milrinone
    D. Start an infusion of epinephrine

26. A pulmonary artery catheter is placed to help guide management of an obese patient with a known history of poorly controlled obstructive sleep apnea who is admitted with refractory hypotension. Cardiac output and pulmonary artery occlusion pressures are markedly decreased, while central venous and pulmonary artery pressures are markedly increased. Of the options listed below, the most beneficial intervention at this time would be to

   A. Administer volume
   B. Begin diuresis
   C. Start an infusion of milrinone
   D. Start an infusion of epinephrine

27. Normal systemic vascular resistance ranges between _____ (dynes)(s)/cm^5:

   A. 50 and 150
   B. 300 and 600
   C. 900 and 1500
   D. 1800 and 2100

28. Normal pulmonary vascular resistance ranges between _____ (dynes)(s)/cm^5:

   A. 50 and 150
   B. 300 and 600
   C. 900 and 1500
   D. 1800 and 2100

29. The cardiac index in a healthy adult ranges between _____ L/min/m^2:

   A. 0.8 and 1.2
   B. 1.4 and 2.0
   C. 2.2 and 4.2
   D. 4.4 and 6.0

30. Serious complications with transesophageal echocardiography (TEE), such as oral or pharyngeal injury or esophageal rupture, have an incidence as high as

   A. 0.01%
   B. 0.1%
   C. 1%
   D. 10%

31. When evaluating regurgitant lesions with transesophageal echocardiography, the Nyquist limit should be set between _____ cm/s:

   A. 30 and 40
   B. 40 and 50
   C. 50 and 60
   D. 60 and 70

32. When evaluating flow at a specific point during echocardiography, you would use

   A. Continuous-wave Doppler
   B. Pulse-wave Doppler
   C. Color Doppler
   D. Pulse-wave or continuous-wave Doppler

33. Pulse oximetry illuminates tissue samples with two wavelengths of light in order to calculate oxygen saturation. These wavelengths are _____ nm:

   A. 540 and 780
   B. 660 and 940
   C. 720 and 960
   D. 480 and 720

34. The accuracy of pulse oximetry can be significantly reduced by all of the following, except

   A. Intravenous bolus of methylene blue
   B. Intravenous bolus of heparin
   C. Severe acidosis
   D. Low blood flow

35. A patient with carboxyhemoglobin will have a pulse oximetry reading that

   A. Converges around a saturation of 85%
   B. Converges around a saturation of 65%
   C. Converges around a saturation of 45%
   D. Varies widely

36. A patient with methemoglobinemia will have a pulse oximetry reading that

   A. Converges around a saturation of 85%
   B. Converges around a saturation of 65%
   C. Converges around a saturation of 45%
   D. Varies widely

37. For the removal of a complex spinal cord tumor, the surgeon expresses concern of damage to the anterior spinal artery. The monitoring that would be helpful to determine viability of the anterior spinal cord intraoperatively would include

   A. Electroencephalography
   B. Motor-evoked potentials
   C. Somatosensory-evoked potentials
   D. Bispectral index or Sedline monitoring

38. A sudden drop in somatosensory-evoked potentials (SSEPs) would cause you to be worried about

   A. Damage to the anterior spinal artery
   B. Damage to the posterior spinal arteries
   C. An insufficient depth of anesthesia
   D. The inadvertent administration of a neuromuscular blocking agent

39. During cervical spine surgery for the resection of an intradural mass, the patient begins to cough. The concentration of isoflurane is subsequently increased. With respect to somatosensory-evoked potential (SSEP) monitoring, you would expect

   A. Amplitude and latency to decrease
   B. Amplitude and latency to increase
   C. Amplitude to decrease and latency to increase
   D. Amplitude to increase and latency to decrease

40. While monitoring somatosensory-evoked potentials, an increase in amplitude is noted. Of the options listed below, the most likely medication to have caused this increase in amplitude would be

   A. Etomidate
   B. Propofol
   C. Midazolam
   D. Sevoflurane

41. If somatosensory-evoked potentials change significantly, the anesthesia provider should consider

   A. Increasing blood pressure
   B. Hyperventilating the patient
   C. Cooling the patient
   D. Hemodilution

42. In the capnogram below, the segment that correlates with the exhalation of anatomic dead space is represented by points

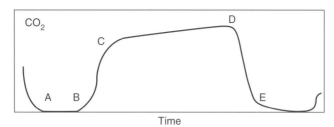

Figure 4-2.

A. A to B
B. A to C
C. C to D
D. D to E

43. In the capnogram (Fig. 4-2), the segment correlating with inspiration is represented by points

A. A to B
B. A to C
C. C to D
D. D to E

44. Capnography can help detect all of the following, except

A. Endobronchial intubation
B. Esophageal intubation
C. Bronchospasm
D. Pulmonary embolism

45. The capnograph depicted in Figure 4-3 is most likely a result of

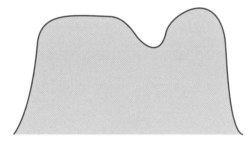

Figure 4-3.

A. Pulmonary embolism
B. Bronchospasm or airway obstruction
C. Esophageal intubation
D. Elimination of neuromuscular blockers

46. Approximately 30 minutes after the induction of general anesthesia in a healthy adult patient, you notice that core body temperature has dropped by a full degree Celsius. This is most likely due to

A. Conduction
B. Convection
C. Redistribution
D. Radiation

47. According to the American Society of Anesthesiologists, temperature monitoring is

    A. Always required
    B. Never required, but recommended
    C. Required for all general anesthetics, however not required for sedation
    D. Up to the discretion of the anesthesia provider

48. Detrimental effects of hypothermia include all of the following, except

    A. Increasing cerebral oxygen consumption
    B. Increasing surgical site infections
    C. Impairment of platelet function
    D. Increasing the duration of action of muscle relaxants

49. During a complex mitral valve replacement, it is determined that the patient will benefit from brief protective hypothermia. Of the options listed below, core temperature is best measured via the

    A. Tympanic membrane
    B. Bladder
    C. Nasopharnyx
    D. Rectum

50. While monitoring a patient for return of neuromuscular function after using rocuronium, you notice the patient has regained four twitches using train of four stimulations. With four twitches on train of four stimulations, the patient may still have blockage of acetylcholine receptors of up to

    A. 25%
    B. 50%
    C. 75%
    D. 90%

CHAPTER 4 ANSWERS

1. **D.**   ASA standards mandate the use of pulse oximetry, capnography, an oxygen analyzer in the breathing system, disconnect alarms, a visual display of an ECG, systemic blood pressure and heart rate monitoring, and temperature monitoring (when clinically indicated) for all cases. The use of a peripheral nerve stimulator is not a mandated monitor.

2. **B.**   During the delivery of anesthesia, the current standard of care is to measure systemic blood pressure and heart rate every 5 minutes at a minimum. The clinical scenario and phase of the operation may mandate more frequent monitoring, which is up to the judgment of the anesthesia provider.

3. **B.**   Lead I correlates with the placement of the negative electrode on the right arm and the positive electrode on the left arm. Lead II correlates with the placement of the negative electrode on the right arm and the positive electrode on the left leg. Lead III correlates with the placement of the negative electrode on the left arm and the positive electrode on the left leg.

4. **C.**   The understanding of coronary anatomy and regions of ischemia on an ECG is fundamental. The right coronary artery provides perfusion to the inferior of the heart in approximately 80% of patients who are considered to be right-dominant (the posterior descending artery is supplied by the right coronary artery in a right-dominant system). This inferior distribution is represented by leads II, III, and AvF. The anterior wall is supplied by the left anterior descending artery, and is represented roughly by leads V1–V4. The lateral wall of the heart is supplied primarily by the left circumflex artery, and is represented by I, AvL, V5, and V6.

5. **C.**   The use of the V5 lead results in the detection of 75% of ischemic episodes. This can be increased to 90% with the addition of the V4 lead, and up to 96% with the addition of leads II and V4.

6. **B.**   A properly-sized noninvasive blood pressure cuff should encompass 40% of the circumference of the arm. A cuff that is too small will result in a reading that is incorrectly high, whereas a cuff that is too large will result in a lower-than-accurate pressure. This is particularly worrisome in this patient when considering her cerebral perfusion pressure, since she already has a history of carotid artery disease and is in the beach chair position.

7. **B.**   When using the oscillometric method to measure blood pressure, the cuff is inflated until no oscillations on the sphygmomanometer are seen. The cuff is then slowly deflated until oscillations are seen, which represents the systolic blood pressure. As the cuff continues to be deflated, you note the point where maximal oscillations occur. This point of maximal oscillation represents the mean arterial pressure. It is not possible to measure a diastolic blood pressure with the oscillometric method.

8. **A.**   The DINAMAP (device for indirect noninvasive automatic mean arterial pressure) method for measuring blood pressure uses an automated cuff that measures oscillometric variations with reduction in cuff pressure to calculate systolic, mean, and diastolic pressures. In general, diastolic measurements with DINAMAP are about 10 mm Hg higher with automated as opposed to direct arterial measurement, whereas systolic and mean pressures tend to correlate well.

9. **D.**   Korotkoff sounds are used to interpret blood pressure when using a stethoscope and a noninvasive blood pressure cuff, and is described in 5 phases of sound. Phase 1 heralds the onset of the first sound heard and correlates with the systolic blood pressure. Phase 5 occurs

at the cuff pressure at which the sound first disappears, and is the phase recommended by the American Heart Association to correspond most reliably with the diastolic heart sound. In cases where Phase 5 does not occur (the sound never fully disappears), Phase 4 is then used to represent the diastolic blood pressure, and is described as a thumping or muting of the sound just before diastole. Phases 2 and 3 have no clinical significance.

10. **C.**   Both pulse oximetry and noninvasive blood pressure cuffs require pulsatile blood flow in order to obtain measurements. These monitors will not be effective during CPB when blood flow is artificially sustained with a more continuous flow. This can also be the case with some patients on left ventricular assist devices, and venous to arterial extracorporeal membrane oxygenation devices, where pulsatile flow is minimal.

11. **C.**   Complications from arterial cannulation include distal ischemia (<0.1%), infection, and hemorrhage. Common sites for cannulation include radial, brachial, axillary, dorsalis pedis, and femoral arteries. Common indications for direct blood pressure monitoring include cardiopulmonary bypass, when wide swings in BP are expected, when rigorous control of BP is necessary, and when there is need for multiple arterial blood gas measurements.

12. **D.**   The ulnar artery is the principal source of blood flow to the hand. Hence radial artery cannulation is much more commonly used for invasive blood pressure monitoring. Cannulation of the brachial artery risks damage to the median nerve. The femoral artery is often used in emergencies, since it is a large vessel and can still be identified in low flow states. Cannulation of the femoral artery risks both local and retroperitoneal hematoma. Dorsalis pedis artery cannulation, while not ideal since it is far from the central circulation, can reliably measure mean arterial pressure.

13. **A.**   Systolic blood pressures are generally higher and diastolic blood pressures are generally lower the further you are from the heart when using direct invasive arterial measurement. For example, when comparing a dorsalis pedis arterial measurement to a femoral arterial measurement, the dorsalis pedis will record higher systolic and lower diastolic pressures compared to the femoral line. However, the mean arterial pressures will be approximately the same. A noninvasive automated blood pressure cuff will tend to correlate with systolic arterial blood pressures, but the diastolic pressure will be approximately 10 mm Hg lower when measured via the direct invasive arterial monitor. An over dampened arterial line tracing will tend to reduce systolic pressures and increase diastolic pressures.

14. **D.**   For every 30 cm in height that a transducer is moved up and down, there is a corresponding change of 22 mm Hg in the blood pressure reading (1 cm H_2O = 0.74 mm Hg).

15. **C.**   Risks and benefits of different central cannulation sites are important for an anesthesia provider to understand. The internal jugular approach has good landmarks, predictable anatomy, and the convenience of being easily accessible at the head of the bed. Disadvantages include risk of carotid artery puncture, trauma to the brachial plexus, and risk of pneumothorax with lower placements. The left internal jugular vein carries the added risk of damage to the thoracic duct, and can be more difficult to pass a pulmonary artery catheter when needed. The external jugular vein can also be cannulated, and its superficial location makes it an easy target, but it can be more difficult to thread a catheter centrally. The subclavian approach has the benefit of also having good landmarks, as well as remaining relatively patent in a hypovolemic patient. The subclavian however does carry the highest risk of pneumothorax, and can be difficult to compress if a hematoma or laceration occurs.

16. **C.**   In the CVP waveform depicted below, the A wave represents atrial contraction, the C wave represents bulging of the tricuspid valve into the atrium during the beginning of systole, the X decent occurs during systole and corresponds to atrial relaxation, the V wave

represents filling of the atrium while the tricuspid valve is closed, and the Y descent occurs when the tricuspid valve opens and the atrium starts to empty.

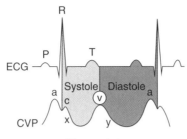

Figure 4-4.

17. B.   In the CVP waveform depicted in Figure 4-4, the A wave represents atrial contraction, the C wave represents bulging of the tricuspid valve into the atrium during the beginning of systole, the X decent occurs during systole and corresponds to atrial relaxation, the V wave represents filling of the atrium while the tricuspid valve is closed, and the Y descent occurs when the tricuspid valve opens and the atrium starts to empty.

18. B.   During systole in a patient with tricuspid regurgitation, part of the ejected volume flows backward into the atrium. Instead of seeing a small C wave that normally represents the bulging of the tricuspid valve, a much larger C wave would be seen as blood flows retrograde into the right atrium and toward the transducer. This retrograde blood flow would continue throughout the systole, and would, therefore, also increase the V wave size, since this is a systolic component of the CVP trace. During cardiac tamponade, there will be elevated pressures throughout the entire waveform, as well as loss of the Y descent. In patients with atrial fibrillation, there will be a loss of the A wave, since there is no longer a uniform atrial contraction, and an overall increase in the C wave size, since filling pressures elevate to compensate and improve ventricular filling. With AV dissociation, there are large and exaggerated A waves (often called "cannon" A waves), which represent atrial contraction against a closed tricuspid valve.

19. A.   See the answer explanation of Question 18. It would be highly unlikely to have elevated filling pressures in a bleeding trauma patient who has not yet been resuscitated. Aortic dissections can cause cardiac tamponade, but only if they involve the aortic root and then extend into the pericardium.

20. B.   While the incidence of complications is infrequent, some of the complications can carry severe morbidity and mortality risks. In addition to universal complications associated with central line placement, some additional pulmonary artery catheter complications include dysrhythmias (most common), catheter knotting, cardiac valve injury, pulmonary artery rupture, development of complete heart block in a patient with preexisting left bundle branch block, pulmonary thromboembolism or air embolism, bacteremia, endocarditis, and sepsis.

21. B.   As well as knowing some valuable indications, it is important to know some of the limitations of a pulmonary artery catheter before subjecting a patient to risks. For example, the measurement of cardiac output in patients with tricuspid regurgitation or ventricular septal defects is inaccurate due to dilution of the injectate. Pulmonary artery occlusion pressure can also inaccurately represent left ventricular end diastolic pressure in patients with mitral stenosis, left atrial myxomas, pulmonary venous obstruction, elevated alveolar pressures, and decreased left ventricular compliance. Other common errors in measurement that are not patient dependent can include an inaccurate volume or temperature of the injectate solution.

22. B.   A pulmonary artery catheter is placed while monitoring the pressure changes measured at the tip of the catheter. The first section shows a traditional CVP waveform measured in the right atrium. As the catheter is advanced, a systolic step-up is seen when entering the right ventricle, a diastolic step-up when entering the pulmonary artery, and a return to a traditional CVP waveform when entering the wedge position.

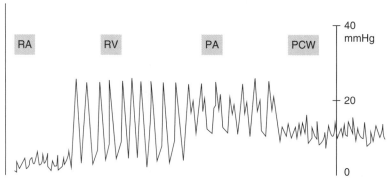

Figure 4-5.

23. **C.**   The tip of the pulmonary artery catheter typically enters the pulmonary artery at around 35 to 45 cm. This can vary from patient to patient, especially with patients at the extremes of height.

24. **B.**   Mixed venous oxygen tension can provide valuable information on the balance between oxygen consumption and delivery. Typical mixed venous oxygen tension in a healthy adult is 40 mm Hg, yielding a saturation of approximately 75%. Reduction in oxygen delivery can be due to a reduction in oxygen content per deciliter leaving the left ventricle, or a reduction in overall cardiac output. Increased oxygen consumption (low mixed venous oxygen) occurs during periods of elevated metabolic states, such as during vigorous exercise or sepsis.

25. **A.**   In the clinical scenario, low central venous, pulmonary artery, and pulmonary artery occlusion pressures support the diagnosis of hypovolemia. Increasing intravascular volume would be the most beneficial intervention at this time.

26. **C.**   The patient's history and clinical scenario suggest right heart failure due to pulmonary hypertension. Milrinone may be beneficial in decreasing pulmonary vascular resistance as well as increasing cardiac output.

27. **C.**   Interpreting physiologic data from a pulmonary artery catheter and guiding therapy requires having an intimate knowledge of baseline values. On average, normal physiologic vascular resistance falls between 900 and 1500 $(dynes)(s)/cm^5$.

28. **A.**   Normal pulmonary vascular resistance ranges between approximately 50 and 150 $(dynes)(s)/cm^5$.

29. **C.**   Normal cardiac index in a healthy adult ranges between 2.2 and 4.2 $L/min/m^2$. Cardiac index is often used over cardiac output in estimating cardiac function, since it is more reliable with extremes of height.

30. **B.**   Serious complications with TEE have been reported in approximately 0.1% of cases, or approximately 1 in 1,000 patients. Strict contraindications to TEE include but are not limited to esophageal spasm, esophageal stricture, esophageal laceration, esophageal perforation, and esophageal diverticulum. Relative contraindications include but are not limited to upper GI bleed, dysphagia or odynophagia, mediastinal radiation, large diaphragmatic hernias, atlantoaxial disease, and difficult intubation due to possibility of unintentional extubation with probe manipulation.

31. **C.**   The current guidelines recommend a Nyquist limit of 50 to 60 cm/s when evaluating regurgitant lesions. Setting the limit to low could result in overestimating the regurgitant lesion, and setting the limit to high could result in underestimating the regurgitant lesion.

32. B. Pulse-wave Doppler is used to capture flow at a specific point. During pulse-wave Doppler, a single crystal is used to both emit and receive ultrasound energy, and the location of the signal can be calculated. Continuous-wave Doppler, on the other hand, uses two separate crystals to send and receive ultrasound energy. This allows the echo machine to detect higher velocities and energy shifts; however, the exact location of the signal cannot be determined. Color-wave Doppler is used to examine regurgitant lesions.

33. B. Pulse oximetry uses two wavelengths of light to calculate oxygen saturation. These wavelengths are 660 nm of red light (well absorbed by oxygenated hemoglobin) and 940 nm of infrared light (well absorbed by deoxygenated hemoglobin).

34. B. The accuracy of pulse oximetry can be affected by many factors. These include but are not limited to low blood flow conditions, patient movement, ambient light, dysfunctional hemoglobin molecules, dyes such as methylene blue and indigo carmine, and altered relationships in the hemoglobin dissociation curve (severe acidosis). Intravenous heparin bolus is not known to distort the accuracy of pulse oximetry.

35. D. Many different clinical situations will cause pulse oximetry to read in characteristic patterns. Methemoglobinemia absorbs both wavelengths of light and tends to converge around a saturation of 85%. Carboxyhemoglobin only absorbs red light, but not infrared light, and can vary widely in saturation readings. Methylene blue, a common dye used during surgery, tends to cause saturations to converge around 65%.

36. A. Many different clinical situations will cause pulse oximetry to read in characteristic patterns. Methemoglobinemia absorbs both wavelengths of light and tends to converge around a saturation of 85%. Carboxyhemoglobin only absorbs red light, but not infrared light, and can vary widely in saturation readings. Methylene blue, a common dye used during surgery, tends to cause saturations to converge around 65%.

37. B. The corticospinal tracts responsible for motor function travel along the anterior spinal cord, and can be monitored using motor-evoked potentials. Sensory tracts, on the other hand, travel along the posterior spinal cord, and can be monitored using somatosensory-evoked potentials. Electroencephalography is commonly used to measure cerebral activity during neurovascular surgeries, such as carotid endarterectomies, looking for decreased cerebral blood flow. Bispectral index or Sedline monitoring is somewhat controversial, but is used to monitor the adequacy of depth of anesthesia.

38. B. SSEPs monitor the posterior spinal column, which would be affected by damage to the posterior spinal arteries or compression of the posterior spinal cord. A light plane of anesthesia would not cause a drop in SSEPs, nor would the administration of a neuromuscular blocking agent (the latter would hinder the use of motor-evoked potentials).

39. C. Halogenated anesthetics as well as nitrous oxide (especially when combined together) can decrease amplitude and increase latency. For this reason, it is recommended to minimize the use of volatile anesthetics to below 1 MAC, or to use a total intravenous technique when monitoring SSEPs.

40. A. Etomidate is known to increase the amplitude of somatosensory-evoked potentials (SSEPs), and can sometimes be dramatic. Propofol is considered to have minimal to no effect on amplitude, and is commonly used as an infusion for the maintenance of anesthesia when monitoring SSEPs. Midazolam has been shown to decrease amplitude, and this should be kept in mind when used for premedication. As discussed in the previous question, sevoflurane would be expected to decrease amplitude and increase latency of SSEPs.

41. A. Medications are not the only variables that affect somatosensory-evoked potentials, as changes in physiology can also alter latency and amplitude. Amplitude decreases during episodes of hypotension, hypoxia, and hyperthermia. Latency can be increased during hypothermia, hypocarbia, and hemodilution/anemia.

42. **A.**   A to B occurs during exhalation of anatomic dead space, B to C occurs during mixing of exhaled dead space and alveolar gas, C to D reflects the exhalation of alveolar gas, with point D correlating with end-tidal carbon dioxide, and D to E represents the beginning of inspiration.

43. **D.**   A to B occurs during exhalation of anatomic dead space, B to C occurs during mixing of exhaled dead space and alveolar gas, C to D reflects the exhalation of alveolar gas, with point D correlating with end-tidal carbon dioxide, and D to E represents the beginning of inspiration.

44. **A.**   It is important to remember that capnography will show a normal capnograph and end-tidal CO_2 immediately following endobronchial intubation. Anesthesia providers must be vigilant to always listen for bilateral breath sounds and observe bilateral chest rise to confirm tracheal intubation.

45. **D.**   The classic image above is commonly referred to as a curare cleft, and occurs when a patient begins to attempt inspiration during the expiratory phase of mechanical ventilation. This is one of the indications that neuromuscular function is returning.

46. **C.**   On average, core temperature declines by approximately 1 to 1.5°C after the induction of general anesthesia. This initial drop in core body temperature is primarily due to redistribution (core to periphery) from the vasodilating properties of many anesthetics. Temperature may continue to drop as processes of heat loss, such as conduction, convection, radiation, and evaporation, occur (as opposed to redistribution).

47. **D.**   The current recommendations from the American Society of Anesthesiologists state that temperature monitoring is required "when clinically significant changes in body temperature are intended, anticipated, or suspected." In addition to considering the surgical procedure, it is also important to consider at risk populations such as the elderly, infants, burn patients, and patients with autonomic dysfunction.

48. **A.**   Uncontrolled hypothermia has many detrimental effects, including increased oxygen utilization through shivering, impaired platelet function and coagulation, delayed wound healing and increasing surgical site infections, as well as potential for serious dysrhythmias. Cerebral oxygen consumption, however, decreases by approximately 7% per degree Celsius decrease in temperature.

49. **A.**   Numerous sites can be used to monitor temperature in the operating room. Of the most common, tympanic membrane (perfused by carotid artery) and pulmonary artery measurements tend to be the best reflectors of core temperature, followed by bladder temperatures. Rectal temperatures overall tend to be a poor substitute, while axillary and skin temperatures are highly prone to error.

50. **C.**   Understanding the limitations of neuromuscular twitch monitoring devices is fundamental for an anesthesia provider. At the point the fourth twitch reappears, still up to 75% to 80% of acetylcholine receptors may be blocked. Adequate reversal (neostigmine–glycopyrrolate) should be given, and clinical signs for return of neuromuscular function should be used to gauge readiness for extubation.

Fluid Management and Blood Transfusion

Rebecca Kalman and Edward Bittner

1. All of the following are signs of dehydration, except

   A. Progressive metabolic acidosis
   B. Urinary specific gravity > 1.010
   C. Urine osmolality < 300 mOsm/kg
   D. Urine sodium < 10 mEq/L

2. Regarding central venous pressure (CVP) monitoring

   A. Low values of <5 mm Hg may be considered normal in the absence of other signs of hypovolemia
   B. CVP readings can be interpreted independently of the clinical setting
   C. CVP monitoring is never indicated in patients with normal cardiac and pulmonary function
   D. In a patient with right ventricular dysfunction, a CVP of 10 mm Hg should be considered elevated

3. In healthy patients, the lactate in lactated Ringer solution

   A. Causes a lactic acidosis
   B. Is converted to bicarbonate by the liver
   C. Is rapidly bound by albumin
   D. Causes a hyperchloremic metabolic acidosis

4. All of the following fluids are generally considered to be isotonic, except

   A. Lactated Ringer
   B. Normal saline
   C. D5 normal saline
   D. D5¼ normal saline

5. All of the following statements regarding dextran solutions are true, except

   A. Dextran 40 may improve blood flow through the microcirculation
   B. Dextrans may have antiplatelet effects
   C. Large-volume infusions of dextrans have been associated with renal failure
   D. Dextran 40 is a better volume expander than dextran 70

6. Which of the following statements is true regarding fluid loss?

   A. Substantial evaporative losses can be associated with large wounds and are directly proportionate to the surface area exposed
   B. Internal redistribution of fluids, "third spacing," cannot cause massive fluid shifts
   C. Traumatized, inflamed, or infected tissues can only sequester minimal amounts of fluid in the interstitial space
   D. Cellular dysfunction as a result of hypoxia usually produces a decrease in intracellular fluid volume

7. The probability of developing anti-D antibodies after a single exposure to the Rh antigen is

   A. <1%
   B. 5% to 10%
   C. 50% to 70%
   D. >80%

8. In a conventional crossmatch

   A. Donor cells are mixed with recipient serum
   B. Recipient cells are mixed with donor serum
   C. Donor serum is tested against red cells of known antigenic composition
   D. None of the above

9. A leftward shift of the oxyhemoglobin dissociation curve may be related to

   A. Low levels of 2,3-DPG in packed red blood cells
   B. Hypothermia resulting from transfusion of blood
   C. Both A and B
   D. None of the above

10. Which of the following statements regarding fresh-frozen plasma (FFP) is correct?

   A. Contains all of the clotting factors except factor VIII
   B. Should not be used in patients with antithrombin III deficiency
   C. Carries the same infection risk as a unit of whole blood
   D. Is contraindicated in the case of isolated-factor deficiencies

11. The most common cause of an acute hemolytic transfusion reaction is

   A. An error during type and screen
   B. An error during type and crossmatch
   C. Misidentification of the patient, blood specimen, or transfusion unit
   D. Defective blood filter

12. Evidence for the fact that leukocyte-containing blood products appear to be immunosuppressive includes all of the following, except

   A. Preoperative blood transfusions appear to improve graft survival in renal transplant patients
   B. Recurrence of malignant growths may be more likely in patients who receive a blood transfusion during surgery
   C. Transfusion of allogeneic leukocytes can activate latent viruses in a recipient
   D. Blood transfusion may decrease the incidence of serious infection following surgery or trauma

13. Bacterial infection due to a contaminated blood product is most likely with transfusion of

   A. Packed red blood cells
   B. Fresh-frozen plasma
   C. Platelets
   D. Cryoprecipitate

14. All of the following qualities are advantages of crystalloid solutions, except

   A. Nontoxic
   B. Reaction-free
   C. Relatively inexpensive
   D. Have the ability to remain in the intravascular space for a relatively long amount of time

15. Administration of large volumes of normal saline can lead to

   A. A metabolic alkalosis
   B. A hyperchloremic-induced nongap metabolic acidosis
   C. An anion gap lactic acidosis
   D. None of the above

16. All of the following solutions contain potassium, except

   A. Lactated Ringer solution
   B. PlasmaLyte
   C. Hespan
   D. Packed red blood cells

17. The storage time for packed red blood cells at temperatures of 1 to 6°C is

   A. 7 to 10 days
   B. 21 to 35 days
   C. 60 to 80 days
   D. 120 days

18. Which of the following statements regarding transfusion of packed red blood cells is most correct?

   A. The hematocrit of 1 unit is usually 30% to 40%
   B. Transfusion of a single unit will increase an adult's hemoglobin concentration about 4 g/dL
   C. May cause clotting if the transfused packed red blood cells are mixed with lactated Ringer solution
   D. Their principle use as that of a volume expander

19. Blood products are tested for all of the following, except

   A. Hepatitis C
   B. HIV
   C. West Nile virus
   D. Herpes virus

20. Regarding assessment of surgical blood loss

   A. Both surgeons and anesthesiologists tend to underestimate blood loss
   B. Measurement of blood in the surgical suction container is all that is necessary to estimate blood loss
   C. The use of irrigating solutions does not complicate assessment of blood loss
   D. A soaked "lap" pad can hold 10 to 15 mL of blood

21. The most common nonhemolytic reaction to transfusion of blood products is

   A. Allergic
   B. Febrile
   C. Anaphylactoid
   D. Urticarial

22. Types of autologous blood transfusion include all of the following, except

    A. Predeposited donation
    B. Intraoperative blood salvage
    C. Normovolemic hemodilution
    D. Donor-directed transfusion

23. A patient with type O blood will have which of the following plasma antibodies?

    A. Anti-A
    B. Anti-B
    C. Both anti-A and anti-B
    D. None

24. After blood is collected, the preservative CPDA-1 is commonly added. This contains all of the following, except

    A. Citrate
    B. Phosphate
    C. Dextrose
    D. Potassium

25. A 51-year-old patient was an unrestrained driver in a motor vehicle crash in which he sustained multiple traumatic injuries. He is on mechanical ventilation, and has received 8 units of packed red blood cells, 4 units of fresh-frozen plasma, and 6 units of platelets. His arterial blood gas reveals a metabolic alkalosis. The most likely explanation for this finding is

    A. Metabolism of citrate to bicarbonate
    B. Under-resuscitation
    C. Continued bleeding
    D. Hypoventilation

26. A 70-year-old patient with chronic renal failure is in the operating room undergoing a kidney transplant. There has been more blood loss than expected, and he has received 6 units of packed red blood cells and 3 units of fresh-frozen plasma. The surgeons still complain that the patient "won't clot." All of the following are potential contributors to his coagulopathy, except

    A. Temperature of 34.9°C
    B. Uremia
    C. Dilutional thrombocytopenia
    D. Fibrinogen level of 250 mg/dL

27. The estimated maintenance fluid requirement for a 9-year-old, 35-kg patient is

    A. 50 mL/h
    B. 75 mL/h
    C. 100 mL/h
    D. 20 mL/h

28. Which of the following patients is *least* likely to need calcium supplementation due to citrate-induced hypocalcemia related to blood transfusion?

    A. A 30-year-old trauma patient receiving massive blood transfusion through a rapid transfuser at a rate of 75 mL/min
    B. A patient with end-stage liver disease undergoing a complicated open shunt procedure, who is hypothermic and has received greater than 2 blood volumes of transfusion
    C. A neonate undergoing congenital diaphragmatic hernia repair
    D. A 50-year-old patient with coronary artery disease undergoing an open femoral popliteal bypass procedure, who has received 3 units of packed red blood cells

29. A medical student asks you if "young" blood is better for critically ill patients. Which of the following statements regarding "young" blood is most correct?

    A. Fresher blood has better ability to deliver oxygen to tissues
    B. Blood from younger donors has lower risk of immunosuppression than blood donated by the elderly
    C. Older blood has a lower potassium content
    D. Fresher blood can be transfused more rapidly than older blood

30. You are caring for an 18-year-old female trauma patient who was emergently transported to the operating room for control of massive bleeding. Due to the acuteness of the patient's bleeding, there was no time for blood typing and she has received 3 units of O-negative packed red blood cells. The blood bank notifies you that the patient's blood type is A-positive. If the patient requires further transfusion, which of the following should be administered?

    A. A-positive RBCs
    B. A-negative RBCs
    C. O-negative RBCs
    D. RhoGAM

CHAPTER 5 ANSWERS

1. C.   When dehydrated, patients with normal renal function will retain sodium and produce a concentrated urine. Urine osmolality is typically greater than 450 mOsm/kg in this setting. Urine sodium will be low, and specific gravity will be high.

2. A.   CVP measurements must be evaluated in context of the clinical setting. Factors such as underlying cardiopulmonary disease, patient position, and anatomy can affect the values. A CVP of <5 mm Hg can be normal in a healthy patient without signs of hypovolemia. For surgical cases during which large fluid shifts are expected, placement of a CVP monitor may be indicated. Patients with compromised right ventricular function generally have high CVPs, and thus, a CVP of 10 mm Hg should be considered normal to low depending on the degree of dysfunction.

3. B.   In healthy patients the lactate in lactated Ringers solution is rapidly converted to bicarbonate by the liver and does not cause a lactic acidosis. Administration of a large volume of normal saline can cause a hyperchloremic metabolic acidosis. Lactate is not bound by albumin.

4. C.   An intravenous solution's effect on fluid movement depends in part on its tonicity. This term is sometimes used interchangeably with osmolarity, although they are subtly different. Osmolarity is the number of osmoles or moles of solute per liter of solution. Tonicity is the effective osmolality and is equal to the sum of the concentrations of the solutes which have the capacity to exert an osmotic force across the membrane. A solution is isotonic if its tonicity falls within (or near) the normal range for blood serum—from 275 to 295 mOsm/kg. A hypotonic solution has lower osmolarity (<250), and a hypertonic solution has higher osmolarity (>350) (Table 5-1).

Table 5-1 Osmolarity and tonicity of commonly used crystalloid solutions

Fluid	Mosm/L	Tonicity
Lactated Ringers	273	Isotonic
Normal saline	305	Isotonic
D5 normal saline	586	Hypertonic
D5¼ normal saline	355	Isotonic

5. D.   While dextran 40 has a molecular weight of 40,000, dextran 70 has a molecular weight of 70,000, and therefore, the latter is broken down more slowly, lasts longer, and is a better volume expander. Dextran 40 appears to improve blood flow through the microcirculation, and all dextrans may have antiplatelet effects. Infusion of large volume of dextran (>20 mL/kg/day) has been associated with renal failure.

6. A.   Substantial evaporative losses can be associated with large wounds and are directly proportionate to the surface area exposed. Third spacing can cause massive fluid shifts, and traumatized, inflamed, or infected tissue can sequester large amounts of fluid. Cellular dysfunction as a result of hypoxia usually produces an increase in intracellular fluid volume.

7. C.   The Rh blood group is second in importance only to the ABO blood group in the field of transfusion medicine. It has remained of primary importance in obstetrics, being the main cause of hemolytic disease of the newborn. The significance of the Rh blood group is related to the fact that the Rh antigen (D antigen) is highly immunogenic. In the case of the D antigen, individuals who do not produce the D antigen will produce anti-D if they encounter the D antigen when transfused with RBCs (causing a hemolytic transfusion reaction). For this reason, the Rh status is routinely determined in blood donors, transfusion recipients, and mothers-to-be.

8. **A.** A crossmatch mimics a transfusion, where donor cells are mixed with the recipient's serum. This has three purposes: (1) confirms ABO/Rh typing, (2) detects recipient antibodies to other blood group systems, and (3) detects antibodies in low titers or those that do not agglutinate easily. Choice C describes an antibody screen.

9. **C.** The level of 2,3-DPG in stored blood is reduced, causing decreased oxygen unloading to the tissues. Hypothermia also causes a leftward shift of the oxyhemoglobin dissociation curve (Fig. 5-1).

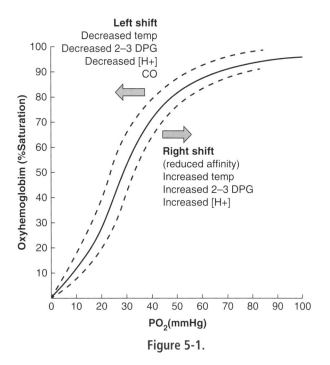

Figure 5-1.

10. **C.** FFP is the fluid portion obtained from a single unit of whole blood that is frozen within 6 hours of collection. All coagulation factors, except platelets, are present in FFP, which explains the use of this component in the treatment of hemorrhage. FFP is also indicated in antithrombin III deficiency and isolated-factor deficiencies. A transfusion of FFP carries the same risk of infection as transfusing a whole blood.

11. **C.** Hemolytic reactions occur when the wrong blood type is administered to a patient. The immediate signs of acute hemolytic transfusion reactions include lumbar and substernal pain, fever, chills, dyspnea, flushing of the skin, and hypotension. The appearance of free hemoglobin in plasma or urine is presumptive evidence of a hemolytic reaction. Acute renal failure reflects precipitation of stromal and lipid contents (not free hemoglobin) of hemolyzed erythrocytes in distal renal tubules. Acute hemolytic transfusion reactions are usually due to ABO blood incompatibility, and the most common cause is misidentification of the patient, blood specimen, or transfusion unit (clerical error).

12. **D.** Blood transfusion suppresses cell-mediated immunity, which may place surgical patients at risk for postoperative infection. The association with long-term prognosis in cancer surgery is unclear, but there is a suggestion of a correlation between tumor recurrence and blood transfusions. Removing most of the white blood cells from blood and platelets (leukoreduction) reduces the incidence of nonhemolytic febrile transfusion reactions and the transmission of leukocyte-associated viruses. Preoperative blood transfusions appear to improve graft survival in renal transplant patients.

13. **C.**   One of the leading causes of transfusion-related fatalities in the United States is bacterial contamination, which is most likely to occur in platelet concentrates. Platelet-related sepsis can be fatal and occurs as frequently as 1 in 5,000 transfusions. Platelets are stored at 20 to 24°C instead of 4°C, which probably accounts for the greater risk of bacterial growth than with other blood products. Any patient in whom a fever develops within 6 hours of receiving platelet concentrates should be considered to be possibly manifesting platelet-induced sepsis, and empirical antibiotic therapy should be instituted.

14. **D.**   Advantages of crystalloid solutions are that they are nontoxic, reaction-free, and inexpensive. Colloid solutions are composed of large-molecular-weight substances that remain in the intravascular space longer than crystalloids, and typically, the initial volume of distribution is equivalent to the plasma volume. The synthetic colloids and processed albumin have minimal or no risks of infection. Colloids are more expensive than crystalloids, but have fewer risks than blood products.

15. **B.**   Normal saline (0.9% NaCl) is slightly hypertonic and contains more chloride than extracellular fluid. Administration of large volumes of normal saline solution can lead to a hyperchloremic non–anion gap metabolic acidosis. Administration of large amounts of lactated Ringer solution may result in a metabolic alkalosis because of increased bicarbonate production from the metabolism of lactate.

16. **C.**   Hespan is colloid containing starch and saline. All of the other options contain potassium. Many patients with hyperkalemia, including patients with renal failure, routinely receive normal saline because it contains no potassium.

17. **B.**   The storage time (70% viability of transfused erythrocytes 24 hours after transfusion) is 21 to 35 days, depending on the storage medium. Changes that occur in blood during storage reflect the length of storage and the type of preservative used.

18. **C.**   Mixing of packed red blood cells with lactated Ringer solution can cause clotting as the citrate in the blood product can bind with calcium in the lactated Ringer. The other options are all false. The hematocrit of 1 unit of packed red blood cells is 70% to 80%. Transfusion of a single unit will increase an adult's hemoglobin concentration by about 1 g/dL. The objective in transfusion of packed red blood cells is to increase the blood's oxygen-carrying capacity. Although transfusion of packed red blood cells increases intravascular fluid volume, they should not be used routinely for this purpose given the risks associated with transfusion.

19. **D.**   The incidence of infection from blood transfusions has markedly decreased. Although many factors account for the marked decreased incidence of transmission of infectious agents via blood transfusion, the most important one is improved methods for testing of donor blood. Currently, hepatitis C, HIV, and West Nile virus are tested by nucleic acid technology.

20. **A.**   Both surgeons and anesthesiologists tend to underestimate blood loss. Measurement of blood in the surgical suction container is only one component of estimating blood loss. Blood lost in sponges, "lap" pads, and occult bleeding under the drapes must be accounted for. The use of irrigating solutions often complicates the assessment of blood loss. A soaked "lap" pad can hold up to 100 to 150 mL of blood.

21. **B.**   Febrile reactions are the most common adverse nonhemolytic reaction and occur with 0.5% to 1% of transfusions. The most likely cause is an interaction between the recipient's antibodies and the antigen present on the leukocytes of platelets of the donor. The patient's temperature rarely increases above 38°C, and the condition is treated by slowing the infusion and administering antipyretics. Severe febrile reactions accompanied by chills and shivering may require discontinuation of the blood transfusion.

22. **D.**   A directed (or designated) blood donation is one in which a patient selects his/her own blood donor(s) for an anticipated, nonemergency transfusion. The donor is typically a friend or relative to the patient. Patients undergoing elective procedures with a high probability of blood transfusion can donate their own blood 4 to 5 weeks prior to surgery, and this is referred to as a predeposited donation. Blood salvage refers to the collection of shed blood intraoperatively, which is then concentrated, washed, and transfused back to the patient. For normovolemic hemodilution, blood is removed just prior to surgery and replaced with crystalloid or colloid. The blood is stored for up to 6 hours, and then be given back to the patient after blood loss.

23. **C.**   Routine typing of blood is performed to identify the antigens (A, B, Rh) on the membranes of erythrocytes. Naturally-occurring antibodies (anti-B, anti-A) are formed whenever erythrocyte membranes lack A or B antigens (or both). These antibodies are capable of causing rapid intravascular destruction of erythrocytes that contain the corresponding antigens.

24. **D.**   CPDA-1 is the most commonly added preservative added to blood products. It contains citrate as an anticoagulant, phosphate as a buffer, dextrose as a red blood cell energy source, and adenine needed for the maintenance of red cell ATP levels. The potassium found in blood comes from the breakdown of red blood cells.

25. **A.**   The citrate in the blood preservative is metabolized to bicarbonate by the liver and can cause a metabolic alkalosis following a large-volume transfusion. Under-resuscitation and bleeding are likely to cause a metabolic acidosis, whereas hypoventilation causes a respiratory acidosis.

26. **D.**   Hypothermia, uremia, and dilution from massive transfusion are all potential reasons for coagulopathy in this patient. A fibrinogen greater than 150 mg/dL should be adequate for clotting.

27. **B.**   According to the "4-2-1 rule," 75 mL/h would be the maintenance rate. This is calculated as 40 + 20 + 15 = 75 mL/h (Table 5-2).

Table 5-2 Formula for calculation of maintenance fluid requirement

Weight up to 10 kg	4 mL/kg/h
11–20 kg	Add 2 mL/kg/h
21 kg and above	Add 1 mL/kg/h

28. **D.**   Hypocalcemia as a result of citrate binding of calcium is rare because of mobilization of calcium stores from the bone, and the ability of the liver to rapidly metabolize citrate to bicarbonate. Therefore, arbitrary administration of calcium in the absence of objective evidence of hypocalcemia is not indicated. Supplemental calcium may be needed when (1) the rate of blood infusion is more rapid than 50 mL/min, (2) hypothermia or liver disease interferes with the metabolism of citrate, or (3) the patient is a neonate.

29. **A.**   Fresher blood (<5 days of storage) has been recommended for critically ill patients in an effort to improve the delivery of oxygen (2,3-diphosphoglycerate concentrations are better maintained with fresher blood). More recently, some evidence suggests that administration of younger blood (i.e., stored <14 days) is associated with better outcomes including decreased mortality rate and fewer postoperative complications, especially with major surgery.

30. **C.**   In an emergency situation that requires transfusion before type and compatibility testing can be performed, O-negative packed red blood cells may be administered. Even if the patient's blood type becomes known and available, after 2 units of type O-negative packed red blood cells have been transfused, subsequent transfusions should continue with O-negative blood. RhoGAM is not indicated since the patient's blood type is Rh+.

Anesthetic Pharmacology

Mian Ahmad and Ashish Sinha

1. Correct statement about metabolism of drugs by the liver is

    A. For drugs with low extraction ratio, liver blood flow is the rate-limiting step in their metabolism
    B. For drugs with high extraction ratio, the capacity of the liver to metabolize the drug is the rate-limiting step
    C. Cytochrome P450 system is highly drug-specific
    D. Removal of the drug from the blood by hepatic clearance is directly proportional to hepatic blood flow and intrinsic clearance

2. When asked to describe the symptoms of her allergy to a local anesthetic that a 26-year-old female had at the dentist's office, the patient describes a feeling of light-headedness, palpitations, and flushing. This reaction is most likely caused by

    A. Methylparaben reaction
    B. Vasovagal reaction
    C. Para-aminobenzoic acid allergy
    D. Epinephrine in the local anesthetic

3. All of the following drugs increase the mean arterial blood pressure, except

    A. Dopamine
    B. Norepinephrine
    C. Epinephrine
    D. Isoproterenol

4. All of the following drugs increase cardiac output, except

    A. Dopamine
    B. Epinephrine
    C. Dobutamine
    D. Norepinephrine

5. In general, norepinephrine causes increase in all of the following, except

    A. Mean arterial blood pressure
    B. Heart rate
    C. Cardiac dysrhythmias
    D. Systemic vascular resistance

6. Stimulation of α_2 receptors causes

    A. Hypertension
    B. Bradycardia
    C. Salivation
    D. Anxiety

7. Labetalol is relatively contraindicated for

    A. Treatment of hypertension in aortic dissection
    B. Treatment of hypertension in preeclampsia
    C. Hypertensive emergencies after cardiac surgery involving second-degree heat block
    D. Hypertension secondary to clonidine withdrawal

8. The best initial treatment for anaphylaxis during general anesthesia is

    A. Methylprednisolone
    B. Famotidine
    C. Diphenhydramine
    D. Epinephrine

9. Compared with thiopental, etomidate causes

    A. Less nausea
    B. Increased seizure threshold
    C. Greater myoclonic activity
    D. Greater histamine release

10. Compared with propofol, ketamine causes

    A. More depression of respiratory drive
    B. More depression of airway reflexes
    C. More bronchodilation
    D. Less analgesia

11. A 65-year-old African American patient is undergoing laparoscopic repair of inguinal hernia under general anesthesia. He has a history of hypertension, diabetes, and depression. His medication list includes lisinopril, hydrochlorothiazide, metformin, and phenelzine. Intraoperative hypotension develops secondary to injury to inferior epigastric artery. Which of the following medications is relatively contraindicated to treat this hypotension?

    A. Epinephrine
    B. Norepinephrine
    C. Ephedrine
    D. Phenylephrine

12. True statement regarding flumazenil is

    A. It binds irreversibly with benzodiazepine receptor
    B. It causes hypertension and tachycardia
    C. It has a shorter duration of action than midazolam
    D. It reverses opioid-induced respiratory depression

13. Midazolam can be administered through all of the following routes, except

    A. Oral
    B. Sublingual
    C. Transcutaneous
    D. Transnasal

14. When sodium bicarbonate is added to lidocaine, more rapid onset of action of lidocaine occurs because of

    A. Increased nonionized lidocaine concentration
    B. Increased ionized lidocaine concentration
    C. Decreased extracellular pH
    D. Increased intracellular pH

15. Which of the following findings suggests current use of cocaine in a patient undergoing preoperative evaluation?

    A. Bradycardia
    B. Hypertension
    C. Pinpoint pupils
    D. Hypothermia

16. Which of the following local anesthetics is an ester?

    A. Lidocaine
    B. Prilocaine
    C. Mepivacaine
    D. Cocaine

17. Which of the statements among the following is true?

    A. Ropivacaine is more potent than bupivacaine
    B. Ropivacaine causes more motor than sensory block
    C. Bupivacaine causes more vasoconstriction than ropivacaine
    D. Ropivacaine is an S-enantiomer of bupivacaine

18. A 75-year-old patient is shivering and has chest pain in the recovery room following exploratory laparotomy for a rupture-obstructed hernia. His heart rate is 123/min, blood pressure is 200/100 mm Hg, and SpO_2 is 97% on 2 L of oxygen via nasal cannula. An EKG shows ST-T wave changes, which are treated with nitroglycerine with no effect. Which of the following is the most appropriate next step?

    A. Administration of hydralazine
    B. Administration of nitroprusside
    C. Administration of esmolol
    D. Application of a warming blanket

19. Which of the following statements about the local anesthetics is false?

    A. They are weak bases
    B. They contain either ester or amide linkage
    C. It is their charged form that interacts with the receptor
    D. They bind the receptor inside the cell

20. Local anesthetics cause their effects by

    A. Increasing the threshold potential
    B. Altering the resting membrane potential
    C. Increasing the rate of depolarization
    D. Decreasing the rate of depolarization

21. Lipid solubility of local anesthetics

    A. Generally correlates directly with the time to onset of action
    B. Increases as the fraction of ionized form of the local anesthetic increases
    C. Increases as the fraction of unionized form of the local anesthetic increases
    D. May be different in in vivo or in vitro systems

22. Which is the correct expected duration of anesthesia after infiltration with the following local anesthetics?

    A. Lidocaine   60 to 120 minutes

    B. Mepivacaine   120 to 240 minutes

    C. Ropivacaine   120 to 180 minutes

    D. Bupivacaine   120 to 180 minutes

23. Use of which of the following local anesthetics for spinal anesthesia is controversial?

    A. Ropivacaine

    B. Bupivacaine

    C. Tetracaine

    D. Lidocaine

The following three questions belong to this clinical situation:

During placement of an interscalene block utilizing 0.5% bupivacaine, a 62-year-old patient suddenly starts experiencing seizures and loses consciousness.

24. Which of the following statements regarding local anesthetic toxicity is correct?

    A. Seizure is a sign of neurotoxicity from high dose of local anesthetic

    B. Loss of consciousness is a sign of low-dose local anesthetic neurotoxicity

    C. The seizure threshold is increased by the administration of thiopental

    D. Seizure may have been caused by injection of the local anesthetic into cervical nerve root

25. Which of the following statements is *false*?

    A. Seizure may have happened secondary to the injection of local anesthetic into vertebral artery

    B. Loss of consciousness may be secondary to high epidural anesthesia

    C. Loss of consciousness may be secondary to high spinal anesthesia

    D. In general, decreased local anesthetic protein-binding decreases potential CNS toxicity

26. Which of the following statements is false?

    A. Repeated attempts at aspiration would have prevented this complication

    B. Addition of epinephrine to the local anesthetic may have helped to prevent this complication

    C. Loss of consciousness means that patient has developed cardiac arrest

    D. Amiodarone is the first line of treatment for cardiovascular toxicity caused by bupivacaine

27. During induction of anesthesia for cesarean delivery in a 22-year-old female, rocuronium is inadvertently substituted for succinylcholine. The neonate does not show any sign of muscle relaxation because rocuronium is

    A. Highly protein bound

    B. "Unaffected by ion trapping"

    C. Lipid soluble

    D. Highly ionized

28. All of the following can lead to hyperkalemic response to the administration of succinylcholine, except

    A. Burn injury

    B. Spinal cord injury

    C. Prolonged ICU stay

    D. Cerebral palsy

29. The dibucaine number in a patient having heterozygous type of plasma cholinesterase will be

    A. 20% to 30%
    B. 30% to 40%
    C. 60% to 80%
    D. 50% to 60%

30. Which of the following muscle relaxants is eliminated mostly by the kidneys?

    A. Rocuronium
    B. Succinylcholine
    C. Vecuronium
    D. Pancuronium

31. The correct recommended intubating dose among the following muscle relaxants is

    A. Vecuronium   0.08 to 0.1 mg/kg
    B. Pancuronium   0.05 to 0.07 mg/kg
    C. Succinylcholine 0.5 to 0.07 mg/kg
    D. Cisatracurium   0.5 to 0.8 mg/kg

32. Which of the following drugs is able to cross the blood–brain barrier?

    A. Physostigmine
    B. Neostigmine
    C. Pyridostigmine
    D. Glycopyrrolate

33. All of the following are side effects of anticholinesterase drugs, except

    A. Excessive salivation
    B. Increased bowel motility
    C. Bradycardia
    D. Bronchodilation

34. Which of the following characteristics of electrical stimulation is the correct representation of the stimulus generated by the nerve stimulator used for monitoring the neuromuscular blockade?

    A. Tetany: A sustained stimulus of 50 to100 Hz, usually lasting 2 seconds
    B. Twitch: A single pulse 0.5 second in duration
    C. Train of four: A series of four twitches in 2 seconds (2-Hz frequency), each 0.2 ms long
    D. Double-burst stimulation: Three short (0.2 ms) high-frequency stimulations separated by a 30-ms interval and followed 1 second later by two or three additional impulses

35. Which of the following antibiotics augments the action of nondepolarizing muscle relaxants?

    A. Penicillin
    B. Cephalosporin
    C. Erythromycin
    D. Streptomycin

36. Immediately after induction of general anesthesia for hip replacement surgery, a 56-year-old patient with severe mitral stenosis and a normal ejection fraction develops a blood pressure of 70/35 mm Hg with a heart rate of 90 bpm. Which of the following is the most appropriate initial treatment?

    A. Dobutamine
    B. Epinephrine
    C. Phenylephrine
    D. Milrinone

37. Mechanism of action of droperidol involves antagonism at all of the following receptors, except

  A. Serotonin
  B. Dopamine
  C. α-Adrenergic
  D. Glutamate

38. Which of the following is *not* seen in acute cyanide poisoning?

  A. Metabolic acidosis
  B. Cardiac arrhythmias
  C. Tolerance to the antihypertensive effect of nitroprusside
  D. Decreased mixed venous oxygen saturation

39. Which of the following medications is associated with extrapyramidal effects?

  A. Midazolam
  B. Glycopyrrolate
  C. Metoclopramide
  D. Famotidine

40. Which of the following medications should be discontinued before the elective surgery?

  A. Metoprolol
  B. Monoamine oxidase inhibitors
  C. Atorvastatin
  D. Ranitidine

41. Administration of magnesium sulfate for preeclampsia results in a decreased dose requirement for each of the following, except

  A. Succinylcholine
  B. Rocuronium
  C. Desflurane
  D. Lidocaine

42. Benefits of epinephrine 1:200,000 added to lidocaine for an epidural injection include all of the following, except

  A. Prolongation of duration of action of lidocaine
  B. Better quality of block
  C. Prophylactic treatment of hypotension associated with the bolus administration of lidocaine
  D. Delayed absorption into systemic circulation, thereby decreasing probability of local anesthetic toxicity

43. Which of the following choices is correct regarding the blood gas partition coefficient?

  A. Nitrous oxide 0.47
  B. Desflurane 0.62
  C. Isoflurane 2.4
  D. Sevoflurane 0.85

44. The use of neostigmine to reverse residual neuromuscular block may slow the metabolism of which of the following drugs administered subsequently?

  A. Rocuronium
  B. Cisatracurium
  C. Pancuronium
  D. Succinylcholine

45. A 45-year-old patient with history of hypertrophic subaortic cardiomyopathy becomes hypotensive. Which of the following drugs is *most* appropriate for treatment of hypotension?

   A. Ephedrine
   B. Amrinone
   C. Phenylephrine
   D. Nitroglycerine

46. Factors that contraindicate ketorolac administration include all of the following except

   A. Renal insufficiency
   B. Factor VIII deficiency
   C. Active peptic ulcer disease
   D. Daily ingestion of aspirin

47. After receiving massive blood transfusion, a patient anesthetized with isoflurane, fentanyl, and nitrous oxide develops acute pulmonary edema. The drug most likely to help him acutely is

   A. Isoflurane
   B. Nitroglycerine
   C. Digoxin
   D. Morphine

48. A 22-year-old college athlete with a history of prolonged QT syndrome presents for an inguinal hernia repair. Which of the following agents would be least likely to further lengthen the QT interval?

   A. Ondansetron
   B. Metoclopramide
   C. Succinylcholine
   D. Propofol

49. Which of the following statements concerning naloxone is true?

   A. Elimination half-life is longer than most of the μ-receptor opioids
   B. It has mixed agonist–antagonist activity
   C. It relieves opioid-induced spasm of the sphincter of Oddi
   D. It does not cross the placenta

50. Which of the following drugs is most likely to cause tachycardia?

   A. Fentanyl
   B. Meperidine
   C. Morphine
   D. Sufentanil

51. Addition of fentanyl to epidural bupivacaine will cause

   A. No change in duration of analgesia
   B. More rapid onset of analgesia
   C. Increased vagal activity
   D. Increased sensory block

52. Compared with sufentanil, alfentanil is characterized by

   A. Higher pK_a
   B. Larger unionized fraction at physiologic pH
   C. Less protein-binding
   D. Greater lipid solubility

53. An inhaled anesthetic has blood/gas partition coefficient of 14.8. Recovery time primarily depends on

   A. Oil/gas solubility of the agent
   B. Cardiac output
   C. Duration of administration
   D. MAC of the drug

54. Nitroprusside therapy for hypertension should be discontinued in the presence of

   A. Acute myocardial infarction
   B. Increasing metabolic acidosis
   C. Mitral regurgitation
   D. Renal failure

55. A 24-year-old man is apprehensive of general anesthesia and prefers a regional anesthetic. Decision is made to conduct spinal anesthesia for the repair of inguinal hernia along with midazolam and fentanyl to allay anxiety. During the procedure, he suddenly loses consciousness. There is profound hypotension with systolic blood pressure of 44 mm Hg and a heart rate of 28 bpm. Cardiopulmonary resuscitation is started. The next most appropriate intervention is administration of

   A. Atropine
   B. Ephedrine
   C. Epinephrine
   D. Flumazenil

56. The effect of gentamycin at the neuromuscular junction is

   A. Prevented by pretreatment with magnesium
   B. Potentiated by anticholinesterases
   C. Decreased by depolarizing relaxants
   D. Partially reversed by calcium

57. Compared with lorazepam (Ativan), midazolam (Versed)

   A. Has a shorter elimination half-life
   B. Has more rapid clearance
   C. Has a larger volume of distribution
   D. Undergoes slower hepatic metabolism

58. The drug that causes dose-dependent EEG evidence of both central nervous system excitation and depression is

   A. Thiopental
   B. Lidocaine
   C. Isoflurane
   D. Midazolam

59. Normal pseudocholinesterase

   A. Is produced primarily at nerve terminals
   B. Is antagonized by acetyl cholinesterase
   C. Resists dibucaine inhibition more than atypical pseudocholinesterase
   D. Metabolizes succinylcholine by Hofmann elimination

60. Succinylcholine has prolonged action in patients carrying homozygous pseudocholinesterase. Which of the following best explains this phenomenon?

   A. Diffusion away from the neuromuscular junction is slow
   B. Hepatic clearance of succinylcholine is reduced
   C. Succinylmonocholine induces neuromuscular block
   D. An increased proportion of succinylcholine reaches the neuromuscular junction

61. Opioid analgesics cause all of the following effects except

    A. Contraction of smooth muscle of the gallbladder
    B. Contraction of detrusor muscle of the urinary bladder
    C. Depress cellular immunity
    D. Delayed gastric emptying

62. Opioids may have more pronounced action in all of the following except

    A. In men compared to women
    B. In older than in younger patients
    C. During liver transplant surgery
    D. In kidney failure

63. Which of the following drugs decreases lower esophageal sphincter tone?

    A. Succinylcholine
    B. Glycopyrrolate
    C. Metoclopramide
    D. Neostigmine

64. A 28-year-old burn patient needs daily wound debridement. Which of the following agents is *not* appropriate to provide a short duration of anesthesia?

    A. Nitrous oxide
    B. Ketamine
    C. Etomidate
    D. Midazolam

65. Eutectic mixture of local anesthetics (EMLA cream) is sometimes used to numb the skin before attempting an intravenous access in pediatric patients. Which of the following local anesthetics is combined with prilocaine to produce this cream?

    A. Bupivacaine
    B. Lidocaine
    C. Mepivacaine
    D. Ropivacaine

66. A 76-year-old man with history of hypertension and cancer of the colon had colectomy under general anesthesia 24 hours ago. He is receiving an epidural infusion of fentanyl at the rate of 100 micro symbol g/h. Which of the following is least likely?

    A. Nausea
    B. Pruritus
    C. Respiratory depression
    D. Hypotension

67. Which of the following may help in mapping of a seizure focus under general anesthesia by enhancing the EEG activity or inducing the seizure?

    A. Thiopental
    B. Ketamine
    C. Diazepam
    D. Isoflurane

68. Which of the following anesthetic agents is contraindicated for use in patients with intermittent porphyria?

    A. Ketamine
    B. Etomidate
    C. Isoflurane
    D. Thiopental

69. Replacing 10 mg of morphine with 30 mg of ketorolac can increase the risk of

    A. Respiratory depression
    B. Analgesia
    C. Nausea
    D. Bleeding

70. The minimum anesthesia concentration (MAC) of desflurane is decreased by

    A. Chronic alcohol use
    B. Respiratory alkalosis
    C. Chronic anemia with hemoglobin of 7.5 gm/dL
    D. Hypothermia to 34°C

71. A 45-year-old woman has been using heroin for last 20 years. Use of which of the following drugs will cause acute withdrawal symptoms?

    A. Butorphanol
    B. Nalbuphine
    C. Buprenorphine
    D. Naltrexone

72. Ketamine administered in anesthetic doses

    A. Decreases intracranial pressure
    B. Causes respiratory depression
    C. Is metabolized by the liver
    D. Increases bronchomotor tone

73. Which of the following drugs is the most appropriate agent for acute treatment of hypertension in a preeclamptic patient?

    A. Magnesium
    B. Labetalol
    C. Lisinopril
    D. Nitroglycerine

74. Which of the following provides the best estimate of complete reversal of neuromuscular blockade?

    A. Double-burst ratio of 1
    B. Train-of-four-ratio of 1
    C. Absence of fade on tetanic stimulation at 50 Hz
    D. Absence of fade of single twitch

75. Which of the following is contraindicated in a patient with Guillain–Barré syndrome?

    A. Intrathecal opioids
    B. Nondepolarizing muscle relaxant
    C. Epidural local anesthetics
    D. Succinylcholine

76. Which of the following drugs is the most appropriate for management of anesthesia in a patient who needs emergency surgery and admits to using cocaine in last 3 hours?

    A. Labetalol before induction
    B. Ketamine for induction
    C. Propofol for induction
    D. Ephedrine for treatment of hypotension

77. During general anesthesia, which of the following agents is most appropriate to treat an acute episode of cyanosis in a child with tetralogy of Fallot?

    A. Atropine
    B. Epinephrine
    C. Phenylephrine
    D. 100% oxygen

78. Rebound hypertension is most likely after sudden discontinuation of which of the following classes of antihypertensive drugs?

    A. Thiazide diuretics
    B. Calcium channel blockers
    C. α-Agonist
    D. Angiotensin-converting enzyme inhibitors

79. A 65-year-old man has nausea and vomiting in the post–anesthesia care unit, needing anti-emetic therapy. He develops involuntary facial movements, difficulty swallowing, and torticollis. Which of the following drugs is most likely to be the cause of these symptoms?

    A. Promethazine (Phenergan)
    B. Diphenhydramine (Benadryl)
    C. Metoclopramide (Reglan)
    D. Granisetron (Kytril)

80. Which of the following statements about ketamine is true?

    A. Tolerance may develop after repeated administration
    B. It is extensively bound to plasma protein
    C. Primary site of action is GABA receptor
    D. Kidney is the primary route of elimination

81. Which of the following statements about etomidate is most likely *true*?

    A. It causes significant dose-dependent respiratory depression
    B. It causes cerebral vasodilatation
    C. It increases frequency of excitatory spikes on the EEG more than thiopental
    D. Most of the administered dose is excreted unchanged by the kidney

82. The MOST likely analgesic mechanism of action of gabapentin for neuropathic pain is

    A. Antagonism at the GABA receptor
    B. NMDA receptor inhibition
    C. Sodium channel blockade
    D. Calcium channel modulation

83. Which of the following properties of local anesthetics is *most* likely a primary determinant of potency?

    A. Vasodilation
    B. pK_a
    C. Protein-binding
    D. Lipid solubility

84. Which of the following statements about etomidate is *most* likely true?

    A. It is water soluble at an acidic pH and lipid soluble at physiologic pH
    B. It may be used as an infusion for sedation in the ICU
    C. It is related to propofol in its chemical structure
    D. Awakening from induction dose is secondary to very rapid liver metabolism

85. A 64-year-old man is scheduled for an open abdominal aortic aneurysm surgery. Anesthetic plan includes placement of an epidural catheter for postoperative pain relief. On review of his medication list, it is noted that he has been taking clopidogrel for a coronary artery stent that was inserted 2 years ago. Which of the following statements about clopidogrel is *most* likely true?

    A. The American Society for Regional Anesthesia recommends that clopidogrel be stopped 3 days before neuraxial anesthesia
    B. A single dose of clopidogrel may have a clinically significant effect on platelet function
    C. Clopidogrel is associated with pancytopenia
    D. Inhibition of platelet function by clopidogrel is reversible

86. Which of the following statements about ketamine is *most* likely true?

    A. Analgesic efficacy of epidural ketamine is equivalent to epidural morphine
    B. Ketamine decreases the duration of action of nondepolarizing neuromuscular-blocking drugs
    C. Ketamine is a direct myocardial depressant
    D. Ketamine decreases the cortical amplitude of somatosensory-evoked potentials

87. A patient has a history of an allergic reaction to a local anesthetic but does not recall the name. Which of the following local anesthetics will *most* likely be the cause of a true allergic reaction?

    A. Procaine
    B. Lidocaine
    C. Mepivacaine
    D. Bupivacaine

88. Which of the following is *most* likely the (analgesic) mechanism of action of lidocaine when used for neuropathic pain?

    A. Inhibition of G-protein–coupled receptors
    B. Antagonism of NMDA receptors
    C. Calcium channel blockade
    D. Sodium channel blockade

89. A 45-year-old farmer is brought into the emergency room. He is agitated and confused. On examination, he has dry skin with fever and rapid heart rate. Anticholinergic poisoning is suspected. Which of the following medications is *most* appropriate to treat his condition?

    A. Neostigmine
    B. Pyridostigmine
    C. Edrophonium
    D. Physostigmine

90. Which of the following medications will prolong the neuromuscular blockade produced by vecuronium?

    A. Carbamazepine
    B. Clindamycin
    C. Quinidine
    D. Verapamil

91. The shorter duration of action of remifentanil compared with fentanyl is primarily due to its

    A. Rapid redistribution
    B. Renal elimination
    C. Metabolism by esterases
    D. Hepatic extraction ratio

92. Which of the following statements about dexmedetomidine is most likely true?

    A. It has more α_2 selectivity than clonidine
    B. It can increase opioid-induced rigidity
    C. Context-sensitive half time increases markedly after prolonged infusion of dexmedetomidine
    D. It has no effect on systemic vascular resistance

93. Which of the following can precipitate an episode of myotonia in a patient with myotonic dystrophy?

    A. Lidocaine administration
    B. Neostigmine administration
    C. Nondepolarizing neuromuscular-blocker administration
    D. Hypothermia

94. A 50-year-old woman had cholecystectomy done under general anesthesia. Rocuronium was used as muscle relaxant, and a combination of anticholinergic and anticholinesterase was used for reversal of muscle-relaxant action. The patient is now bradycardic. The combination of reversal agents most likely to cause the bradycardia is

    A. Atropine and edrophonium
    B. Glycopyrrolate and edrophonium
    C. Atropine and neostigmine
    D. Glycopyrrolate and neostigmine

95. A 68-year-old man is undergoing exploratory laparotomy for intestinal obstruction. Cause of obstruction is found to be an ileal carcinoid tumor. Suddenly, the patient develops broncho-spasm, and the peak airway pressure increases from 24 to 45 cm of H_2O. Which of the following is the best treatment for the bronchospasm in this situation?

    A. Dexamethasone
    B. Sevoflurane
    C. Ketamine
    D. Somatostatin

96. A 15-year-old boy has severe gastroenteritis with nausea, vomiting, and diarrhea for last 3 days. A CT scan of the abdomen shows intussusceptions, which needs exploratory lapa-rotomy for relief of intestinal obstruction. The patient's systolic blood pressure is 78 mm Hg and heart rate is 112 bpm. Thiopental is selected as the induction agent for general anesthesia. A decreased dose of this agent is recommended in patients with hypovolemic shock primarily because

    A. Delivery of the drug to the brain is increased
    B. Hepatic clearance is decreased
    C. Thiopental is a myocardial depressant
    D. Thiopental is a vasodilator

97. A 75-year-old woman is scheduled for mitral valve repair. High-dose fentanyl is used to induce anesthesia. In order to counteract the bradycardia caused by fentanyl, pancuronium is administered. Pancuronium blocks the bradycardia caused by fentanyl by acting on which of the following?

    A. β-Adrenergic receptors
    B. Cardiac muscarinic receptors
    C. Carotid baroreceptors
    D. Central vagal nuclei

98. Which of the following medications would be *most* appropriate to treat symptomatic bradycardia 1 month after cardiac transplant?

   A. Glycopyrrolate
   B. Phenylephrine
   C. Atropine
   D. Isoproterenol

99. Which of the following statements about propofol infusion syndrome is *most* likely false?

   A. Mortality rate in an established case is very high
   B. Rhabdomyolysis is one of the diagnostic criteria
   C. Tachycardia is an early sign of this syndrome
   D. Cardiac dysfunction is very common in this condition

100. A patient is undergoing resection of a supratentorial brain tumor. He is normocarbic, and his mean blood pressure is 70 mm Hg. Administration of which of the following is most likely to decrease cerebral blood volume?

   A. Nitrous oxide at 0.5 minimum alveolar concentration (MAC)
   B. Desflurane at 1 MAC
   C. Thiopental 2 mg/kg
   D. Phenytoin 15 mg/kg

101. Which of the following classes of drugs is most likely to be responsible for an anaphylactic reaction during general anesthesia?

   A. Neuromuscular-blocking drugs
   B. Opioids
   C. Antibiotics
   D. Radio contrast dyes

CHAPTER 6 ANSWERS

1. **D.**   Clearance of drugs that are mainly metabolized in the liver is a function of the amount of drug brought into the liver by its blood flow multiplied by ability of the hepatocytes to clear the blood of that drug. For drugs that have a high extraction ratio, the liver removes the entire drug entering the liver in one pass. Lidocaine and propranolol are examples of this kind of clearance. Alfentanil, on the other hand, has a low extraction ratio, and liver blood flow does not really affect its clearance. Instead, it is the intrinsic ability of the liver to clear the blood of this drug that determines alfentanil's clearance. Cytochrome P450 system can metabolize a wide variety of drugs by a single group of enzymes.

2. **D.**   Many patients believe that they are allergic to local anesthetic. Questioning them about it is important; otherwise, options for safe delivery of anesthesia can get challenging. Dentists usually add epinephrine to the local anesthetic to decrease the bleeding associated with the dental procedure. If any epinephrine gets access to the vascular system, it can cause transient tachycardia and hypertension that patient may describe as palpitations, flushing, and dizziness. If labeled as an allergic reaction, it may limit anesthetic options for the patient in the future. In an emergent situation where a spinal anesthetic could have been possible, one may have to utilize general anesthesia and risk airway complications. It is important to elucidate the real allergic reaction for an elective case by subjecting the patient to allergy testing. Serum testing is available. Skin testing is not indicated because of the risks involved. Most of the allergic reactions observed with local anesthetics are not due to the local anesthetic molecule but either to para-aminobenzoic acid, a metabolite of ester local anesthetics, or to methylparaben and metabisulphite, which are both preservatives. True type 1 allergic reaction with local anesthetic is extremely rare but will present as anaphylaxis with hypotension and respiratory symptoms. Vasovagal response usually manifests as pale skin with very low heart rate and blood pressure. Although this patient did have light-headedness, she also had flushing and palpitation which is not consistent with vasovagal reaction.

3. **D.**   Effect of sympathomimetic drugs on the mean arterial blood pressure is mediated through their effect on the adrenergic receptors they stimulate. Ultimate effect is generated through complex interaction of different factors based on baseline sympathetic tone, patient's volume status, and condition of the heart. Although isoproterenol increases contractility through its action on β_2 receptors, it also stimulates β_1 receptors in big vascular beds like muscle, causing vasodilatation and decreasing the systemic vascular resistance. So despite increasing contractility of the heart and increasing the cardiac output, the mean arterial blood pressure can decrease with administration of this drug. Other medications increase the mean arterial blood pressure by their effect on α_1 and β_1 receptors.

4. **D.**   All of these catecholamines cause stimulation of β_1 receptors, thus increasing cardiac contractility, but norepinephrine also has a very strong effect on α_1 receptors, thus increasing afterload to such a degree that cardiac output may actually decrease after administration of this drug.

Cardiac output = Systemic blood pressure/Systemic vascular resistance

According to this formula, systemic vascular resistance (SVR) is inversely related to cardiac output; thus, an increase in the SVR may decrease the cardiac output. Other drugs have more effect on cardiac contractility than on SVR, and thus, cardiac output increases with their administration.

5. **B.**   Effect of norepinephrine is on α_1 receptors and systemic vascular resistance, and thus on systemic mean arterial blood pressure may be so pronounced that there may be a decrease in heart rate secondary to baroreceptor response. It does increase the likelihood of cardiac dysrhythmias in the presence of some older anesthetics like halothane as well as in hypoxia and hypercarbia.

6. B.   Stimulation of α_2 receptors causes inhibition of release of norepinephrine, thus decreasing the activity of the sympathetic nervous system. Hypotension and bradycardia are side effects that sometimes limit the use of medications like clonidine and dexmedetomidine. In the past, these drugs were used mainly as antihypertensives, but applications based on their sedative, anxiolytic, and analgesic properties are becoming increasingly common. Dry mouth may also result from the use of dexmedetomidine.

7. C.   Labetalol is a competitive antagonist at the α_1 and β adrenergic receptors. It is a useful agent in the perioperative period because vasodilatation caused by α_1 blockade is not accompanied with tachycardia with its attendant risks. It is a particularly useful drug in hypertensive patient with diagnosis of aortic dissection as it decreases the sheer force across the dissection. It does not cross the placenta and does not decrease the uterine blood flow even when patient is hypotensive, so it is used in obstetric patients with preeclampsia to control their blood pressure. Clonidine is a stimulant of α_2 receptors, thus decreasing sympathetic activity, and its long-term administration leads to up regulation of adrenergic receptors. Sudden withdrawal of this medication leads to overactivity of the sympathetic system and a β-blocker antagonist is very helpful in controlling the manifestations of this overactivity. Abnormalities of cardiac conduction system are a relative contraindication to the administration of labetalol as it may worsen the degree of conduction blockade.

8. D.   Although all of these medications may be useful in the event of anaphylaxis during a general anesthetic, epinephrine is considered to be the drug of choice and is indicated as the first line of treatment. Dose depends on the severity of the reaction and may be anywhere from 10 μg to 1 mg if cardiac arrest develops. Its α_1 action counteracts the severe vasodilatation, which is the hallmark of this condition. Its β_2 action helps treat bronchoconstriction while β_1 action helps support the cardiac output. H_1- and H_2-blockers are also indicated in the treatment of anaphylaxis and help mitigate the effects of type 1 antigen antibody reaction on mast cells and other mediators, causing vascular dilatation and increased capillary permeability, but their actions are neither as rapid nor as profound as epinephrine. Steroids stabilize the cell membranes of mast cells and eosinophils, thus decreasing the intensity of the immunologic response, but their action takes 4 to 6 hours to develop, and there is little evidence to support the use of steroids for the acute treatment of anaphylaxis.

9. C.   Etomidate actually causes a decrease in the seizure threshold, and is thus useful in cases of electroconvulsive therapy for severe depression. Spontaneous movements characterized as myoclonus occur in more than 50% of patients receiving etomidate and may be associated with seizure-like activity on the EEG. Another side effect is an increased incidence of nausea and vomiting in the postoperative period. It does not cause histamine release in contrast to thiopental, which has been shown to release histamine in vitro.

10. C.   Ketamine differs from other induction agents used in contemporary practice of anesthesia in many important ways. Instead of acting directly on the reticular-activating system (RES), it causes dissociation of thalamus (which relays sensory information from the RES to cerebral cortex) from the limbic cortex (which is involved with the awareness of sensation). In sharp contrast to other anesthetic agents, it increases blood pressure, heart rate, and cardiac output by central stimulation of sympathetic system and inhibition of uptake of norepinephrine. In the same vein, its effect on the ventilator drive and airway reflexes is minimal, if any. It is an excellent bronchodilator and analgesic. Thiopental, propofol, and etomidate, on the other hand, may be anti-analgesic.

11. B.   Phenelzine inhibits monoamine oxidase, an enzyme that metabolizes catecholamines, allowing their levels to build up in the adrenergic neurons. Ephedrine has both direct and indirect actions on adrenergic system. Indirect action involves release of exaggerated amounts of norepinephrine from the adrenergic neurons leading to catastrophic increase in blood pressure. More direct-acting medication like phenylephrine is a better choice in a patient using monoamine oxidase inhibitors.

12. **A.** Flumazenil is useful as a specific reversal agent for benzodiazepine overdose. It has minimal intrinsic activity on this receptor, but because of similarity in the chemical structure, it acts as a competitive antagonist in the presence of agonist at the receptor site. Duration of action is short (60–90 minutes), so repeated doses or infusion is required if recurrence of sedation is desired. Reversal of benzodiazepine action does not lead to cardiovascular side effects or evidence of acute stress response. It does not have any effect on opioid receptor, so is not useful to reverse respiratory depression caused by narcotic overdose.

13. **C.** Although most common route of administration of midazolam in anesthesia is intravenous, this drug can be given via many routes. Midazolam oral suspension is used routinely in pediatric anesthesia. Intramuscular injection can be painful, but intranasal route utilizing mucosal atomization device may be useful to treat seizure activity. Bioavailability of sublingual midazolam is much better than orally administered drug. Exposure of the acidic midazolam preparation to the physiologic pH of blood causes a change in the ring structure that renders the drug more lipid soluble, thus speeding its passage across the blood–brain barrier. There is no preparation available for transcutaneous delivery of this drug in comparison to fentanyl.

14. **A.** Since local anesthetics are weak bases, they exist largely in the ionic form, making it difficult for them to cross the cell membrane, thus delaying their local anesthetic action. Addition of sodium bicarbonate promotes nonionized fraction of local anesthetic, promoting more rapid onset of its action. Depending on the amount injected, the local pH may increase, but effect on the intracellular pH is minimal, if any.

15. **B.** Cocaine inhibits reuptake of catecholamines into preganglionic nerve terminal; it has a sympathomimetic effect, causing tachycardia, hypertension, pupillary dilatation, and increased skin temperature. Chronic use may lead to cardiomyopathy and depletion of catecholamine stores with unpredictable manifestations during anesthesia.

16. **D.** There are important differences between the two classes of local anesthetics. Ester local anesthetics are metabolized by plasma cholinesterase, and so patients with atypical variety of enzyme is liable to develop local anesthetic toxicity because of slow metabolism. They are metabolized to para-aminobenzoic acid (PABA), and individuals known to have allergy to this substance should not be given ester kind of local anesthetic. Commercial multidose preparations of amides often contain methylparaben, which has a chemical structure similar to that of PABA. This preservative may be responsible for most of the rare allergic responses to amide agents. Amide local anesthetics are metabolized by liver, and decreased liver blood flow or history of liver failure may lead to toxicity even when less-than-maximum-recommended dose is used. All of the local anesthetics included in this question have amide structure in their molecule, except cocaine.

17. **D.** Ropivacaine is less lipid soluble, and thus less potent than bupivacaine. For a given dose, the sensory block is more than the motor block. Part of the reason ropivacaine may be less cardio toxic than bupivacaine is that it causes vasoconstriction in the tissues, thus decreasing the rate of absorption into systemic circulation.

    Enantiomers are stereoisomers that exist as mirror images. Enantiomers have identical physical properties except for the direction of the rotation of the plane of the polarized light. Ropivacaine is an S-enantiomer of mepivacaine and bupivacaine.

18. **C.** Oxygen demand of the myocardium increases with increase in heart rate and blood pressure. Esmolol will decrease both the heart rate and blood pressure rapidly, thus decreasing the oxygen demand. Hydralazine will decrease the blood pressure but may make the tachycardia worse. Same is true for nitroprusside. Shivering increases oxygen demand and needs to be treated promptly. Application of warming blanket may be effective if patient is hypothermic, but it may take a while for the body temperature to improve. It may not be effective in this patient if his temperature is normal and if the mechanism of shivering involves inhibition of thermoregulatory mechanisms of the body by the residual anesthetic.

Esmolol is a short-acting β-blocker that will decrease the heart rate and myocardial contractility through its inhibition of β₁ receptors, thus decreasing the myocardial oxygen demand. Improved heart rate will also help with improved supply of oxygen to the myocardium by increasing the diastolic time during which most of the left-ventricular myocardium gets its oxygen.

19. **C.**   Local anesthetics exert their electrophysiologic effects by blocking sodium ion conductance. This effect is primarily mediated by interaction with specific receptors that are within the inner vestibule of the sodium ion channel.

20. **D.**   Local anesthetics decrease the rate of depolarization of the cell membrane when a nerve impulse arrives and changes the resting membrane potential of the neuron. Normally, this potential is −90 mV inside the cell. When an impulse reaches the cell, it increases the inflow of sodium into the cell, causing this potential to move toward a positive value. If this change is enough to reach a critical level called the threshold potential, an action potential is generated; otherwise, the impulse dies down. Local anesthetics decrease the rate of change of this potential so that it does not reach the threshold level. They do not change the threshold potential or resting membrane potential per se.

21. **D.**   Lipid solubility of a local anesthetic is directly proportional to its potency. It is ordinarily expressed as a partition coefficient, which is determined by comparing the solubility in aqueous phase, generally water or buffered solution. Since the site of action of the anesthetic molecule is inside the nerve cell, higher the proportion of neutral base or the unionized form, higher the lipid solubility and higher the potency. Ionization makes it more resistant to enter the cell and decreases its potency.

It is important to appreciate that measures of anesthetic activity may be affected by the in vitro and in vivo system in which these effects are determined. For example, tetracaine is 20 times more potent than bupivacaine when studied in isolated nerve tissue but has equivalent potency compared with bupivacaine when tested in intact in vivo systems. The effect actually may vary even in different areas of the body like epidural space vs. peripheral nerve block because of secondary effects such as the inherent vasoactive properties of the anesthetic.

22. **A.**   Infiltration of local anesthetic in peripheral tissues is different from injection into a nerve sheath for a peripheral nerve block. Duration of anesthesia after infiltration is much less than after a nerve block. Anesthesia after ropivacaine and bupivacaine lasts 4 to 8 hours, while lidocaine is effective only from 1 to 2 hours. Mepivacaine is in between with duration of action from 90 to 180 minutes.

23. **D.**   Use of many local anesthetics for spinal anesthesia is still evolving. Lidocaine was introduced into clinical practice in 1946. It was commonly used for spinal anesthesia until reports of transient neurologic symptoms (TNS) started appearing in the literature. Incidence of TNS is relatively high with up to one-third of patients complaining of pain and dysesthesia 12 to 24 hours after the surgery. Although symptoms are transient, pain sometimes is so severe that it may exceed the pain of surgery and may necessitate readmission into the hospital. This issue has raised questions regarding the advisability of continued use of lidocaine for spinal anesthesia.

24. **A.**   If central nervous system toxicity was to happen from slow absorption of local anesthetic or injection into a vein, symptoms are usually milder to begin and escalate finally to the seizure level. Early symptoms of local anesthetic toxicity may manifest as circumoral numbness, metallic taste in the mouth, and tremors. As the serum levels of the local anesthetic increase further, seizure may result due to excitation of some focus in the central nervous system. Further increase in these levels leads to depression of the nervous system manifesting as lethargy and coma.

Direct injection into a nerve usually causes a shooting pain along the length of the nerve with involuntary withdrawal of the limb in an awake patient, not a seizure. It is recommended to avoid performance of a nerve block under general anesthesia so that patient could point to this, and thereby avoidance of nerve injury. Treatment is supportive. Specific treatment for the seizure is either benzodiazepine or barbiturates that increase the seizure threshold. It is important to control the seizure because intense muscular activity increases oxygen utilization and carbon dioxide production, causing both metabolic as well as respiratory acidosis. If the dose of bupivacaine that gained access to vascular system is high, the major danger is cardio toxicity that is made much worse and is extremely difficult to treat in the presence of acidosis.

25. **D.**   It is recommended that the needle used for interscalene block should be of appropriate length for the given patient. Nerve roots in this region are very superficial and if a longer needle is used, a medially directed needle may end up in either epidural or intrathecal space leading to high epidural or intrathecal block respectively. This usually presents as catastrophic hypotension, respiratory distress followed by cardiovascular collapse depending on the dose injected. Seizure is not a presentation of high epidural or intrathecal injection. Higher protein-binding decreases the chance of neurotoxicity by decreasing the free fraction of the drug available for absorption into the circulation.

26. **D.**   Frequent attempts at aspiration are recommended whenever large dose and volume of local anesthetic is injected for epidural or peripheral nerve block to avoid injecting the local anesthetic in the vascular or intrathecal space. Cases of local anesthetic toxicity have been reported even when aspiration was negative for blood or CSF.

    Addition of a dilute concentration of epinephrine to local anesthetic is helpful as it may alert the practitioner to inadvertent vascular injection of the local anesthetic by increase in the heart rate. It also helps delay the systemic absorption of local anesthetic, thus keeping the maximum serum concentration lower.

    It is possible that loss of consciousness is secondary to cardiac arrest, but it may also be secondary to high-dose CNS toxicity, respiratory arrest, or high neuraxial anesthesia.

    Amiodarone was the drug of choice to treat cardiovascular toxicity of bupivacaine in the past, but now 20% intralipid has replaced this drug. Recommended dosage for cardiovascular collapse secondary to bupivacaine toxicity is 1.5 mL/kg bolus, followed by 0.25mL/kg/min for the next 10 minutes. Oxygenation, ventilation, and good basic and advanced life support are extremely essential as bupivacaine toxicity is adversely affected by hypercarbia, acidosis, and hypoxia.

27. **D.**   Neuromuscular-blocking drugs (NMBDs) are highly charged molecules because of the presence of a quaternary ammonium group in their structure. This makes them poorly lipid soluble so that they do not cross biologic membranes like blood–brain barrier, renal tubular epithelium, and placenta. Administration of these drugs thus does not produce central nervous system effects; renal tubular reabsorption is minimal, and maternal administration does not adversely affect the fetus. Issue of ion trapping can only develop if a drug gets trapped in the acidic environment of fetal blood after it has crossed the placenta.

28. **D.**   Any time prolonged skeletal muscle inactivity or extensive muscle damage exists, patient may be susceptible to hyperkalemia after the administration of succinylcholine and is dependent on development of extrajunctional atypical receptors. In some patients, potassium levels may exceed 10 mEq/L. This can lead to serious cardiac arrhythmias and even cardiac arrest. The duration of susceptibility to the hyperkalemic response to succinylcholine is unknown but probably decreases after 3 to 6 months of denervation injury.

    Although cerebral palsy seems to be a muscular problem, consensus is that it is safe to use succinylcholine for these patients if airway management will be facilitated by its use.

29. **B.**   Atypical plasma cholinesterase lacks the ability to hydrolyze ester bonds in drugs such as succinylcholine and remifentanil. Diagnosis of presence of atypical enzyme can be made by measuring the ability of dibucaine, a local anesthetic, to inhibit the activity of this enzyme. A normal enzyme gets inhibited the most (80%), while atypical homozygous type is minimally inhibited (20%). Heterozygous variety has lesser inhibition.

In clinical terms, this leads to prolonged paralysis following administration of succinylcholine, with duration ranging from 5 to 10 minutes with normal enzyme to 60 to180 minutes for patients having homozygous atypical variety of enzyme.

30. **D.**   Choice of the muscle relaxant for any given anesthetic depends on many factors like duration of surgical procedure, comorbidities of the patient, required speed of onset, route of elimination, duration of action, and associated side effects like tachycardia or hyperkalemia. Out of these factors, the duration of action depends on the dose, presence of associated conditions like hypothermia, concomitant use of drugs that influence the muscle relaxation like magnesium or calcium channels blockers, and the presence of hepatic or renal disease. Intermediate acting neuromuscular blockers like rocuronium and vecuronium undergo primarily hepatic metabolism and biliary excretion with minimal renal excretion (10%–25%).

Many of the long-acting neuromuscular blockers are excreted by the kidney, and their use in patients with renal failure may lead to prolonged neuromuscular blockade. Pancuronium is one of these long-acting agents, and 80% of its administered dose is excreted by the kidney. As discussed in the previous question, succinylcholine is metabolized by the plasma cholinesterase and only a fraction of the administered dose reaches the neuromuscular junction.

31. **A.**   Onset and duration of action are largely dependent on the dose administered. Although smaller doses can be effective, the recommended intubating dose is usually two to four times higher than ED_{95}. This provides a higher incidence of better and earlier intubating conditions than would be possible with ED_{95}. Higher doses do lead to longer duration of action so that the return of the first twitch on train of four, a prerequisite before a reversal agent can be administered, is delayed.

32. **A.**   Anticholinesterases are used to reverse the effects of nondepolarizing neuromuscular-blocking agents (NMBDs). Selection of these drugs depends on many factors. One of the considerations is the ability of the selected drug to cross the blood–brain barrier. As NMBDs do not cross the blood–brain barrier, there is no effect on the central nervous system. Using an anticholinesterase with only peripheral action thus makes sense because central nervous system side effects of a drug like physostigmine can be avoided. These effects can be very pronounced in elderly patients, leading to confusion and agitation in the recovery room. Neostigmine and pyridostigmine, with their quaternary ammonium structure and consequent inability to cross the blood–brain barrier, are thus preferred agents to reverse the actions of NMBDs than physostigmine which crosses that barrier readily. Same principle applies to anticholinergic agents that are administered along with anticholinesterase drug to counteract the surge of acetylcholine causing bradycardia. Atropine and scopolamine, with their tertiary character, may cross the blood–brain barrier and may cause central nervous system effects. Glycopyrrolate, on the other hand, has quaternary structure and lacks central nervous system effects and has largely replaced atropine for blocking the adverse muscarinic effects.

33. **D.**   Administration of anticholinesterase agent leads to accumulation of acetylcholine, manifesting increased cholinergic actions in the body. Vagal stimulation causes bradycardia and, if not antagonized by concomitant administration of a cholinergic agent, may lead to cardiac standstill. Antisialagogue actions of these agents are also helpful in reducing the excessive salivation induced by parasympathetic overactivity of acetylcholine generated by inhibition of cholinesterase. Disruption of gastrointestinal anastomosis is another consideration, secondary to increased peristalsis of the bowel. Cholinergic activity may also lead to bronchospasm and not bronchodilation.

34. **C.**   Impulses generated by the nerve stimulator are standardized to ensure uniformity of monitoring. Out of the different patterns described in the question, only the characteristic of train of four is correct. Although this mode is used more often in modern clinical practice of anesthesia, in fact the absence of fade—a hallmark of nondepolarizing block—is a more reliable indicator of reversal of neuromuscular blockade with tetanic or double-burst

stimulation. A depolarizing block is characterized by absence of fade but takes on characteristics of a nondepolarizing block if enough depolarizing agent is administered.

35. **D.** Many physiologic factors and anesthetic and nonanesthetic drugs interact with nondepolarizing muscle relaxants (NDMRs). Volatile and local anesthetics potentiate, while depolarizing muscle relaxants antagonize the effects of these drugs. Intravenous anesthetic agents do not have any appreciable muscle-relaxant effect in normal doses. Aminoglycoside antibiotics potentiate the effects of NDMRs, while penicillin, cephalosporins, erythromycin, and tetracycline are devoid of neuromuscular effects. Streptomycin belongs to aminoglycoside family, and thus augments the effects of NDMRs.

36. **C.** Induction of anesthesia in a patient with severe valvular stenosis can lead to decreased ventricular filling secondary to vasodilatation and decreased venous return. Increase in the heart rate is very poorly tolerated as the ventricular filling is impaired because of decreased diastolic time. In the presence of normal ejection fraction, augmentation of cardiac contractility with administration of milrinone, epinephrine, or dobutamine may not be needed. Administration of phenylephrine will cause venoconstriction through stimulation of α_1 receptors and increase the left-ventricular filling pressure, thus increasing the cardiac output and blood pressure. Increase in blood pressure will cause baroreceptor-induced decrease in heart rate, allowing more time in diastole, improving the left-ventricular filling. Increasing afterload with phenylephrine will decrease abnormal transmitral valvular pressure gradient that will help with restoration of perfusion pressure.

37. **D.** Droperidol is a butyrophenone and is structurally related to haloperidol. It affects many receptors in the central nervous system, including dopamine receptors in the caudate nucleus and the medullary chemoreceptor trigger zone. The latter effect explains its ability to counteract nausea and vomiting. Apart from that it also interferes with transmission mediated by serotonin, norepinephrine, and GABA. The net effect is appearance of tranquility and sedation in patients premedicated with this drug, but they are often extremely apprehensive and fearful. For this reason, droperidol has fallen into disfavor as a sole premedication. Peripherally, droperidol causes α blockade. Administration of droperidol may lead to hypotension in a hypovolemic patient. It may also cause prolongation of QT interval and torsades de pointes, and because of this, the US Food and Drug Administration has associated a black box warning with droperidol. Prior to use of droperidol, a 12 lead should be recorded, and in the presence of QT interval being more than 440 ms in men and more than 450 ms in women, droperidol should not be given.

38. **D.** A healthy adult can eliminate cyanide via the liver at a rate equivalent to cyanide production during sodium nitroprusside (SNP) infusion at the rate of 2 μg/kg/min. When the rate of SNP infusion exceeds that or when sulfur donors and methemoglobin are exhausted, cyanide toxicity may develop. Free cyanide radical binds with inactive tissue cytochrome oxidase and prevent oxidative phosphorylation. This may cause tissue anoxia, metabolic acidosis, and increased oxygen saturation of venous blood because of inability of the cells to extract oxygen from arterial blood. Ultimately, cardiac arrhythmias may develop. Cyanide toxicity must be suspected earlier than that stage in any patient who develops resistance to the hypotensive action of a maximum dose of SNP.

39. **C.** Dopamine is a major neurotransmitter in extrapyramidal system. Drugs that antagonize dopamine and are able to cross the blood–brain barrier may lead to extrapyramidal symptoms, which may manifest as torticollis, oculogyric crisis, and agitation. List of drugs that can precipitate these symptoms is long, but important ones in the perioperative period are droperidol, metoclopramide, haloperidol, and promethazine. Fortunately, it is readily treated by administration of diphenhydramine. Midazolam is also helpful in treating this condition. Famotidine and glycopyrrolate are not associated with any extrapyramidal effects.

40. B.   All of the medications mentioned in the question should be continued in the perioperative period, *except* monoamine oxidase inhibitors. By decreasing the metabolism of catecholamines, these medications cause an increase in the amount of norepinephrine available at the presynaptic adrenergic nerve ending. Use of indirect-acting sympathomimetic drug like ephedrine to treat hypotension will lead to exaggerated response with severe degree of hypertension and cardiac arrhythmias. Recommendation is to stop these agents at least 2 weeks before the planned surgery. Since this can cause problem in a patient who is dependent on this medication, this group of medication is falling out of favor.

There is strong evidence to continue the use of β-blockers, cholesterol-lowering agents, and H$_2$-blockers. Most hospitals have policies to ensure that patients using long-term β-blockers receive them in the perioperative period. Similarly, there is evidence that perioperative continued use of statins leads to better outcomes.

41. D.   Dose of magnesium sulfate used to treat preeclampsia is high and can interfere with the effects of many medications used in anesthesia. It decreases the MAC of volatile anesthetics and potentiates the muscle relaxation caused by both depolarizing as well as the nondepolarizing muscle relaxants. The doses of these agents need to be reduced, and the ability of the patient to breathe spontaneously the end of general anesthetic where muscle relaxant was used needs to be assessed very carefully. Magnesium does not affect the dose of local anesthetic.

42. C.   The absorption of the epinephrine from the epidural space into systemic circulation is too slow for it to counteract the hypotension which is caused by a bolus of lidocaine. Local vasoconstriction by epinephrine slows down the systemic absorption of lidocaine, leading to lower serum levels, decreasing the chance of local anesthetic toxicity as well as prolongation of the block by allowing the lidocaine to work longer on the neuronal tissue. Epinephrine improves the quality of block by acting on the analgesic adrenergic receptors in the spinal cord.

43. A.   The relative solubility of an anesthetic in air, blood, and tissues is expressed as partition coefficients. Each efficient is the ratio of the concentration of the anesthetic gas in each of the two phases at equilibrium. Lower the partition coefficient, higher the rate of equilibration. In other words, for an anesthetic with a lower alveolar to blood partition coefficient, the rate of rise of alveolar concentration, and thus alveolar partial pressure, will be higher than an anesthetic with higher partition coefficient. Since it is the alveolar partial pressure that determines the partial pressure in the brain, more rapid rise of alveolar pressure is translated into faster anesthetic induction. Another factor that plays a role in this regard is the concentration effect. Nitrous oxide, being a less potent anesthetic with a MAC of 104, is administered in much larger quantities to induce anesthesia than a potent agent like sevoflurane. The massive inflow (higher concentration) of nitrous oxide leads to higher rate of rise of alveolar concentration (FA) of with a blood gas partition coefficient of 0.46 compared with desflurane with partition coefficient of 0.42.

44. D.   Neostigmine causes inhibition of plasma cholinesterase. As succinylcholine is metabolized by this enzyme, administration of succinylcholine after the use of neostigmine for reversal of neuromuscular blockade may lead to longer-than-expected duration of action of succinylcholine. In this situation, continue to mechanically ventilate the patient until the patient meets extubation criteria. Rocuronium is mainly metabolized by liver and excreted into bile, cisatracurium via Hofmann elimination and pancuronium via kidney. Neostigmine does not interfere with any of these processes.

45. C.   Patients with hypertrophic cardiomyopathy behave as if they have aortic stenosis except that the left-ventricular outflow obstruction is dynamic instead of being fixed. Decreased afterload under general anesthesia causes the gradient between the left-ventricular pressure and the aortic pressure to increase, leading to collapse of the left-ventricular outflow tract, increasing the obstruction, and decreasing the cardiac output. Restoration of the afterload with administration of phenylephrine reverses this effect. It also decreases the heart rate, allowing more time for left-ventricular perfusion to take place during the diastole. Decreasing the cardiac contractility may also be helpful as that will prevent the opposing walls of the outflow tract to come together relieving the obstruction. Amrinone will actually increase the contractility while reducing the afterload: both effects being undesirable in this clinical situation. Ephedrine will increase the heart rate as well as cardiac contractility, thus making the situation worse as described above. Nitroglycerine may worsen the hypotension and may not be a good choice for a hypotensive patient.

46. **D.** Ketorolac is a valuable nonsteroidal analgesic with modest anti-inflammatory action. It was the sole nonsteroidal anti-inflammatory drug available in intravenous form prior to the availability of IV ibuprofen. Thirty milligrams of ketorolac is equivalent in potency to 100 mg of meperidine or 10 mg of morphine. Unfortunately, it has many side effects that limit its use in the perioperative period. Inhibition of prostaglandin which is part of its analgesic mechanism of action leads to afferent arteriolar constriction.

47. **B.** As the clinical situation seems to indicate the need for an agent that is potent and extremely fast in its onset of action, nitroglycerine will be more helpful in this situation. Nitroglycerine is converted into nitric oxide, which is a very potent vasodilator increasing the venous capacitance. This action of nitroglycerine helps relocate the intravascular volume into peripheral compartment, thus unloading the central compartment and allowing the pulmonary edema fluid to be reabsorbed into the circulation.

48. **D.** Ondansetron has been shown to increase the QT interval. This response is comparable to that occurring with droperidol. Although there is no clear association between torsades de pointes and this drug, it is recommended that this drug be avoided in patients with congenital prolonged QT syndrome. Metoclopramide has a similar effect. Succinylcholine administration can prolong QT interval possibly from potassium efflux and by its effect on the autonomic nervous system. Propofol, on the other hand, has been shown to be safe in patients with this condition and may actually decrease the QT interval increase induced by sevoflurane.

49. **C.** Naloxone is a nonselective opioid antagonist at all three μ-receptors. It does not seem to have any agonist activity at the opioid receptors. Unfortunately, half-life is shorter (30–45 minutes) than most commonly used opioids. So renarcotization is a possibility. It is useful in the treatment of opioid-induced spasm of the sphincter of Oddi. Naloxone easily crosses the placenta. For this reason, administration of naloxone to an opioid-dependent parturient may produce acute withdrawal in the neonate.

50. **B.** Opioids usually cause bradycardia. This effect is mediated through central nervous system. They also have direct effect on the cardiac pacemaker cells. Morphine causes vasodilatation, and in the presence of preexisting hypovolemia, it may lead to decreased blood pressure and baroreceptor-induced tachycardia. Meperidine is an exception; it has intrinsic atropine-like activity that may cause tachycardia after its administration.

51. **B.** Opioid receptors are found inside substantia gelatinosa in the spinal cord. Addition of fentanyl to local anesthetic injected in the epidural space decreases the onset of analgesia time. Since epidural bupivacaine has a longer duration of action than epidural fentanyl, the duration of block may not be prolonged. Epidural fentanyl has no effect on the vagus nerve. Degree of analgesia is enhanced by addition of fentanyl to epidural local anesthetic, but the effect on the sensory and motor block is not augmented.

52. **B.** Alfentanil has a fast onset of action compared with sufentanil because of a very high proportion of it being unionized at physiologic pH: 90% vs. 20%. This is explained by the lower pK_a of alfentanil (6.5) vs. sufentanil (8.0). So its penetration into brain is much faster than sufentanil. Its protein-binding is comparable to sufentanil, while lipid solubility is much less, leading to lower total volume of distribution.

53. C. Higher oil/gas partition coefficient means higher proportion of inhaled agent is in soluble form in blood before enough partial pressure is achieved at the alveolar, and finally in the brain, to anesthetize the patient. Same process is reversed at the time of awakening. With increased time of administration, so much anesthetic is found in the tissues in a soluble form that all other factors become much less important as determinants of recovery time. Higher cardiac output may slow down the recovery time, but its effect will be smaller than the effect of duration of administration. MAC of the drug in itself does not determine the time of induction or recovery.

54. D. Hallmark of nitroprusside poisoning is increasing metabolic acidosis secondary to impaired oxidative phosphorylation in the cell because of accumulation of cyanide ions. Acute myocardial infarction is not a contraindication in itself of nitroprusside therapy as long as it is needed to treat high blood pressure. Same is true for mitral regurgitation, and in fact, nitroprusside may be helpful as it may increase the cardiac output in this condition by decreasing the afterload.

Renal failure may increase the availability of sulfate ion, which allows production of more thiosulfate to act as a donor and thus convert cyanide to thiocyanate. Prolonged administration of high doses of nitroprusside may lead to thiocyanate accumulation and toxicity.

55. C. Spinal anesthesia is rarely associated with dramatic drop of heart rate and blood pressure in young individuals. The mechanism is poorly understood. Proposed mechanism includes preexisting hypovolemia, unrecognized hypoxemia secondary to sedation, or a high spinal with inhibition of cardioacceleratory sympathetic nerves arising from T1 to T4 segments of the spinal cord.

In the clinical scenario described, atropine in itself may not be able to correct the hemodynamics, and the situations call for initiation of measures required in advanced cardiac life support. If there is no pulse, chest compressions along with administration of epinephrine may be the best course of action.

56. D. Gentamycin is an aminoglycoside antibiotic that enhances neuromuscular blockade action of muscle relaxants used in anesthesia. Magnesium in itself potentiates neuromuscular-blocking agents' action and so acts synergistically to prolong the neuromuscular blockade. Anticholinesterases increase the amount of acetylcholine available at the neuromuscular junction by inhibiting the enzyme that metabolizes it. Succinylcholine-induced neuromuscular blockade enhances the weakness produced by aminoglycoside antibiotics.

Proposed mechanism of action of these antibiotics in causing the potentiation of action of neuromuscular-blocking agents is the inhibition of release of acetylcholine at the prejunctional site. Calcium antagonizes this action of antibiotics, and at least temporarily reverses their effect on enhancement of neuromuscular-blocking action of these antibiotics. But since calcium also stabilizes the postjunctional membrane to the effect of acetylcholine, sometimes the effect of calcium on antagonism of antibiotic-induced enhancement of neuromuscular blockade produced by nondepolarizing neuromuscular-blocking agents is unpredictable.

57. A. Lorazepam is conjugated in the liver with glucuronic acid to produce inactive metabolites, but this process is much slower than the metabolism of midazolam. As a result, the elimination half-life of lorazepam is much longer (10–20 hours) compared with midazolam (1–4 hours). Similarly, the clearance of midazolam is six to eight times that of lorazepam. Volume of distribution of lorazepam is comparable to midazolam.

58. B. Volatile anesthetics cause characteristic dose-dependent changes in the EEG. Increasing depth of anesthesia with isoflurane from the awake state is characterized by increased amplitude and synchrony. Periods of electrical silence begin to occupy a greater portion of the time as depth increases (burst suppression). Midazolam and thiopental both increase the inhibitory action of GABA receptor and slow down the EEG. Lidocaine, on the other hand, has a biphasic action. At a lower serum level, it causes restlessness, tremor, tinnitus, and vertigo culminating in tonic–clonic seizure, which reflects inhibition of cortical inhibitory neurons. Larger doses inhibit both inhibitory and excitatory neurons, leading to central nervous system depression and coma.

59. **B.** Plasma pseudocholinesterase or nonspecific cholinesterase is an enzyme with molecular weight of 320,000. It is found in plasma and most tissues but not in red blood cells. It degrades acetylcholine released at the neuromuscular junction. It is primarily produced in the liver, so end-stage liver disease may decrease plasma cholinesterase activity. Normal plasma pseudocholinesterase does not resist dibucaine inhibition, while the abnormal one does. So the dibucaine number is a good estimation of the degree of qualitative abnormality of the enzyme. Acetylcholinesterases antagonize this enzyme. Metabolism of succinylcholine by pseudocholinesterase is a two-step process of hydrolysis. First step converts succinylcholine to succinylmonocholine, and the second step to succinic acid.

60. **D.** As mentioned in the previous discussion pseudocholinesterase metabolizes the injected succinylcholine before it reaches neuromuscular junction. This process is so fast that only 5% of injected succinylcholine reaches the neuromuscular junction. In the presence if atypical pseudocholinesterase, this metabolism is slow, and greater quantity of succinylcholine reaches neuromuscular junction, leading to prolonged apnea, following the standard dose of succinylcholine. Diffusion away from the neuromuscular junction stays the same whether the patient has normal or atypical enzyme and does not contribute much to the cessation of action of succinylcholine. Succinylcholine is not metabolized in the liver, although pseudocholinesterase is produced in the liver. Liver disease has to be severe before decreases in plasma pseudocholinesterase production sufficient to prolong succinylcholine-induced neuromuscular block will occur because an increased proportion of succinylcholine reaches the neuromuscular junction.

61. **B.** Effects of narcotics on smooth muscles are variable in different areas of the body. It causes contraction of the smooth muscle of the gastrointestinal tract, causing variety of side effects like constipation, biliary colic, and delayed gastric emptying. Increased biliary pressure occurs when the gallbladder contracts against a closed or narrowed sphincter of Oddi. Urinary urgency is produced by opioid-induced augmentation of detrusor tone, but, at the same time, the tone of the bladder sphincter is enhanced, causing urinary retention. Opioids alter the development, differentiation, and function of immune cells. Chronic rather than acute use of opioids is associated with immunosuppression, and withdrawal from opioids can also increase the degree of immunosuppression.

62. **A.** Morphine exhibits greater analgesic potency and slower onset of action in women than men. Older individuals are also more prone to the sedative effect of opioid drugs compared with younger individuals. Liver disease does not seem to affect the sensitivity of the individual to opioid administration except during liver transplant surgery; when in anhepatic phase, the effect of opioids may be enhanced. Morphine-6-sulfate may accumulate in cases of renal failure, causing unexpected ventilatory depressant effects from even a small dose of morphine.

63. **B.** Lower esophageal sphincter mechanism consists of the intrinsic tone of the intrinsic smooth muscle of the distal esophagus and the skeletal muscle of the diaphragm. Under normal circumstances, the lower esophageal sphincter is approximately 4 cm long. Muscle tone in the lower esophageal sphincter is the result of neurogenic and myogenic mechanisms. A substantial portion of the neurogenic tone in the humans is due to cholinergic innervation via the vagus nerve. The presynaptic neurotransmitter is acetylcholine, and postsynaptic neurotransmitter is nitric oxide. The normal lower esophageal sphincter pressure is 10 to 30 mm Hg at end exhalation. Succinylcholine increases intragastric and lowers esophageal pressures. Neostigmine also increases this sphincter's tone by increasing the concentration of acetylcholine. Metoclopramide also increases lower esophageal sphincter tone and is helpful in treating the symptoms of gastroesophageal reflux and associated esophagitis. Glycopyrrolate, on the other hand, relaxes the smooth muscle of this sphincter.

64. C. All of the agents mentioned in this question can be used to anesthetize a patient for a short duration of time on frequent basis except for etomidate as its adrenal suppressive action will impair the ability of the patient to mount a stress response, which this patient will need on an ongoing basis.

65. B. Eutectic mixture is a combination of two substances whose melting point is lower than that of either of the constituents. EMLA cream is a eutectic mixture of lidocaine (2.5%) and prilocaine (2.5%) with a melting point of 180°C so that the mixture is an oily liquid at body temperature.

Five percent EMLA cream is applied to dry intact skin and covered with an occlusive dressing for at least an hour. It provides topical anesthesia for 1 to 2 hours. The amount of drug absorbed depends on application time, dermal blood flow, skin thickness, and total dose administered. Some patients may dislike the tingling feeling that is produced by this drug. It should not be applied to broken skin or mucous membranes. Side effects include skin blanching, erythema, edema, and methemoglobinemia. The last side effect is secondary to metabolism of prilocaine O-toluidine and may be more common if the patient is concurrently taking sulfonamides and other methemoglobin-inducing drugs.

66. D. Epidural opioids can cause nausea, pruritus, and respiratory depression. Biggest advantage of these agents over epidural administration of local anesthetics is the hemodynamic stability, as there is no inhibition of sympathetic system. Hypotension is highly unlikely with epidural fentanyl administration.

67. B. Intractable seizures are sometimes treated with excision of the seizure focus in the brain. Anesthesiologist is sometimes asked in these cases to help locate the focus through enhancing the EEG activity or actually inducing the seizure during the anesthetic. Some anesthetic agents are known to increase the seizure activity and can be utilized for that purpose. Etomidate, methohexital, older inhaled anesthetic enflurane, and, to some degree, ketamine can be helpful in this regard. Other anesthetics actually increase the seizure threshold and make it difficult for the surgeon to find the area of interest.

68. D. All the porphyrias result from a defect in heme synthesis. Heme is an essential component of hemoglobin, myoglobin, and cytochromes, that is, compounds involved in the transport and activation of oxygen and the electron transport chain. For anesthesiologists, porphyria can be divided into inducible and noninducible. Inducible ones are those that are triggered by an exogenous factor like administration of a drug. Drugs that induce cytochrome enzymes like barbiturates and phenytoin can precipitate an episode of porphyria. Signs and symptoms depend on the type of porphyria, but anesthesiologist is usually involved in a case where patient is brought to the operating room for exploratory laparotomy secondary to nausea, vomiting, and pain in the abdomen. No organic cause of these symptoms is found, and patient may then develop other signs of porphyria postoperatively like neurologic signs of hemiplegia, quadriplegia, psychiatric disturbances, and alteration of consciousness or pain.

Inhaled anesthetics, nitrous oxide, induction agents other than barbiturates, and opioids are all safe to use in these patients. Elicitation of family history and past history of similar episodes can help with the diagnosis. Perioperatively, disturbances of autonomic system and electrolyte imbalance are common and need to be addressed.

69. D. Ketorolac is a nonsteroidal anti-inflammatory analgesic that is available in parenteral form. Administration of this medication will help avoid side effects that are associated with the use of morphine, such as nausea and respiratory depression. Ketorolac 30 mg produces equivalent analgesia compared with 10 mg of morphine. Since it is devoid of action on the sphincter of Oddi, it is a useful drug in patients who have pain secondary to biliary spasm. Like any other nonsteroidal anti-inflammatory drug, it does carry the side effect of inhibition of platelet function and increasing the chance of bleeding postoperatively.

70. D.   MAC is defined as the dose of an anesthetic at which 50% of patients do not move in response to a surgical incision. Different drugs and physiologic and pathologic states can affect the MAC of an anesthetic. Chronic alcohol use increases the MAC, while acute intoxication decreases it. Respiratory alkalosis does not seem to have any effect. Chronic anemia decreases MAC, but it seems to do so only if hemoglobin level is below 5 gm/dL. Hypothermia decreases the MAC, while hyperthermia increases it.

71. D.   All of the drugs mentioned in the question are agonist–antagonist at different opioid receptors except naltrexone, which is a pure antagonist. Use of naltrexone in this patient who has been using heroin for such a long time will precipitate withdrawal symptoms, which include body aches, runny nose, excessive tearing and salivation, diarrhea, mood swings, and, in some cases, high blood pressure, tachycardia, and increased temperature. Severity and duration of these symptoms vary.

72. C.   Ketamine causes minimal to no respiratory depression when used to induce general anesthesia. The ventilatory response to carbon dioxide is maintained, and the $Paco_2$ is unlikely to increase more than 3 mm Hg. It is a potent vasodilator of cerebral vessels, and patients prone to have increased intracranial pressure (ICP) may show a sustained rise in ICP after induction of anesthesia with ketamine despite normocapnia.

   Ketamine has bronchodilator activity and is at least as effective as halothane in preventing experimentally induced bronchospasm in dogs. It has been used in subanesthetic doses to treat bronchospasm in the operating room and ICU. It is readily metabolized in the liver by the cytochrome P450 system of enzymes to form norketamine, which is one-fifth to one-third as potent as ketamine.

73. B.   Treatment of hypertension in a preeclamptic patient aims at decreasing the risk of cerebral hemorrhage while maintaining and even improving tissue perfusion. Nitroprusside, a potent vasodilator of resistance and capacitance vessels with an immediate but evanescent action, is useful in preventing dangerous elevations in systemic and pulmonary artery blood pressure during laryngoscopy, and is ideal for treatment of hypertensive emergencies. Its infusion can be titrated to effect. Labetalol and hydralazine can be used to provide a longer lasting control of blood pressure but may not be fast enough in their action to control a sudden acute rise of blood pressure that is associated with this condition. Magnesium is primary therapy to prevent seizures in this condition. It is a smooth-muscle relaxant and helps with control of high blood pressure but in itself is not good enough to control the elevation of blood pressure in preeclampsia. Lisinopril is an angiotensin-converting enzyme inhibitor, which is contraindicated during pregnancy because of the risk of fetal abnormalities.

74. B.   The response of the nerve to electrical stimulation depends on three factors: the current applied, the duration of the current, and the position of the electrodes. These factors can be modified in different ways to take advantage of the characteristic features of the nondepolarizing neuromuscular blockade: fade and post-tetanic facilitation with high-frequency stimulation. When stimulation is applied at a frequency of ≥30 Hz, the mechanical response of the muscle is the fusion of individual twitch responses. In the absence of neuromuscular-blocking drugs, no fade is present and the response is sustained. During nondepolarizing block, the response achieves a peak and then fades. Higher the frequency, more useful it is to detect residual blockade, although sometimes there may be fade after stimulation with 100 Hz in the absence of a neuromuscular block. On the other hand, with train of four when 2-Hz stimulation is used, the mechanical or electrical response decreases little after the fourth stimulus, and the degree of fade is similar to that found at 50 Hz. Problem with train of four is the difficulty to evaluate by visual or tactile means the difference between the height of first and the fourth twitch. Irrespective of the experience, it is difficult for anesthesiologists to detect train-of-four fade when actual train-of-four ratio is 0.4 or greater, meaning thereby that residual paralysis may go undetected. This shortcoming may be overcome, to some extent by applying two short tetanic stimulations (three impulses at 50 Hz, separated by 750 ms), and by evaluating the ratio of the second to the first response.

75. D. Guillain–Barré syndrome is the most common cause of acute flaccid paralysis. It is an autoimmune disease triggered by bacterial or viral infection. Paralysis leads to proliferation of extrajunctional acetylcholine receptors with risk of hyperkalemia if succinylcholine is used. These patients may show a range of sensitivity to nondepolarizing muscle relaxants from extreme sensitivity to resistance. Use of these agents although is not contraindicated as long as caution is practiced in assuring return of normal muscular power at the end of the procedure before extubation is performed. If the circumstances allow, intrathecal opioids and epidural local anesthetics may actually be a better way to provide anesthesia for these patients.

76. C. Sympathetic stimulation at the time of intubation may cause an exaggerated sympathetic response and needs to be considered in this situation. Blockade of α receptors by labetalol may be helpful under this condition, but its concomitant blockade of β receptors may pose problem. Intense increase in the afterload secondary to exaggerated release of norepinephrine may not be tolerated by the heart that is inhibited by labetalol. Direct vasodilators like nitroglycerine and nitroprusside are more suitable for this situation than a nonselective β-blocker agent. As ketamine can stimulate sympathetic discharge, it is not an appropriate induction agent for this patient. Ephedrine may also increase the release of norepinephrine from the stored site and cause profound hypertension and cardiac dysrhythmias. Propofol does not have any such action, and it is appropriate for use in this case. As mentioned earlier, cocaine inhibits reuptake of norepinephrine into the presynaptic nerve, thus making it accumulate in these nerve endings.

77. C. An acute of episode of cyanosis in a child with history of tetralogy of Fallot signifies more right-to-left shunt because of decreased systemic vascular resistance. Phenylephrine may be an appropriate agent for this situation, as it will increase the systemic vascular resistance through its action on α_1 receptors, thus decreasing the shunt. As more blood flows through the lungs before returning to the heart, more oxygen will be available to the peripheral tissues improving the cyanosis.

Oxygen in this situation may not be helpful as not enough of the blood is flowing through the lungs. Other options also may help treat the primary problem. Children with this condition learn to treat these episodes, called "tet spells," by squatting down, thus increasing their systemic vascular resistance and venous return to the heart.

78. C. Clonidine has been in clinical use for over two decades now. It is a very potent antihypertensive and is very useful to control high blood pressure in some patients with a very resistant kind of disease. Unfortunately, oral dose requires repeated doses, and omission of a dose, as will happen if a long surgical procedure was scheduled, may lead to severe rebound hypertension. Availability of transcutaneous patch has helped decrease this problem. A differential diagnosis in a patient with hypertension in the recovery room should always include possibility of rebound hypertension secondary to omission of a dose of an α agonist like clonidine.

Other antihypertensive agents mentioned in the question do not lead to rebound hypertension, although hypotension during anesthesia associated with perioperative use of drugs causing angiotensin-converting enzyme blockade can be difficult to manage.

79. C. Postoperative nausea and vomiting (PONV) is one of the most disliked side effects of anesthesia and surgery. Efforts to treat it sometimes lead to troublesome side effects which look alarming at the time of presentation but are easy to treat. Dystonic reactions, including tardive dyskinesia, torticollis (commonly called oculogyric crisis), dysphagia, and excessive salivation, are some of the manifestations of this pseudoparkinsonian syndrome. Butyrophenones, phenothiazines, gastrointestinal prokinetics, and lithium are some of the etiologic agents.

Although promethazine can cause these reactions, the incidence is much lower than with metoclopramide. Granisetron is a 5-HT$_3$-receptor antagonist similar to ondansetron. The 5-HT$_3$-receptor antagonists have become the most frequently administered prophylaxis and treatment for PONV due to their efficacy. Central nervous symptoms occur in less than 8% of patients treated with this group of drugs. Intravenous diphenhydramine provides excellent relief of these neurologic symptoms.

80. **A.** Repeated administration of ketamine may necessitate increased dose to achieve the same effect. This phenomenon could partly be explained by the fact that chronic administration of ketamine stimulates the liver enzymes that metabolize it. It exerts its primary anesthetic and analgesic action through NMDA receptor, although it is found to interact with many other receptors in the central nervous system. Primary site of metabolism of ketamine is liver. It is not significantly bound to plasma proteins and thus is readily available for distribution into the tissues.

81. **C.** Etomidate cannot be used as an infusion because of its suppressive action on the adrenal gland; otherwise, it would be an ideal sedative agent for procedure that needs moderate sedation as it does not depress respiration even when used in induction doses. It is a potent cerebral vasoconstrictor and causes decrease in cerebral metabolism as well as cerebral blood flow. In comparison to thiopental it increases the excitatory spikes on the EEG and is a good agent for anesthesia for electroconvulsive therapy and mapping for seizure focus if EEG activity needs to be facilitated. An administered dose of etomidate is almost completely metabolized by the liver, and very little of the parent molecule is found in the urine.

82. **D.** Gabapentin has become a first-line treatment for neuropathic pain. This action is not mediated through GABA receptors as would be expected from the name. Instead, it modulates voltage-gated calcium channels which get activated in an injured nerve. Inhibition of this channel leads to decreased influx of calcium into the nerve cell, decreasing neuronal transmission responsible for causing pain.

    Gabapentin has not been found to interact directly with NMDA receptor. Gabapentin's role in treatment of neuropathic pain has not been linked with any interaction with sodium channel.

83. **D.** Lipid solubility of a local anesthetic is most closely related to its potency, while pK_a determines the onset of action. As a result, more lipid-soluble local anesthetics like tetracaine and bupivacaine are more potent (needing less dose) than less lipid-soluble local anesthetics like lidocaine. The pH at which the charged and uncharged forms of the drug exist in equal concentration is pK_a. As it is the uncharged form that crosses the neuronal membrane, local anesthetics with a pK_a farther from the physiologic pH have more of the drug in ionized (charged) form delaying their onset of action. This is not the only determinant of the onset of action, though chloroprocaine has a very short onset of action despite having a pK_a of 8.7. Reason is that the quantity of the drug injected is so high with chloroprocaine that more of its molecules are available in its uncharged form despite the low percentage of the drug found in uncharged form. Protein-binding of the local anesthetic determines its duration of action as the receptors are proteins, and a drug with a higher affinity for protein will latch on to these receptors longer than a drug with less affinity for protein-binding. Intrinsic property of a drug to cause vasodilatation causes the drug to get absorbed in the systemic circulation, reducing its duration of action at the site of injection compared to a local anesthetic which causes vasoconstriction.

84. **A.** Etomidate is a carboxylated imidazole. It resembles midazolam in its pharmacokinetics, in that it is water soluble in acidic form and would be useless as an induction agent, except that it changes its characteristics in the body and becomes lipid soluble on exposure to physiologic pH. Unlike propofol, it is not useful for sedation of the patients in the ICU because of its action on adrenal glands. It inhibits 11-β-hydroxylase, thus causing inhibition of conversion of cholesterol to cortisol. Patients experiencing sepsis or hemorrhage, and who might require an intact cortisol response, would be at risk if etomidate is administered to them. Even a single dose may lead to a prolonged depressant effect (4–8 hours) on the adrenal gland. As propofol is a substituted isopropyl phenol, it is very dissimilar in its chemical structure to etomidate. Like other induction agents, awakening from an induction dose of etomidate is secondary to redistribution of the drug. Liver metabolism of etomidate is very complete but not fast enough that that action will lead to awakening from an induction dose of this agent.

85. **A.**   Clopidogrel binds to ADP receptors on the surface of platelets. This action leads to inhibition of activation, aggregation, and degranulation of platelets. Clopidogrel modifies the ADP receptor irreversibly, resulting in its inhibition for the lifetime of the platelet, which is up to 7 days. So recommendation from ASRA is to avoid performing a neuraxial block for 7 days even if only a single therapeutic dose of clopidogrel was used by the patient. Clopidogrel may cause neutropenia, thrombotic thrombocytopenic purpura, and hepatic dysfunction but has not been associated with pancytopenia.

86. **C.**   NMDA receptors have been documented in the spinal cord, and epidural ketamine does have some analgesic action but much less than morphine. Of all the anesthetics available, ketamine maintains the muscle tone the most, and so it does not decrease the duration of action of nondepolarizing neuromuscular-blocking agents. Although in vivo ketamine has been shown to maintain the stroke volume, in vitro studies with isolated myocardial cell show that ketamine leads to decrease in the force of contraction of myocardial cell. In vivo finding is explained by the ability of ketamine to stimulate sympathetic system, which counteracts its myocardial depressant action. This action of ketamine can get unmasked in a patient with chronic congestive heart failure, that is, already using maximum sympathetic activity to maintain his or her cardiac output. Ketamine does not decrease the amplitude of the cortical sensory–evoked potentials.

87. **A.**   True allergic reaction to a local anesthetic is very rare, but is more common with ester local anesthetics compared with amide local anesthetics. Procaine is the only ester local anesthetic among the choices given in this question. All others are amides. So it is probably from procaine.

88. **A.**   Lidocaine has been in use for treating a myriad of pain conditions involving neuropathic pain. Although primary mechanism of its analgesic action may be through blockade of the sodium channel, it acts on many other channels including calcium and G-protein–coupled receptors. So the mechanism of its analgesic action may be more complicated than simple blockade of sodium channel. Although lidocaine has been found to inhibit NMDA receptor in supra clinical levels, activation of this receptor would not lead to analgesia.

89. **D.**   Belladonna alkaloids found in the nature sometimes lead to manifestations of anticholinergic syndrome. Factors that need to be taken into consideration for treatment of this condition include whether there is CNS involvement or not. In this case, it seems that manifestations of CNS involvement are obvious. Neostigmine, pyridostigmine, and edrophonium have quaternary ammonium ion in their chemical structure, making them unable to cross the blood–brain barrier. Physostigmine being a tertiary compound is able to cross this barrier and is able to antagonize the central actions of these anticholinergic agents.

90. **D.**   Many physiologic factors and medications are associated with potentiation of action of neuromuscular blockers. Calcium channel blockers like verapamil lead to decreased sarcoplasmic concentration of calcium, which may potentiate the muscle weakness as well as prolong the duration of action of neuromuscular-blocking agents.

    Carbamazepine was originally used as anticonvulsant but has been found to be useful in many other conditions. It is not associated with prolonged action of neuromuscular-blocking agents.

    Many antibiotics, notably aminoglycosides, prolong the actions of these drugs, but clindamycin is safe to use and has not been shown to have any deleterious effect when used concomitantly with drugs like vecuronium.

91. **C.**   Remifentanil is metabolized by nonspecific esterases found in blood and tissues. This metabolism is so rapid that action of remifentanil is terminated without the need for redistribution or hepatic extraction. There is no accumulation of the drug in patients with renal failure. Elimination half-life (6 minutes) is not prolonged even after a prolonged infusion. Hypothermia during cardiac bypass does prolong its elimination time up to 20%.

92. **C.**   Dexmedetomidine is an α_2-agonist, which acts centrally to inhibit sympathetic nervous system activity. Clonidine belongs to the same group of medicines. Dexmedetomidine

actually sometimes is used to treat spasm observed in cerebral palsy patients. Its effect in opioid-induced rigidity is not well studied. Decay time of the serum levels of dexmedetomidine after a short duration of infusion is very fast, but if it used for longer time, for example, 10 hours, as it is sometimes used in intensive care unit setting, the sedative action may take a long time to dissipate. Dexmedetomidine decreases systemic vascular resistance, and that is one of its mechanism by which it may cause a decrease in blood pressure.

93. **D.** Myotonia is characterized by continued involuntary contraction of a group of muscles. So once triggered, muscles fail to relax. Myotonic dystrophy is the most common form. Succinylcholine can cause severe hyperkalemia and is contraindicated in this condition. Nondepolarizing muscle relaxants may not be able to reverse this spasm. As neostigmine can also trigger myotonic episode, its use for reversal of muscle relaxants is not indicated. For that reason, it is prudent to avoid using longer-acting nondepolarizing agents that may require reversal agents.

   Hypothermia can trigger this condition, so precautions need to be taken to avoid it during any anesthetic. Best treatment to relieve the spasm is to inject local anesthetic into the muscle.

94. **C.** Administration of anticholinesterase agents to reverse the action of nondepolarizing agent allows the acetylcholine levels to build up not only in neuromuscular junction of the skeletal muscle but also at the level of muscarinic receptors. That leads to the problem of bradycardia if not effectively counterbalanced by administration of an anticholinergic agent. Finding the best combination of these agents is of great importance to an anesthesiologist. Older anticholinesterase agent edrophonium causes the cholinesterase activity to increase in cardiac muscarinic receptors, while neostigmine was found to have additional direct action on these cardiac receptors. Despite that finding, neostigmine-induced bradycardia is effectively prevented by administration of anticholinergic agent compared with edrophonium, where this effect is not as predictable. Another factor to consider is the onset of action of these drugs. Atropine and edrophonium are very fast-acting, while neostigmine and glycopyrrolate are slower in onset. As a result, if glycopyrrolate is injected to counteract the cholinergic response induced by edrophonium, the chance of development of bradycardia is greatest with this combination, as glycopyrrolate will take much longer and may not reverse all of the cholinergic effect produced by edrophonium.

95. **D.** Carcinoid syndrome can be precipitated in the operating room when the carcinoid tumor is manipulated by the surgeon. Cause is the release of massive amount of hormones made by the carcinoid tumor into the systemic circulation. Signs and symptoms during anesthesia may include flushing of head, neck, and upper thorax, bronchospasm, and hypo or hypertension. Many carcinoid tumors contain somatostatin receptors: a gastrointestinal regulatory peptide that reduces the production and release of gastro pancreatic hormone. Somatostatin infusion can avoid and treat the manifestation of this syndrome in the perioperative period. A synthetic analogue: octreotide is used more often in contemporary practice. It is recommended to be started 2 weeks prior to the scheduled surgery and continued in the postoperative period. Ketamine is not indicated in this condition, as it may increase the sympathetic nervous system discharge and worsen the situation. Sevoflurane is helpful to treat bronchospasm acutely but is not specific for this condition and may not be potent enough to treat bronchospasm induced by these hormones. Dexamethasone is not indicated for the acute treatment of bronchospasm, as its onset of action measures in hours and not in minutes.

96. **D.** This patient seems to be in hypovolemic shock. Body's response to such a state is to redirect the intravascular volume to vital organs like brain and heart by causing peripheral vasoconstriction through activation of the sympathetic system. Thiopental is a known vasodilator. Mechanism of this action includes barbiturate-induced depression of the medullary vasomotor center and decreased CNS outflow from the CNS. This vasodilatation will cause peripheral pooling of blood. This may cause catastrophic drop in blood pressure, which this patient may not be able to tolerate. Metabolism of thiopental by the liver is slow and does not contribute appreciably to the termination of effect of this drug. Thiopental does have negative inotropic effects on the heart, although this effect is normally masked by baroreceptor-mediated responses.

97. D.   Patients with valvular heart disease are sometimes extremely sensitive to abrupt changes in the heart rate. High-dose fentanyl has been shown to cause bradycardia through its effect on the vagus nerve. To some extent, this may be desirable in a patient with stenotic valvular lesion. In case of regurgitant lesions, this may lead to critical decrease in cardiac output. In order to counteract this bradycardia action of the fentanyl, some anesthesiologists like to use a muscle relaxant that causes tachycardia. Pancuronium and an older nondepolarizing muscle-relaxant gallamine were used for this purpose. Effect of pancuronium on the heart rate is elicited at the level of sinoatrial node by blockade of the muscarinic receptors. On the other hand, effect of fentanyl that caused bradycardia was more through central nuclei of the vagus nerve. Carotid baroreceptors and β adrenergic receptor are not involved in induction of tachycardia noticed after administration of pancuronium.

98. D.   Different surgical techniques are used to suture the donor heart to the cuff of the recipient heart. In any case, donor sinoatrial (SA) node is severed of its autonomic nervous system connections. As a result, all of the drugs that use SA node and normal conduction system of the heart to produce their cardiac effects fail to produce their effects in a transplanted heart. Although α_1 receptors are found in the heart, their stimulation with phenylephrine is not associated with chronotropic effects.

Only drugs that are able to directly stimulate the adrenergic receptors found in the myocardium are useful in treating bradycardia in a transplanted heart. Isoproterenol being a direct β_1 stimulant is the drug of choice to treat an episode of bradycardia under these circumstances.

99. C.   Propofol infusion syndrome was first described in pediatric intensive care units, but quite a few adult cases have been reported now. Earliest sign of syndrome is metabolic acidosis because of impairment oxidative phosphorylation in the mitochondria, anaerobic metabolism, and accumulation of lactic acid. Cardiac dysfunction is also an early sign, which manifests early on as bradycardia, and right-heart block is very common. Rhabdomyolysis is a hallmark of this condition, and free myoglobin precipitates in the renal tubules, leading to kidney failure. In an established case, the mortality rate is extremely high, in excess of 80%. Higher cumulative dose of propofol over a relatively longer period of time seems to be associated with higher incidence of this condition. This has led to a drop in the popularity of this drug in the pediatric intensive care setting.

100. C.   Generally, cerebral blood flow is related to cerebral metabolic rate with factors that decrease cerebral metabolic rate decrease the cerebral blood flow. This coupling effect is preserved during anesthesia, but the degree of the coupling may be altered by anesthetic agents where inhalational agents have relatively higher cerebral blood flow for any degree of cerebral metabolic rate. This variation is different for different inhalational agents and also at different doses of the same agent. At 1.5 MAC, the overall effect of desflurane is cerebral vasodilatation and increased blood flow.

Although nitrous oxide has been shown to have species-specific action on cerebral vasculature, it is clear that in humans, it is a cerebral vasodilator with potential of increasing the cerebral blood flow and intracranial pressure. Phenytoin is an anticonvulsant, which has many central nervous system effects but has not been shown to be a cerebral vasodilator. Pentothal decreases cerebral metabolic rate and is known to preserve the normal coupling between the metabolism and blood flow. So administration of this agent will decrease the cerebral blood flow.

101. A.   Anaphylactic reaction during anesthesia is estimated to occur between 1 in 5,000 and 1 in 25,000 cases. Neuromuscular-blocking drugs seem to be the most common agents causing this reaction. Incidence is far too low to determine the relative frequency of occurrence with individual neuromuscular blocker. Latex, antibiotics, and induction agents are much less common etiologic agents in anesthesia. Opioids extremely rarely cause anaphylactic reactions.

7

Spinal and Epidural Anesthesia

Thomas Halaszynski

1. A spinal neuraxial anesthetic was given 20 minutes earlier to a 28-year-old G3P2 parturient scheduled for repeat cesarean section. Alcohol swab exam revealed that she has lost temperature sensation up to T2 level. At what level do you anticipate the block will reach to provide adequate pain control?

   A. T2
   B. T3
   C. T4
   D. T5

2. You have just administered a bolus of 2% lidocaine (25 mL) through an epidural catheter that has been working well for labor analgesia in preparation for emergency cesarean section for fetal distress in an otherwise-healthy 35-year-old woman. Shortly after administration of lidocaine, the patient complains of nausea, and you notice that her heart rate has decreased from 99 to 38 bpm. The most likely cause is

   A. Anaphylactic reaction to lidocaine
   B. Pneumothorax
   C. Epidural level is higher than T4
   D. Amniotic fluid embolus

3. Contraindication(s) for neuraxial blockade include(s)

   A. Severe aortic stenosis
   B. Severe bleeding tendency
   C. Existing severe hypotension
   D. All of the above

4. During epidural placement using a midline approach, the epidural needle penetrates all the following anatomical layers, except

   A. Ligamentum flavum
   B. Subarachnoid membrane
   C. Supraspinous ligament
   D. Intraspinous ligament

5. Major benefits of a neuraxial block in a Whipple procedure include all the following, except

   A. Decreases the incidence of atelectasis
   B. Leads to earlier return of GI function
   C. Decreases the risk of urinary retention
   D. Reduces the risk of pulmonary embolism or deep-vein thrombosis

6. The correct statement for human neuraxial anatomy is

    A. Adult spinal cord ends at L2

    B. Spinal cord in children ends at L3

    C. The dural sac and subarachnoid space in adults end at S1

    D. The dural sac and subarachnoid space in children end at S2

7. Blood supply to the human spinal cord includes all of the following, except

    A. Blood supply to the spinal cord is from a single anterior spinal artery and two posterior spinal arteries

    B. The anterior spinal artery supplies the anterior two-thirds of the spinal cord, and the posterior spinal arteries supply the posterior one-third

    C. Anterior spinal artery originates from the vertebral artery

    D. Posterior spinal artery originates from the posterior cerebral artery

8. The principal site of action of local anesthetics placed into the epidural space is the

    A. Spinal cord

    B. Nerve roots

    C. Epidural space

    D. Subarachnoid space

9. Lidocaine and epinephrine are commonly used together when testing epidural anesthesia because

    A. Lidocaine injection (3 mL of 1.5%) intravascularly will induce local anesthetic toxicity such as perioral numbness

    B. Intrathecal injection of epinephrine will result in a high spinal

    C. Intrathecal injection of lidocaine can cause a low-level spinal anesthesia with some degree of motor block

    D. Intravascular injection of epinephrine (typically 15 µg/3 mL) can cause hypertension more than tachycardia

10. As an adjuvant in epidural anesthesia, epinephrine can

    A. Prolong duration of blockade

    B. Improve the quality of blockade

    C. Decrease the peak plasma levels of local anesthetic concentration

    D. All of above

11. Factors that can affect the level of an epidural anesthetic include

    A. Patient weight, amount of local anesthetic injected, patient position

    B. Patient height, amount of local anesthetic injected, patient position

    C. Patient age, amount of local anesthetic injected, patient position

    D. B and C

12. Addition of sodium bicarbonate to epidural local anesthetics may accelerate the onset of blockade with all of the local anesthetics, except

    A. Lidocaine

    B. Chloroprocaine

    C. Mepivacaine

    D. Bupivacaine

13. Factors influencing the level of spinal anesthesia achieved include all of the following, except

    A. Baricity of anesthetic solution

    B. Patient age

    C. Volume of anesthetic solution injected

    D. Patient gender

14. All of the following factors may influence the spinal level achieved during spinal anesthesia, except

    A. Drug dose
    B. Needle direction
    C. Patient position at the time and immediately following injection
    D. Patient weight

15. Complications from neuraxial blockade may include all of the following, except

    A. Radiculopathy
    B. Anterior spinal artery syndrome
    C. Arachnoiditis
    D. Constipation

16. Neuraxial block complications using local anesthetics alone include all of the following, except

    A. Post–dural puncture headache
    B. Urinary retention
    C. Postoperative cognitive dysfunction
    D. High spinal anesthesia

17. Spinal anesthesia was performed on a 25-year-old healthy male for ureter stent placement. A total of 1.5 mL of 5% preservative-free lidocaine in 7.5% dextrose was injected intrathecally after being mixed with CSF. There was evidence of free CSF flow before and after injection. The surgery was performed in the lithotomy position and was uneventful, but the patient complained of severe buttock pain in the post–anesthesia care unit. A neuro exam was negative for sensory and motor deficits. The most likely diagnosis is

    A. Spinal hematoma
    B. Spinal abscess
    C. Transient neurological symptoms
    D. Radiculopathy

18. You are consulted as to when a patient would be an appropriate candidate for a neuraxial block following administration of the following anticoagulant medications (patient does not have any other coagulopathies, and does not take other medications that could influence coagulation). The most correct statement is

    A. Last dose of ticlopidine (Ticlid) 7 days ago
    B. Last dose of clopidogrel (Plavix) this morning
    C. Last dose of abciximab (ReoPro) 24 hours ago
    D. Last dose of eptifibatide (Integrilin) 12 hours ago

19. You performed an epidural anesthetic for an elective open–abdominal aneurysm repair. You are asked to advise the surgeon when it would be considered safe to administer intraoperative intravenous heparin:

    A. Not at all
    B. One hour after epidural placement
    C. Two hours after epidural placement
    D. Four hours after epidural placement

20. A higher-than-expected spinal level achieved or greater dermatomal spread of local anesthetic can be associated with all of the following clinical situations, except

    A. Pregnancy
    B. Ascites
    C. Elderly
    D. Female gender

21. Commonly used spinal anesthesia adjuvants include all the following, except

   A. Morphine
   B. Clonidine
   C. Dexmedetomidine
   D. Ephedrine

22. A 75-year-old female with ovarian cancer is scheduled for total abdominal hysterectomy/bilateral salpingo oophorectomy and tumor debulking. A thoracic epidural anesthesia was performed using a test dose of 1.5% lidocaine with 1:200,000 epinephrine injected through the epidural Tuohy needle that resulted in no evidence of adverse sequelae. An epidural catheter was then threaded through the needle followed by evidence of negative aspiration through the catheter. A total of 10 mL 0.5% bupivacaine was administered through the epidural catheter. Thirty seconds later, the patient became agitated and complained of lightheadedness, tinnitus, and feeling faint, but still able to move all of her extremities. Her BP decreased from 150/70 to 100/45 mm Hg and her HR decreased from 85 to 55 bpm. The patient maintained spontaneous breathing throughout with an oxygen saturation (SpO$_2$) of 95%. The most likely diagnosis is

   A. Local anesthetic systemic toxicity (LAST)
   B. High epidural anesthesia
   C. Total spinal anesthesia
   D. Anaphylactic reaction

23. All of the following local anesthetic systemic toxicity (LAST) treatment measures should be performed when caring for a patient who may be experiencing toxicity, except

   A. Stop epidural medication administration
   B. Support the airway with 100% oxygen
   C. Administer intravenous epinephrine according to ACLS protocols
   D. Administer an intralipid bolus and continuous infusion

24. You have just placed a lumbar epidural for labor analgesia at L3–L4 interspace in a 34-year-old G2P1 woman of 39 weeks' gestation. The patient is 6-feet tall and weighs 300 pounds. Two hours later, you are called for an emergency cesarean section on the woman. The minimum amount of 2% lidocaine you would need to administer through the epidural catheter in order to achieve a T4 level is

   A. 5 mL
   B. 10 mL
   C. 20 mL
   D. 30 mL

25. The correct statement regarding caudal anesthesia is

   A. Caudal anesthesia is essentially sacral epidural anesthesia
   B. Caudal anesthesia can only be performed in pediatric population
   C. A caudal anesthesia catheter should be positioned without penetrating the sacrococcygeal ligament
   D. The younger the child, the less likely you are to experience an intrathecal injection

26. You just placed a thoracic epidural in a morbidly obese female (5'1" and 350 lb). You quickly administer a total of 20 mL 0.5% bupivacaine through the epidural catheter. As you reposition the patient from the sitting to the supine position, the patient complains of shortness of breath, bilateral arm weakness, and nausea. Her HR has decreased from a baseline of 98 to 41 bpm, and her systolic blood pressure has decreased from a baseline of 140s to 70s mm Hg. The most likely cause is

   A. Accidental intravascular injection of local anesthetic
   B. Local anesthetic systemic toxicity
   C. A high epidural block
   D. Anaphylactic reaction to local anesthetic or latex

27. The most likely reason for dyspnea in a patient experiencing the effects of a high neuraxial blockade is

    A. Phrenic nerve palsy when the neuraxial level reaches T3–T5
    B. Patient is experiencing an anxiety attack
    C. Medullary hypoperfusion
    D. Congestive heart failure

28. In the situation of a high spinal anesthetic, which of the following drug is pharmacodynamically considered the least useful in controlling hypotension

    A. Ephedrine
    B. Atropine
    C. Phenylephrine
    D. Epinephrine

29. During performance of lumbar epidural anesthesia for labor analgesia, you experience free-flowing cerebrospinal fluid (CSF) from the advancing 17G Tuohy epidural needle. The epidural needle is removed and a second attempt is successfully performed with an epidural catheter placed at a different level. Which of the following you would *not* recommend for the patient to practice in the next 72 hours?

    A. Bed rest
    B. Fluid restriction
    C. Increase caffeine intake
    D. Continue with daily stool softener

30. You are consulted by an emergency room (ER) physician to evaluate a patient experiencing a severe and bilateral retro-orbital headache, described as constant, along with diplopia. The ER physician also indicated that the patient presented to the ER 2 days prior with fever, chills, and photophobia when a diagnostic lumbar puncture was performed with a 20G needle. The CSF study proved negative for meningitis, but now the patient has returned to the ER with complaints of a severe headache that has failed therapies of bed rest, caffeine, nonsteroidal anti-inflammatory drugs, and increased fluid intake. The next method of treatment you would suggest is

    A. Repeat the CSF study as one set of negative results is not definitive
    B. Recommend opioids for treatment of the headache
    C. Recommend performing an epidural blood patch
    D. Continue with conservative therapy as it will eventually prevail

31. Incorrect statement regarding neuraxial blockade is

    A. Dermatome level of anesthesia achieved with a spinal anesthetic is often more predictable than following an epidural blockade
    B. Spinal anesthesia can more rapidly and consistently produce denser motor blockade than epidural anesthesia
    C. Local anesthetics administered during epidural anesthesia are typically more volume-dependent, and during spinal anesthesia are more concentration-dependent
    D. Thoracic epidural anesthesia has an increased risk of urinary retention compared to lumbar epidural anesthesia when the same volume of local anesthetic is administered

32. Following performance of spinal anesthesia at the L4–L5 level with 3 mL of 5% lidocaine, you suspect a potential injury to the conus medullaris. Which of the following symptoms is *least* likely to be associated with cauda equina syndrome?

    A. Urinary incontinence
    B. Saddle anesthesia
    C. Quadriceps weakness
    D. Biceps femoris weakness

33. You are called to see a 76-year-old female who had a L3–L4 lumbar epidural placed 3 days prior for postoperative analgesia for a colectomy. The epidural placement was traumatic on the first attempt (at L4–L5 level) with evidence of positive blood aspiration. The patient is now complaining of new onset back pain with radiation to the right lower extremity and right knee weakness that was confirmed by physical exam. The most likely diagnosis and optimal management is

A. Breakthrough pain in a patient who is confused, treat with additional pain medications
B. Stat MRI of the back to rule out neuraxial hematoma
C. Surgical complication, consult orthopedics
D. Symptomatic spinal stenosis, consult neurology for suggestions

CHAPTER 7 ANSWERS

1. **C.** In spinal and epidural anesthesia, differential blockade is frequently reported to observe the "two segments rule," namely, sympathetic block is two segments higher than sensory block, and sensory block is two segments higher than motor block. In this spinal block, alcohol swab tested the level of sensory/sympathetic blockade.

2. **C.** A large local anesthetic bolus to a parturient with an anticipated epidural space reduced in size secondary to engorged epidural veins and enlarged uterus can cause a higher level of epidural blockade than anticipated. If the block level reaches higher than T4 and influences T1–T4 (cardiac accelerator fibers), patients may have bradycardia, hypotension, anxiety on physical exam and report symptoms such as nausea, vomiting, and headache, and even paresthesia in the upper extremities.

3. **D.** Neuraxial block is a great alternative to general anesthesia for many surgical procedures below the diaphragm and an excellent choice for postoperative pain control. However, there are conditions where neuraxial block needs to be used with caution. Neuraxial blocks are associated with a sympathectomy and can therefore worsen existing hypotension and hypovolemia. Hypotension in combination with aortic and/or mitral valve stenosis may not be very well tolerated. Although spinal/epidural hematoma is rare yet possible, the risk of bleeding is significantly higher in patients with a known coagulopathy.

4. **B.** To perform an epidural block, the needle passes through several layers, including skin, subcutaneous tissue, supraspinous ligament, intraspinous ligament, and ligament flavum. To perform a spinal anesthesia, the needle goes deeper to penetrate the dura and frequently the subarachnoid membrane.

5. **C.** Neuraxial blocks in upper abdominal and thoracic procedures offer advantages of decreased pulmonary and cardiac complications in high-risk patient populations, promote peristalsis, and reduce conditions for a hypercoagulation state perioperatively. However, urinary retention is one of the potential major side effects associated with neuraxial blockade.

6. **B.** The spinal cord typically ends around L1 in adults, and around L3 in children. This is the reason why neuraxial blocks are performed below these levels and carry a lower risk of direct spinal cord injury. The dural sac and subarachnoid spaces end at S2 in adults and S3 in children.

7. **D.** Blood supply to the spinal cord is by one anterior spinal artery and two posterior spinal arteries. The anterior spinal artery supplies the anterior two-thirds of the spinal cord, and the posterior spinal arteries supply the posterior one-third. The anterior spinal artery is branched from the vertebral artery, and the posterior spinal artery arises from the posterior inferior cerebellar artery.

8. **B.** Major site of action of neuraxial blockade takes place on the nerve roots. Local anesthetics act on nerve roots in the subarachnoid space in the case of a spinal blockade and on the nerve roots in the epidural space in the case of epidural anesthesia.

9. **C.** A total of 3 mL of 1.5% lidocaine with 1:200,000 epinephrine is commonly used when testing for epidural anesthesia to rule out intrathecal (lidocaine can result in spinal blockade) and/or intravascular injection. Intravascular injection of epinephrine (15 µg) can result in a transient increase in heart rate of 20% or higher, within 30 seconds of injection and without evidence of a BP change.

10. **D.** During epidural anesthesia, epinephrine in the dose of 5 µg/mL will improve the quality of an epidural anesthetic. Additionally, epinephrine can also prolong blockade duration, delays local anesthetic intravascular absorption, and decreases peak plasma local anesthetic concentration(s).

11. **D.**   It is currently believed that body weight alone does not influence the level of an epidural block (although extreme obesity may). Patient height (vertebral levels covered decrease with height) and age (vertebral levels covered increase with age) along with local anesthetic volume (about 1 to 2 mL local anesthetic medication per segment) and patient position (theory of gravity) can play significant roles.

12. **D.**   Addition of a base with acidic local anesthetic medications will increase the amount of uncharged local anesthetic molecules injected and can therefore increase diffusion of local anesthetic molecules through the lipid layer of the cell membrane. However, sodium bicarbonate is not used with bupivacaine as it can precipitate in solutions of a pH above 6.8.

13. **D.**   Major factors influencing the level of spinal anesthesia includes baricity of local anesthetic solution, patient position immediately following spinal block placement, drug dose used, site of injection, patient age and spine anatomy, pH of the CSF, drug volume used, needle orifice direction, patient height, and patients being pregnant.

14. **D.**   Major factors influencing the level of spinal anesthesia includes baricity of local anesthetic solution, patient position immediately following spinal block placement, drug dose used, site of injection, patient age and spine anatomy, pH of the CSF, drug volume used, needle orifice direction, patient height, and patients being pregnant.

15. **D.**   Complications from neuraxial blockade can be diverse and range from death, cardiac arrest, seizures, paraplegia, radiculopathy, anterior spinal artery syndrome, high/total spinal anesthesia, arachnoiditis, post–dural puncture headache, back pain, epidural hematoma, epidural abscess, and urinary retention. However, the complication rates are typically low and may even improve bowel function and decrease constipation.

16. **C.**   Potential complications of neuraxial blockade can be diverse and range from death, cardiac arrest, seizures, paraplegia, radiculopathy, anterior spinal artery syndrome, high/total spinal anesthesia, arachnoiditis, post–dural puncture headache, back pain, epidural hematoma, and epidural abscess. However, complication rates are low and patients do not typically experience delirium unless systemic opioid analgesics have been used.

17. **C.**   Although transient neurological symptoms are usually self-limiting, it can be bothersome to patients. The etiology is mostly likely due to the high concentration of lidocaine; therefore, 5% lidocaine is now avoided in spinal anesthesia when possible.

18. **D.**   According to the ASRA guidelines, waiting period for the commonly used antiplatelet agents are as follows: ticlopidine (Ticlid) 14 days, clopidogrel (Plavix) 7 days, abciximab (ReoPro) 48 hours, and eptifibatide (Integrilin) 8 hours.

19. **B.**   Subcutaneous heparin prophylaxis at once or twice daily is not a contraindication to neuraxial anesthesia placement or prior to epidural catheter removal. Systemic heparin administration can be considered safe if given 1 hour or longer following neuraxial blockade according to the ASRA guidelines.

20. **D.**   Factors associated with a decreased CSF volume include pregnancy, large abdominal tumor, ascites, and the elderly, and can be associated with an exaggerated spread of neuraxial local anesthetic (volume and amount of local anesthetic injected remain constant).

21. **D.**   Adjuvants added to neuraxial local anesthetics may improve quality and/or prolong the duration of spinal anesthesia. Some commonly used agents include the following: opioids such as morphine and fentanyl, α_1 agonist such as epinephrine and α_2 agonists such as clonidine/dexmedetomidine. Indirect-acting vasopressors added to local anesthetic mixtures have not been shown to be effective.

22. **A.** According to ASA closed-claims database, LAST is more common than what is being formally reported. Performing a test dose with epinephrine and aspiration is not always 100% effective. Small and incremental dosing of epidural medications should always be considered as another safety measure to decrease the risk.

23. **C.** In LAST management, steps taken toward advanced life support still need to be followed despite evidence that intralipid administration is the definitive treatment. Administration of epinephrine as well vasopressin in the treatment of LAST should be avoided as it has not been shown to be associated with improved patient outcomes.

24. **B.** Initial vertebral level achieved with epidural anesthesia can be variable and is not as predictable as spinal anesthesia. The generally accepted rule is that 1 to 2 mL of an appropriately selected local anesthetic should be administered for each vertebral level of anesthesia desired in adults.

25. **A.** Caudal anesthesia is a type of epidural anesthesia performed in the sacral region just as lumbar epidural anesthesia is performed in the lumbar region. Caudal anesthesia can also be used in adults, but may be more difficult to perform due to calcification of the sacrococcygeal ligament. Caudal anesthesia needle/catheter placement must penetrate the sacrococcygeal ligament in order to enter the caudal space. Within the sacral canal, the dural sac stops at the first sacral vertebra in adults and approximately around the third sacral vertebra in infants; therefore, the risk of spinal anesthesia is higher in younger children.

26. **C.** Rapid injection of large volumes of local anesthetics either epidurally or intrathecally, especially in short and obese patients can predispose them to higher-than-anticipated levels of neuraxial anesthesia. In this particular situation, the cardiac accelerator fibers were affected, and therefore, the patient experienced bradycardia and hypotension.

27. **C.** Although phrenic nerve palsy may contribute to patient's experiences of shortness of breath and apnea, the most likely reason for dyspnea following a high neuraxial blockade is persistent hypotension-induced brain-stem hypoperfusion. Therefore, airway support is needed and aggressive control of hypotension is important in the management of high neuraxial blockade effects.

28. **C.** Hypotension associated with a high spinal may be worsened as a result of effects on the cardiac accelerator fibers at the T1–T4 levels. Therefore, a vasopressor that can simultaneously increase both HR and BP would be the most ideal medication to administer. All of the above drugs, except phenylephrine, can be used to treat severe bradycardia in the management of a high neuraxial block associated with a decreasing heart rate.

29. **B.** In patients who may experience a "wet tap" during placement of an epidural, conservative therapy should include bed rest and plenty of fluid intake, including caffeine; food diet low in fiber and stool softeners are encouraged to prevent straining.

30. **C.** Initially, a post–dural puncture headache is typically treated conservatively. If there is insufficient or no evidence of symptomatic improvement after 24 to 48 hours, most clinicians may choose to perform an epidural blood patch (if no contraindications) with 15 to 20 mL of autologous blood.

31. **D.** During neuraxial blockade, urinary retention is most often due to the local anesthetic effects on the S2–S4 nerve roots. Opioids can also adversely affect bladder function. Therefore, a lumbar epidural anesthetic has a higher risk of bladder reflex inhibition and urinary retention than a thoracic epidural.

32. C.   Cauda equina syndrome is usually secondary to neurotoxic effects from local anesthetics on the sacral nerve roots. All of above symptoms, with the exception of the quadriceps muscles, could be explained by the cauda equina syndrome (innervated by the sacral plexus). Quadriceps muscles are innervated by lumbar plexus and lumbar nerve roots and are rarely involved in the cauda equine syndrome.

33. B.   Epidural hematoma may present with back pain, focal neurological deficits, and bowel and bladder dysfunction. If a neuraxial hematoma is suspected, emergent intervention needs to be taken to confirm diagnosis and then to perform an emergency decompression as soon as possible to avoid permanent spinal cord/nerve roots injury.

CHAPTER 8

Peripheral Nerve Blocks

Thomas Halaszynski

1. An 85-year-old male is scheduled for a right distal radius and ulnar open reduction interior fixation at the wrist. Medical history is significant for chronic obstructive pulmonary disease dependent on 2 L of oxygen, hypertension, diabetes mellitus, and coronary artery disease with a stent inserted one year ago. Given that the surgeon plans to use a forearm tourniquet, the regional anesthesia technique that would be most appropriate for this patient is

   A. An interscalene brachial plexus block plus an intercostal brachial nerve block
   B. A supraclavicular approach to the brachial plexus plus an intercostal brachial nerve block
   C. An infraclavicular block of the brachial plexus at the cords plus an intercostal brachial nerve block
   D. Superficial cervical plexus blockade plus an intercostal brachial nerve block

2. While performing an axillary brachial plexus block, all of the following nerves are spared, except

   A. Musculocutaneous nerve
   B. Ulnar nerve
   C. Lateral brachial cutaneous nerve
   D. Medial brachial cutaneous nerve

3. Contraindications to safely perform peripheral regional anesthesia include all of the following, except

   A. Patients who may not provide absolute cooperation during nerve block placement (mental retardation) without administration of sedation
   B. Patient refusal
   C. Severe coagulopathy while anticipating a deep nerve plexus blockade
   D. Evidence of infection at injection site

4. While performing a peripheral nerve block in an awake patient, access and/or use of all of the following should be considered mandatory, except

   A. Administer supplemental oxygen
   B. Apply standard ASA monitors
   C. Access to resuscitation medications and equipment
   D. Immediate access to a mechanical ventilator

5. The most correct statement regarding the appropriate use of ultrasound equipment during performance of regional anesthesia is

   A. Higher frequency ultrasound probes are used for deeper penetration
   B. High-frequency ultrasound probes provide for higher image resolution
   C. Liner array probes are typically used for imaging deeper anatomical structures
   D. The curvilinear probe is designed to best image superficial structures

6. Which of the following nerves is typically spared during performance of an interscalene brachial plexus block?

   A. Median
   B. Axillary
   C. Musculocutaneous
   D. Ulnar

7. Following successful performance of a right interscalene block for surgical rotator cuff repair in a 27-year-old patient with no other medical issues, you are called to the recovery room (post–anesthesia care unit) 3 hours later to evaluate the patient. The patient's symptoms include drooping of the right eyelid, redness of the conjunctiva, and pupillary constriction. The most likely diagnosis is

   A. Spinal anesthesia
   B. Subdural injection of local anesthetic
   C. Horner syndrome
   D. Cerebrovascular accident (CVA)

8. A supraclavicular block of the brachial plexus does not provide consistent surgical anesthesia for shoulder surgery secondary to potential sparing of which of the following nerve branches of the brachial plexus?

   A. Musculocutaneous and axillary nerve branches
   B. Axillary and suprascapular nerve branches
   C. Ulnar and axillary nerve branches
   D. Suprascapular and supraclavicular nerve branches

9. Performing an infraclavicular approach for brachial plexus blockade would deposit local anesthetics at which of the following anatomical levels of the plexus?

   A. Trunks
   B. Divisions
   C. Cords
   D. Roots

10. A supraclavicular approach for brachial plexus blockade would deposit local anesthetics at which of the following anatomical levels of the plexus?

    A. Branches
    B. Trunks/Divisions
    C. Cords
    D. Roots

11. When performing an axillary block of the brachial plexus for distal upper extremity surgery, which of the following nerves most often needs to be targeted separately?

    A. Ulnar
    B. Radial
    C. Musculocutaneous
    D. Median

12. Anatomical location of the musculocutaneous nerve in the upper forearm is most frequently found within which of the following muscles?

    A. Triceps brachii
    B. Biceps brachii
    C. Coracobrachialis
    D. Brachialis

13. While performing an ultrasound-guided axillary nerve block along with a nerve stimulator, your needle tip is imaged inferior to the pulsating axillary artery, and you see evidence of flexion of fourth and fifth digits. The stimulating needle tip is in closest proximity to which of the following peripheral nerve branches of the brachial plexus?

    A. Median
    B. Ulnar
    C. Musculocutaneous
    D. Radial

14. During placement of an ultrasound-guided and nerve stimulator–assisted axillary nerve block, your needle tip is imaged superiorly to the axillary artery. You also see pronation of the patient's forearm. The needle tip is in closest proximity to which of the following branches of the brachial plexus?

    A. Median nerve
    B. Axillary nerve
    C. Musculocutaneous nerve
    D. Interscalene nerve

15. While performing an axillary nerve block by both ultrasound guidance and nerve-stimulator assistance, the image of your needle tip is seen posterior to axillary artery, and you observe supination of the forearm. The needle tip is closest to which of the following brachial plexus nerve branches?

    A. Infraclavicular nerve
    B. Ulnar
    C. Intercostal brachial nerve
    D. Radial nerve

16. After performing an axillary peripheral nerve block, your ultrasound probe moves to scan laterally and you see what appears to be an oval and hyperechoic nerve structure within the belly of the coracobrachialis muscle. When the needle tip is advanced closer to this structure and the nerve stimulator is activated, you notice that the elbow begins to flex. The most likely nerve branch that is being stimulated is

    A. Median nerve
    B. Triceps brachii nerve
    C. Musculocutaneous nerve
    D. Radial nerve

17. You successfully perform a right supraclavicular nerve block for a right wrist open reduction interior fixation. You are called to the post–anesthesia care unit 2 hours later because the patient is complaining of pain on the back of the wrist, which extends distal to the index, middle, and ring fingers on the dorsal surface of the hand. You consent the patient to perform a terminal branch nerve block to supplement the initial block. The nerve that would be needed to be blocked is

    A. Median nerve
    B. Radial nerve
    C. Infraclavicular nerve
    D. Interscalene nerve

18. You have just successfully performed a Bier block using 50 mL 0.5% lidocaine for carpal tunnel release surgery in a 45-year-old male (height, 6 ft; weight, 200 lb). The patient was sedated with 2 mg of midazolam upon arrival to the OR. Ten minutes following the local anesthetic placement, the surgeon indicates that the surgery is finished. At the surgeon's request, the nurse releases the tourniquet that was placed on the upper arm. The patient soon becomes agitated, and you notice twitching of the patient's arms and legs. The most likely diagnosis is

    A. Anaphylaxis to midazolam
    B. New-onset seizure disorder
    C. Allergic reaction to the local anesthetic
    D. Local anesthetic systemic toxicity (LAST)

19. A properly performed lumbar plexus block will result in blockade of all the following nerve branches, except

    A. Femoral nerve
    B. Lateral femoral cutaneous nerve
    C. Obturator nerve
    D. Sciatic nerve

20. Electrical nerve stimulation of which of the following nerves will produce quadriceps muscle contraction?

    A. Femoral nerve
    B. Sciatic nerve
    C. Lateral femoral cutaneous nerve
    D. Obturator nerve

21. You have just performed a femoral nerve block in preparation for a tibial plateau fracture repair using 20 mL 0.5% ropivacaine. Three hours postsurgery in the recovery room, the patient complains of lateral thigh pain. Was the femoral nerve block a failure and what would be the most appropriate action?

    A. Yes, repeat the femoral nerve block due to a failed block
    B. No, repeat the femoral nerve block as the effectiveness of the local anesthetic has worn off after 4 hours
    C. No, the pain expressed is not located within the distribution of the femoral nerve, supplement with a lateral femoral cutaneous nerve block
    D. Yes, the pain is due to a failed femoral block, but do not repeat the block as there exists a high risk of nerve injury

22. A properly placed psoas compartment block or posterior lumbar plexus block can be associated with any of the following complications, except

    A. Retroperitoneal hematoma
    B. Spinal anesthesia
    C. Local anesthetic systemic toxicity
    D. Sciatic nerve injury

23. You are consulted on an ASA IV patient for a right-ankle surgery. The patient has a known history of difficult intubation and status post–spinal fusion surgery. The surgeon is requesting for a peripheral nerve block that will provide for surgical anesthesia. Which of the following nerves will need to be blocked in order to provide for complete anesthesia during performance of foot and ankle surgery?

    A. Both sciatic and femoral nerve blockade
    B. Sciatic nerve block alone
    C. Femoral nerve block alone
    D. Sciatic, femoral, and obturator nerve blocks

24. All of the following nerves provide sensory innervation to the foot, except

    A. Lateral femoral cutaneous nerve
    B. Sural nerve
    C. Deep peroneal nerve
    D. Superficial peroneal nerve

25. The most correct statement concerning a unilateral paravertebral block is

    A. Such a block is always associated with a similar degree of sympathectomy as with an epidural block
    B. Such a block is often associated with a higher serum level of local anesthetic than that achieved with an intercostal nerve block due to high vascularity
    C. It is not likely to be associated with a pneumothorax
    D. Such a block may be associated with epidural spread of local anesthetic

26. The most incorrect statement regarding transversus abdominis plane (TAP) block is

    A. TAP blocks can provide analgesia following hernia repair surgeries
    B. TAP blocks can often alleviate both somatic and visceral pain
    C. One potential complication includes liver injury
    D. Unilateral TAP blocks never cross over the midline

27. When performing a transversus abdominis plane (TAP) block, the goal is to deposit/inject local anesthetic between which of the following two muscle layers?

    A. External oblique and internal oblique muscles
    B. Internal oblique and transversus abdominis muscles
    C. Transversus abdominis and external oblique muscles
    D. Rectus abdominis and external oblique muscles

28. While performing the popliteal approach for a sciatic nerve block under ultrasound guidance, you are able to identify the popliteal artery adjacent to two hyperechoic nerve structures that appear to become one nerve structure upon proximal movement of the ultrasound probe placed within the popliteal fossa. The correct identity of the two nerve branches is

    A. The nerve on the lateral side is the common peroneal nerve, and the nerve on the medial side is the tibial nerve (combined nerve is the sciatic nerve)
    B. The nerve on the lateral side is the sciatic nerve, and nerve on the medial side is the deep peroneal nerve (combined nerve is the femoral nerve)
    C. The nerve on the lateral side is the common tibial nerve, and nerve on the medial is the superficial peroneal nerve (combined nerve is the sciatic nerve)
    D. The nerve on the lateral side is the common posterior tibial nerve, and the nerve on the medial side is the superficial peroneal nerve (combined nerve is the femoral nerve)

29. The most appropriate statement regarding the function of the saphenous nerve is

    A. It serves as both a motor nerve and a sensory nerve
    B. It is the motor terminal branch of the femoral nerve
    C. It is the sensory terminal branch of the femoral nerve
    D. It is a sensory terminal branch of the sciatic nerve

30. An interscalene block will typically deposit the local anesthetic between which of the following two muscles?

    A. Anterior and middle scalene muscles
    B. Middle and posterior scalene muscles
    C. Anterior and posterior scalene muscles
    D. Sternocleidomastoid and anterior scalene muscles

31. A 45-year-old healthy male is scheduled for bilateral elbow open reduction interior fixation secondary to a motor vehicle accident. Successful bilateral supraclavicular blocks were planned and performed under ultrasound guidance, with 20 mL 0.5% ropivacaine injected for each block on each side. In the operating room, the patient is receiving 25 µg/kg/min of a propofol infusion and oxygen via a non-rebreather bag. The patient also received 2 mg of midazolam, but no opioids. Thirty minutes after incision, the patient is experiencing progressive respiratory depression, and the oxygen saturation decreases from 100% to 85%. The most likely diagnosis is

    A. Local anesthetic systemic toxicity (LAST)
    B. Dysfunction of the diaphragm (diaphragm palsy)
    C. Methemoglobinemia
    D. Aspiration pneumonia

32. The most appropriate treatment for the patient in the above scenario is

    A. Methylene blue due to local anesthetic systemic toxicity
    B. Flumazenil to antagonize midazolam (oversedation)
    C. Endotracheal intubation to provide respiratory support
    D. Antibiotics to treat aspiration pneumonia

33. A 56-year-old woman is scheduled for a right total knee replacement. She has a medical history of hypertension, diabetes mellitus, obesity, and is status post L1–L5 vertebral fusion. The regional anesthetic technique that will provide her the most optimal perioperative pain management is

    A. A femoral nerve block and an epidural
    B. A femoral and proximal sciatic nerve block
    C. Both a femoral and popliteal sciatic nerve block
    D. A sciatic nerve block and a spinal

34. A 65-year-old female is scheduled for a right total shoulder replacement. Under ultrasound guidance, you perform a right interscalene nerve block and place a catheter for continuous local anesthetic infiltration planned for 3 days. One week later, the patient complains of persistent parasthesia of the entire right arm, including the wrist, hand, and all fingers (from the shoulder to the fingers). An MRI shows a diffuse swelling of the brachial plexus at the level of the cords. The most likely diagnosis is

    A. Direct nerve injury/trauma from the block needle used
    B. Irritation of the brachial plexus at the level of the branches from the continuous peripheral nerve catheter
    C. Surgical trauma/manipulation of the brachial plexus at the level of the cords
    D. Local anesthetic toxicity of the brachial plexus at the level of the roots/trunks

35. The foot is supplied mainly by which of the following nerve(s)?

    A. Sciatic nerve
    B. Obturator and tibial nerves
    C. Femoral and lateral femoral cutaneous nerves
    D. Saphenous and common peroneal nerves

36. The following local anesthetic medication is associated with the highest risk for cardiovascular collapse in the event of local anesthetic systemic toxicity (LAST)

    A. Lidocaine
    B. Bupivacaine
    C. Ropivacaine
    D. Mepivacaine

37. The most appropriate nerve block for pain management in a patient scheduled for a total hip replacement is

    A. Femoral nerve block
    B. Lumbar plexus block
    C. Femoral and obturator nerve block
    D. Femoral and lateral femoral cutaneous nerve block

38. The femoral nerve provides sensory innervation to the

    A. Lower extremity below the knee
    B. Anterior and medial thigh
    C. Posterior and medial thigh
    D. Almost the entire ankle

39. Sciatic nerve blockade provides sensory loss of the

    A. Anterior and lateral thigh
    B. Posterior thigh and majority of the leg below the knee
    C. Medial and posterior thigh
    D. Medial leg below the knee

40. You perform a right-side T3–T5 paravertebral blockade for a patient who is to undergo a right mastectomy with axillary lymph node dissection. Medical history of the patient includes alcohol abuse and panic attacks. After the surgery in the post–anesthesia care unit, the patient complains of a new-onset right-arm paresthesia. Vital signs remain stable along with strong and equal upper extremity bilateral pulses. The most likely diagnosis is

    A. Surgery-related brachial plexus nerve injury and/or positional injury
    B. The patient is experiencing withdrawal from alcohol
    C. Side effects/complications of the paravertebral block on the brachial plexus
    D. Patient is having a panic attack

41. You successfully perform and place a bilateral T8 continuous paravertebral block catheters for an open–partial hepatectomy. Eighteen hours postoperatively, the patient complains of 7/10 pain. To improve postoperative analgesia, 10 mL of 0.2% ropivacaine is administered through each catheter. Twenty minutes later, the patient indicates that the pain has decreased to 4/10. The most likely aspect of paravertebral blockade that can account for the reason why the patient did not achieve a pain-free condition is

    A. The block level was too high; it should have been placed at the T10 level
    B. The block level is too low; it should have been placed at the T6 level
    C. Paravertebral blockade analgesia provides for mostly somatic blockade and does not provide for complete coverage of visceral pain
    D. The local anesthetic volume administered is too small

42. A patient is to undergo surgery to create an arteriovenous fistula for hemodialysis on the antecubital area of the right upper extremity. You perform a right supraclavicular block uneventfully using 20 mL 0.5% ropivacaine. The patient has a medical history significant for hypertension and end-stage renal disease. Three days following the surgery, the patient complains that she has no sensation from the right elbow to the tips of all her fingers, but she can move all of her fingers normally. The most likely etiology is

    A. Neurotoxicity of the trunks/divisions of the brachial plexus secondary to the ropivacaine
    B. Nerve injury secondary to the regional block needle used
    C. Prolonged effect of the local anesthetic secondary to the patient's renal failure
    D. Possible surgery-related injury at the elbow that may warrant an electrophysiology study

43. While performing an axillary brachial plexus blockade, the goal is to deposit local anesthetic medications at what location of the brachial plexus and to target which specific nerve structures?

    A. Level of the branches and targeting the radial, median, and ulnar peripheral nerves
    B. Level of the trunks and targeting the interscalene, radial, and ulnar peripheral nerves
    C. Level of the divisions and targeting the supraclavicular, median, and radial peripheral nerves
    D. Level of the cords and targeting the infraclavicular, ulnar, and radial peripheral nerves

44. Which of the following approaches to blockade of the brachial plexus is associated with the highest incidence of a pneumothorax?

    A. Interscalene and axillary approaches
    B. Supraclavicular and interscalene approaches
    C. Infraclavicular and axillary approaches
    D. Axillary and interscalene approaches

45. All of the following medication adjuvants can be used in combination with local anesthetic solutions during performance of a peripheral nerve blockade to extend the duration/effectiveness of nerve blockade, except

    A. Epinephrine
    B. Ketamine
    C. Dexamethasone
    D. Clonidine

46. While performing a femoral nerve block guided with a nerve stimulator, you observe a strong sartorius muscle twitch that disappears at 0.2 mA. What does this mean and how should you proceed further?

    A. The stimulating block needle tip is in the correct position, and the local anesthetic can be injected
    B. The needle tip is likely superficial to the femoral nerve, and the block needle needs to be readjusted (twitch may not be from stimulation of the femoral nerve) prior to local anesthetic injection
    C. Sartorius muscle twitch indicates that the needle tip is in the correct location, but you need to get closer to the nerve as 0.2 mA stimulus is too high
    D. The block needle needs to be repositioned more medially, and a paresthesia must be elicited prior to local anesthetic injection

47. The trauma team in the ICU did not want a thoracic epidural placed on a trauma patient with bilateral rib fractures secondary to concerns about the potential hemodynamic instability that may result. Therefore, both right T7 and left T5 continuous paravertebral catheters were successfully placed for this patient under ultrasound guidance. Twenty minutes following the administration of 10 mL of 0.2% ropivacaine administered through each catheter (following evidence of negative aspiration), the systolic blood pressure dropped by 50 mm Hg. The most likely diagnosis is

    A. Performance of paravertebral blockade creates identical concerns about potential hemodynamic compromise as do thoracic epidural blocks
    B. Local anesthetic toxicity as the paravertebral space is very vascular
    C. Possible epidural spread of local anesthetics from either one or both the paravertebral catheters
    D. Venous bleeding into the paravertebral space resulting in large volumes of local anesthetic absorption from the paravertebral blocks

CHAPTER 8 ANSWERS

1. **C.** In a patient with severe pulmonary compromise, performing either an interscalene or supraclavicular block of the brachial plexus should be approached with caution secondary to the increased risk of an ipsilateral phrenic nerve palsy. Placement of an interscalene block for wrist surgery may also not be optimal as it may not effectively block the ulnar nerve distribution to the wrist. A superficial cervical plexus block (C1–C4) will not effectively provide anesthesia/analgesia to the wrist. Both infraclavicular and axillary approaches to the brachial plexus would be appropriate for wrist surgery, along with a reduced incidence of adverse effects on the phrenic nerve. Intercostobrachial nerve blockade is added to cover the T2 dermatome distribution that is not included in a properly performed brachial plexus block and will contribute to alleviating tourniquet discomfort in the medial portion of the upper arm.

2. **B.** The musculocutaneous and medial brachial cutaneous nerves branch from the brachial plexus at a more proximal location than can be consistently anesthetized with an axillary nerve block approach of the brachial plexus. Therefore, these nerve branches need to be blocked separately if they innervate the planned surgical area. The lateral brachial cutaneous nerve is a branch of musculocutaneous nerve.

3. **A.** Patient refusal is an absolute contraindication following informed consent. Evidence of anticipated injection-site infection and severe coagulopathy are considered relative contraindications, and risk-to-benefit analysis needs to be carefully considered. Non-cooperative patients can often pose an increased risk to patient/operator safety, but it is not an absolute contraindication to performing regional anesthesia.

4. **D.** Regional anesthesia should be administered in a monitored location where standard ASA monitors. Supplemental oxygen along with resuscitative medications and equipment should be readily accessible and immediately available. However, immediate access to a functioning anesthesia ventilator is not always necessary.

5. **B.** High-frequency ultrasound probes are typically manufactured with a liner probe design and provide high image resolution used for superficial anatomical structures. Low-frequency ultrasound probe equipment is typically produced with a curvilinear probe design and reveals a lower image resolution, but is used for visualizing deeper anatomical structures secondary to better penetration.

6. **D.** The ulnar nerve branch originates from the C8–T1 nerve roots. Properly performed interscalene approach to brachial plexus blockade can provide for a dense blockade of the C5–C7 nerve roots/trunks and less consistent blockade of the C8–T1 nerve roots/trunks. Therefore, an interscalene approach to blockade of the brachial plexus for distal upper extremity surgical procedures may not be the most ideal approach.

7. **C.** A Horner syndrome (miosis, ptosis, and anhidrosis) can be commonly seen following an interscalene block. This syndrome is often due to proximal tracking of local anesthetic and blockade of the sympathetic fibers to the cervicothoracic ganglion. In patients where a CVA may also be within the differential diagnosis, a thorough history and neural exam should always be included.

8. **B.** A supraclavicular approach to brachial plexus blockade does not consistently and reliably provide anesthesia/analgesia to the axillary and suprascapular nerve branches. Therefore, a supraclavicular block can be used for postoperative analgesia, but may not be ideal for surgical anesthesia during invasive shoulder procedures. Sparing of ulnar nerve during a supraclavicular block may also occur that would not provide effective anesthesia for procedures distal to the mid-humerus.

9. **C.**   At the infraclavicular level, the brachial plexus forms three cords in relation to axillary artery and named according to their position around the artery: medial, lateral, and posterior cords.

10. **B.**   Supraclavicular blockade of the brachial plexus is often referred to as the "spinal anesthesia" of the upper extremity. It provides anesthesia of the brachial plexus distal to the roots and proximal to the cords of the plexus. There has been an increased practice of performing the supraclavicular approach to blockade of the brachial plexus secondary to the introduction of ultrasound into clinical practice as anesthesiologists can now appreciate a decreased incidence of pneumothorax under real-time ultrasound guidance.

11. **C.**   The musculocutaneous nerve typically branches off more proximal to the axillary approach of brachial plexus blockade and is frequently not adequately anesthetized with a traditional axillary block of the plexus (local anesthetics are deposited around the axillary artery). Therefore, the musculocutaneous nerve must be targeted separately when performing an axillary block of the brachial plexus for distal upper extremity surgery.

12. **C.**   Although some anatomical variation can be found with the brachial plexus at the level of the axilla, the musculocutaneous nerve is most commonly positioned within the coracobrachialis muscle or between the bellies of the biceps and coracobrachialis muscles.

13. **B.**   Some anatomical variation can exist, but the ulnar nerve is frequently positioned inferior to the axillary artery. Stimulation of the ulnar nerve will cause wrist flexion, flexion of the fourth and fifth digits, and thumb adduction.

14. **A.**   The median nerve is most frequently positioned superior to the axillary artery (with some anatomical variations). Stimulation of the median nerve will cause muscle stimulation, creating wrist flexion, thumb opposition, and forearm pronation.

15. **D.**   Despite some anatomical variations within the nerve-branch distribution of the brachial plexus around the axillary artery, the radial nerve is most frequently positioned posterior to axillary artery. Stimulator of radial nerve will induce digit/wrist/elbow extension and forearm supination.

16. **C.**   Musculocutaneous nerve is frequently found within coracobrachialis muscle and/or between the biceps and coracobrachialis muscles. Stimulation of the musculocutaneous nerve will characteristically cause elbow flexion.

17. **B.**   The sensory distribution on the dorsal surface of the hand described in the question matches the innervation provided by the radial nerve. Therefore, a terminal nerve block anywhere along the distribution of the radial nerve proximal to the wrist would be an appropriate place to supplement the initial brachial plexus block.

18. **D.**   LAST can occur when a large volume of local anesthetic is absorbed into or directly injected into the systemic circulation. A Bier block can provide surgical anesthesia for short procedures of the extremity, lasting 60 minutes or less. However, patients may complain of tourniquet pain that can become evident as early as 20 minutes following block performance. In order to prevent or reduce the incidence of LAST, the tourniquet needs to remain inflated and in position for a minimum of 15 to 20 minutes even if the surgical procedure finishes early. Even after 15 to 20 minutes has elapsed, cautious, intermittent, and slow release of tourniquet is recommended.

19. **D.**   The three major nerve branches of the lumbar plexus that are affected by such a block include femoral, lateral femoral cutaneous, and obturator nerves. Sciatic nerve originates from the sacral plexus and is not part of the lumber plexus.

20. **A.** The femoral nerve provides motor supply to the quadriceps muscles and sensory supply to portion of the medial thigh. The femoral nerve does not have any motor components below the knee (only a sensory branch, saphenous nerve, below the knee).

21. **C.** The lateral femoral cutaneous nerve supplies the lateral portion of the thigh. Blockade of the lateral femoral cutaneous nerve is not always consistently blocked with femoral nerve block approach, but can be blocked separately if/when needed.

22. **D.** A lumbar plexus block is considered a deep block and has been described as an advanced block in regional anesthesia. Some potential complications include retroperitoneal hematoma, local anesthetic systemic toxicity, intrathecal and/or epidural injections of local anesthetics, and renal injury (with potential for subsequent hematoma). The typical approach for lumbar plexus blockade should not cause injury to the sciatic nerve unless an improperly placed or misdirected regional block needle is positioned too caudad that could then result in injury to sacral plexus and the sciatic nerve.

23. **A.** For complete surgical anesthesia of the foot and ankle, both sciatic and femoral/saphenous nerves need to be anesthetized/blocked. The obturator nerve does not provide sensory or motor nerve distribution to foot or ankle.

24. **A.** An ankle block can be performed by providing anesthesia and blocking the five nerves that innervate the foot, namely, the superficial and deep peroneal nerve, saphenous nerve, sural nerve, and posterior tibial nerve.

25. **D.** Advantages of properly placed paravertebral nerve blocks include reduced degrees of local anesthetic–induced sympathectomy compared to epidural or spinal anesthesia and a lower risk of local anesthetic systemic toxicity as compared with intercostal nerve blocks. However, one of the major concerns for potential complications is development of a pneumothorax, and paravertebral blocks can be associated with variable degrees of local anesthetic epidural spread, especially when placing bilateral paravertebral blocks.

26. **B.** TAP blocks can provide analgesia for peripheral somatic pain of the abdomen and can be associated with a low yet potential risk of bowel perforation and liver injury. For midline ventral hernia surgery, performing bilateral TAP blocks are often needed. TAP blocks do not cover crappy, visceral pain.

27. **B.** The subcostal (T12), ilioinguinal (L1), and iliohypogastric (L1), and genitofemoral nerves are targeted when performing a TAP block. These nerves have a typical distribution between the internal oblique and transversus abdominis muscles.

28. **A.** Popliteal approach to the sciatic nerve block is typically performed at the site of bifurcation of the tibial (medial position) and common peroneal (lateral position) nerves. The sciatic nerve is most optimally blocked with local anesthetic at the union (bifurcation) of these two nerves that frequently become one nerve structure approximately 7 to 10 cm proximal to the popliteal crease.

29. **C.** The saphenous nerve is a terminal sensory nerve branch of the femoral nerve with NO motor components. Under certain clinical situations, the saphenous nerve is preferentially blocked to avoid motor blockade of the anterior quad muscles that can result from performance of a femoral nerve block (increased risk of fall).

30. **A.** The brachial plexus nerve root/trunk is usually positioned between the anterior and middle scalene muscles. When local anesthetics are placed between these two muscle bundles, it is commonly referred to as an interscalene block.

31. **B.**   Bilateral supraclavicular blockade can significantly increase the risk of symptomatic phrenic nerve palsy. Methemoglobinemia can happen in patients with certain local anesthetics, but usually not from ropivacaine administration. LAST can occur from administration of toxic doses of any local anesthetic, but is most often an acute event from systemic administration.

32. **C.**   The witnessed respiratory depression is most likely due to diaphragm palsy and the urgent need for ventilation assistance until resolution of phrenic nerve dysfunction. An appropriate option would be to intubate the patient and provide any necessary sedation and then extubation upon evidence of recovery of diaphragm function.

33. **B.**   Femoral and proximal sciatic nerve block together can often provide for excellent perioperative pain control and can facilitate physical therapy with a reduced incidence of interference with ambulation. These peripheral regional techniques can be particularly useful in patients with difficulty or contraindications to neuraxial blockade.

34. **C.**   Shoulder surgery is one of the upper extremity procedures that can often be associated with nerve injuries secondary to patient pathology, surgical manipulation(s), surgical trauma, brachial plexus nerve stretching or compression, etc. If such an injury was due to performance of the peripheral nerve block and/or catheter placement, it often tends to involve more isolated nerve roots/trunks of the brachial plexus from the interscalene approach rather than diffuse influences at more distal levels of the plexus. Surgical complications of the brachial plexus often tend to be more diffuse and less selective. Nerve-conduction studies and EMG should be considered rather than merely delineating an etiology of the injury.

35. **A.**   The sciatic nerve supplies all of the motor innervation and the majority of the sensory innervation to the lower extremities below knee except the medial side of the lower extremity that is innervated by the saphenous nerve.

36. **B.**   Bupivacaine is best known for its high cardiovascular toxicity, although any of the local anesthetic medications listed above can result in LAST. One of the reported advantages of ropivacaine over bupivacaine is its relatively lowered incidence of cardiovascular toxicity. The other listed local anesthetic medications tend to have neurological toxicity prior to progressing toward cardiovascular collapse.

37. **B.**   A femoral block for hip surgical procedures have intrinsic limitations as does not completely cover ALL dermatome distributions of the hip. A properly placed and functioning lumbar plexus blockade/catheter will cover the femoral, obturator, and lateral femoral cutaneous nerve and often provides for better pain control of the hip in conjunction with a sciatic/sacral nerve plexus block.

38. **B.**   The femoral nerve provides sensory innervation to the anterior and medial thigh above the knee, and medial side of the lower extremity below the knee. The femoral nerve innervates and supplies motor control of the anterior quadriceps muscles above the knee and no motor innervation below the knee.

39. **B.**   Sciatic nerve blockade provides sensory loss to the posterior thigh by blocking the posterior cutaneous nerve along with everything below the knee, except for the medical lower leg, which is innervated by the saphenous nerve.

40. **A.**   The most likely cause is secondary to axillary lymph node dissection–related brachial plexus injury. The level of paravertebral blocks was at T3–T5; therefore, the brachial plexus should not be affected (C4–T1) by the paravertebral-injected local anesthetic.

41. C. Paravertebral blockade provides mostly for somatic-induced pain with little visceral pain coverage; therefore, hepatectomy patients need additional pain-management modalities such as opioids.

42. D. Neurologic injuries secondary to positional, compressional, ischemic injury often creates a more diffuse type of an injury pattern similar to the one described in the question. If the neurologic injury were due to complications from placement of a single-shot supraclavicular blockade or local anesthetic used during block placement, then these types of injuries would tend to have a more isolated pattern. Peripheral nerve block injuries from a supraclavicular block would be more likely to result in evidence of an injury pattern isolated to the trunks or divisions of the brachial plexus, and the patient would typically reveal symptoms above elbow as well. Without any adjuvant, ropivacaine block will not last as long as 72 hours.

43. A. Axillary block is typically performed at the level of the individual peripheral nerve branches of the brachial plexus, specifically the radial, median, and ulnar nerves.

44. B. Supraclavicular approach to blockade of the brachial plexus carries a high risk of pneumothorax followed by the interscalene approach. This pneumothorax risk has decreased and is believed to be secondary to the more frequent use of ultrasound-guided regional anesthesia. Now the supraclavicular approach to blockade of the brachial plexus is commonly performed with ultrasound guidance.

45. B. All of the above adjuvant medications, except ketamine, are commonly used in peripheral nerve blocks to improve the density and prolong the duration of nerve blockade efficacy. Ketamine, along with ephedrine, when mixed with local anesthetics during a peripheral nerve block has been studied in animal models and was deemed to offer little to no additional benefits or synergistic effects.

46. B. Sartorius muscle twitch could be secondary to stimulation of a small branch from the femoral nerve that innervates the sartorius muscle or secondary to direct muscle stimulation. The femoral nerve is usually positioned more lateral and deeper to this small branch that originates from the femoral nerve which innervates the sartorius muscle.

47. C. A potential advantage of paravertebral blockade compared to neuraxial blockade is a reduced incidence of creating an intense sympathectomy resulting in hemodynamic compromise. However, when bilateral paravertebral blocks are performed, the potential exists that epidural spread could be significant, resulting in an observation of a moderate BP decrease.

Pain Management

Thomas Halaszynski

1. At what time frame following the postsurgical period does persistent postsurgical pain become defined as being "chronic pain"?

   A. 1 to 2 weeks
   B. 3 to 4 weeks
   C. 1 to 2 months
   D. 6 to 12 months

2. Both surgical trauma and anesthetic administration techniques can modulate which of the following human stress responses?

   A. Neuroendocrine
   B. Metabolic
   C. Inflammatory
   D. All of the above

3. Nonsteroidal anti-inflammatory drugs (NSAIDs) are often used as part of "multimodal" analgesic therapy; some of the potential advantages include all of the following, except

   A. Decreases opioid requirements
   B. Can decrease postoperative pain intensity
   C. Indirect effect of decreasing opioid-related side effects
   D. Can improve wound healing

4. Type(s) of symptomatic pain conditions that best describes "chronic" pain often includes

   A. Neuropathic pain alone
   B. Nociceptive pain alone
   C. Neuropathic or nociceptive pain
   D. Somatic or visceral pain

5. At what levels does the modulation of pain by electrical stimulation result in the activation of inhibitory fibers?

   A. Nociceptor level alone
   B. Spinal cord level alone
   C. Only within the brain
   D. All of the above

6. Activation of which of the following mechanisms and/or pathways best describes "central sensitization" at the level of the spinal cord?

   A. Second-order wide dynamic range neurons
   B. Dorsal horn neuron
   C. Spinal cord reflexes
   D. All of the above

7. A 26-year-old female undergoes a left stellate ganglion block for treatment of complex regional pain syndrome of the left hand. Twenty minutes after the block is placed, skin temperature in the left arm rises from 33 to 36.5°C. Venous engorgement of the left arm and hand, left eye papillary constriction, and drooping of the eyelid are observed. The pain is not relieved. Which of the following can best explain the block failure?

   A. Pain-carrying fibers originated from right stellate ganglion
   B. Pain-carrying fibers originated from middle cervical ganglion
   C. Pain-carrying fibers originated from inferior cervical ganglion
   D. Pain-carrying fibers originated from second thoracic ganglion

8. Chronic pain indications for insertion of a spinal cord stimulator include all of the following, except

   A. Phantom pain
   B. Complex regional pain syndrome
   C. Chronic visceral pelvic pain
   D. Compartment syndrome pain

9. The term used to best describe the PAIN condition "perception toward ordinary non-noxious stimulus as being painful" is

   A. Hyperalgesia
   B. Anesthesia dolorosa
   C. Hypalgesia
   D. Allodynia

10. Incorrect statement related to the definition of an abnormal sensation is

    A. Dysesthesia is an abnormal sensation with or without a stimulus
    B. Paresthesia is abnormal sensation without a stimulus
    C. Neuralgia is due to abnormality in nerve roots
    D. Hyperesthesia is an abnormal sensation of exaggerated response to mild stimulation

11. Which of the following clinical diagnoses best describes deafferentation pain?

    A. Herniated disk
    B. Amputation
    C. Neuropathic pain
    D. Diabetic neuropathy

12. Gasserian ganglion block is most commonly used for neuropathic pain located in which of the following nerve distributions?

    A. Facial nerve
    B. Trigeminal nerve
    C. Glossopharyngeal nerve
    D. Vagal nerve

13. Major excitatory neurotransmitters responsible for pain modulation include all the following, except

    A. Substance P
    B. Glutamate
    C. Somatostatin
    D. Aspartate

14. All the following are inhibitory neurotransmitters in the pain pathway, except

    A. Norepinephrine
    B. Adenosine
    C. Serotonin
    D. Calcitonin gene-related peptide

15. Incorrect statement regarding secondary hyperalgesia is

    A. It is caused by neurogenic inflammation
    B. It is associated with Lewis' triple response
    C. It is increased by injection of local anesthetics
    D. It is increased by application of capsaicin

16. Types of pain disorders that are commonly treated using "sympathetic blockade" include all of the following, except

    A. Complex regional pain syndrome
    B. Phantom limb pain
    C. Postherpetic neuralgia
    D. Acute pain due to pelvic exenteration

17. Systemic responses of the human body that can develop secondary to symptoms of acute pain include all of the following, except

    A. Hypertension and tachycardia
    B. Increased work of breathing
    C. Urinary retention
    D. Increased peristalsis

18. A 56-year-old man presented to his primary care physician with a complaint of right buttock and right leg pain along with numbness and tingling sensations. He was subsequently diagnosed with a piriformis syndrome (trapped nerve). The nerve(s) responsible for this diagnosis is/are

    A. Femoral and saphenous nerves
    B. Ilioinguinal nerve
    C. Sciatic nerve
    D. Obturator and femoral nerves

19. A 56-year-old patient with a past medical history of hypertension, diabetes, and alcohol abuse presents to the operating room for a right-elbow open reduction internal fixation, secondary to a motor vehicle accident that occurred 24 hours ago. On postoperative day 1, the patient complains of right fourth and fifth digit numbness and minor pain. A diagnosis of cubital tunnel syndrome has been made. The nerve most likely to be involved is

    A. Median nerve
    B. Ulnar nerve
    C. Radial nerve
    D. Musculocutaneous nerve

20. Incorrect statement regarding myofascial pain is

    A. Myofascial pain is associated with muscle discomfort (pain, stiffness, weakness, spasm)

    B. Patient may have several trigger points producing pain upon stimulation

    C. Systemic diseases such as connective tissue disease may cause myofascial pain

    D. Myofascial pain is never associated with autonomic dysfunctions

21. The diagnosis of fibromyalgia includes all of the following, except

    A. Minor pain

    B. Pain lasts more than 3 months

    C. No other pathologies can explain or contribute to the pain

    D. Frequent association with psychiatric diagnosis

22. Common causes for lower back pain include all of the following, except

    A. Lumbosacral strain

    B. Degenerative disk disease

    C. Myofascial syndromes

    D. Fibromyalgia syndrome

23. A 68-year-old male presents to his primary care physician's office with a major complain of back pain radiating into the gluteal region and pain in the distribution of the plantar surface of the foot on the same side. The patient's physical examination reveals decreased plantar flexion of the foot. An MRI will most commonly show a herniated disk at

    A. L2–L3

    B. L3–L4

    C. L4–L5

    D. L5–S1

24. Disk herniation at L4–L5 of the vertebral column often presents with all of the following clinical symptoms, except

    A. Diminished dorsiflexion of the foot

    B. Quadriceps femoris muscle weakness

    C. Posterior-lateral thigh pain

    D. Dorsal foot pain between first and second toes

25. Facet syndrome is characterized by all the following, except

    A. Pain relieved by local anesthetic injection of the medial branches of the posterior rami of spinal nerves

    B. Pain relieved by an intra-articular injection of the zygapophyseal joints

    C. Pain can be exacerbated by overextension and lateral rotation of back

    D. Pain is sympathetically mediated

26. Incorrect statement regarding neuropathic pain is

    A. It includes pain associated with stroke, spinal cord injury, and diabetic neuropathy

    B. It is not associated with low back pain or multiple sclerosis

    C. Neuropathic pain can be paroxysmal

    D. Neuropathic pain can be associated with hyperpathia

27. Regarding the treatment of neuropathic pain, the correct statement is

    A. Narcotics is the most effective and "first-line" treatment option

    B. It is most optimally treated with multimodal therapies

    C. Sympathetic blockade will eliminate *all* neuropathic pain

    D. Spinal cord stimulator is not an effective therapy

28. Pathological features of complex regional pain syndrome include all the following, except

    A. It is sympathetically mediated
    B. It is often associated with documented nerve injury
    C. It is only associated with major injuries (never from minor procedures)
    D. It is not associated with evidence of skin color, hair, and temperature changes

29. Incorrect statement regarding treatment of complex regional pain syndrome (CRPS) is

    A. Efficacious treatment with multimodal therapy early in the diagnosis (within 1 month of symptom) is most effective
    B. It responds well to sympathetic blockade
    C. If not treated properly and in a timely fashion, CRPS can result in functional disability
    D. Patients need to refrain from physical therapy until the pain syndrome is resolved

30. Possible complications to disclose when obtaining an anesthesia consent from a patient prior to performance of a celiac plexus block include all of the following, except

    A. Postural hypotension and lightheadedness
    B. Constipation and urinary retention
    C. Vena cava and aortic vascular injury
    D. Retroperitoneal hemorrhage

CHAPTER 9 ANSWERS

1. **C.**   Persistent postsurgical pain is defined as chronic pain that continues beyond the usual recovery period of 1 to 2 months following surgery (well past the normal convalescence period expected for a particular/specific surgical procedure). Chronic pain is defined as pain that has lasted longer than 3 to 6 months, though some other investigators have placed the transition from acute to chronic pain at 12 months. The incidence of persistent postsurgical pain can often exceed an incidence of 30% after certain high-risk/surgically invasive procedures such as amputations, thoracotomy, mastectomy, and inguinal hernia repair. Acute pain will typically last less than 30 days, chronic pain to more than 6 months duration, and subacute pain lasts from 1 to 6 months. A popular alternative definition of chronic pain involving no arbitrarily fixed durations is "pain that extends beyond the expected period of healing."

2. **D.**   Many perioperative factors can produce significant influence toward amplifying or decreasing the surgical stress response(s) such as neuroendocrine, metabolic, and inflammatory changes. These factors can be further modified by patient-specific contributions such as anxiety/depression, surgical history, surgical technique (open vs. laparoscopy), and anesthetic techniques (general vs. regional).

3. **D.**   NSAIDs have not only many of the above-identified advantages, but also several potential side effects that the practitioner must remain cognizant of such as risk of gastrointestinal bleeding, renal injury, and the potential to impair wound healing.

4. **C.**   Chronic pain is most often defined as neuropathic and/or nociceptive in nature. Chronic pain may be divided into nociceptive pain—caused by activation of nociceptors—and neuropathic pain—caused by damage to or malfunction of the nervous system. Neuropathic pain is divided into peripheral (within the peripheral nervous system) and central (originating from the brain/spinal cord). Peripheral neuropathic pain is often described as burning, tingling, electrical, stabbing, and/or pins and needles sensation(s). Nociceptive pain is divided into superficial or deep, and deep pain into deep somatic and visceral pain. Superficial pain is initiated by activation of nociceptors in the skin or superficial tissues. Deep somatic pain is initiated by stimulation of nociceptors in ligaments, tendons, bones, blood vessels, and muscles, and is described as dull, aching, poorly-localized pain. Visceral pain originates in the internal organ system(s) of the body. Visceral pain may be well-localized, but often is difficult to locate, and several visceral regions can produce "referred" pain when damaged or inflamed, where the sensation is located in an area distant from the site of pathology or injury.

5. **D.**   Modulation of pain can happen centrally or peripherally. It can occur at the nociceptor level peripherally or centrally either in the spinal cord or in supraspinal structures. These modulation effects can be either inhibitive or facilitative. In the brain and the spinal cord, much of the information from the nociceptive afferent fibers results from excitatory discharges of multireceptive neurons. Pain information in the central nervous system is controlled by ascending and descending inhibitory pathways (using endogenous opioids or other endogenous substances). In addition, a powerful inhibition of pain-related information occurs in the spinal cord. These inhibitory systems can be activated by brain stimulation and peripheral nerve stimulation. However, pain is a complex perception that is influenced also by prior experience and by the context within which the noxious stimulus occurs. This sensation is also influenced by emotional state.

6. **D.**   Central sensitization is an enhancement in the function of neurons and circuits in nociceptive pathways, caused by increases in membrane excitability and synaptic efficacy as well as reduced inhibition and is a manifestation of the plasticity of the somatosensory nervous system in response to activity, inflammation, and neural injury. Central sensitization is responsible for hyperalgesia and there are three mechanisms that have been identified at the level of spinal cord: (1) windup of second-order wide dynamic range neurons, (2) dorsal horn neuron receptor field expansion, and (3) hyperexcitability of flexion reflexes.

7. **D.** The stellate ganglion (cervicothoracic ganglion or inferior cervical ganglion) is a sympathetic ganglion formed by the fusion of the inferior cervical and first thoracic ganglion. Stellate ganglion is located at the level of C7 (seventh cervical vertebra), anterior to the transverse process of C7, superior to the neck of the first rib, and just below the subclavian artery. Complications of stellate block include intravascular injection, intrathecal/epidural injection, bleeding, pneumothorax, brachial plexus involvement, local anesthetics spread to recurrent laryngeal nerve, and osteomyelitis or mediastinitis (rarely).

8. **D.** A spinal cord stimulator is a device used to exert pulsed electrical signals to the spinal cord to control chronic pain, and additional applications include use in some motor disorders. Spinal cord stimulation is most effective for neuropathic pain, of which some common indications include sympathetically mediated pain, phantom limb pain, ischemic pain due to peripheral vascular disease, peripheral neuropathies, and visceral pain. Compartment syndrome pain often requires urgent evaluation and possible need for emergency fasciotomy.

9. **D.** Hyperalgesia is an exaggerated response to noxious stimuli, an extreme and exaggerated reaction to a stimulus which is normally painful. Anesthesia dolorosa is pain in area that has no sensation, is pain felt in an area (usually of the face) that is completely numb to touch with the pain described as constant, burning, aching, or severe. Hypalgesia equals reduced sensitivity to pain, the opposite of hyperalgesia. Allodynia is defined as pain due to a stimulus that does not normally provoke pain. Temperature or physical stimuli can provoke allodynia (which may feel like a burning sensation) and can often occur after injury.

10. **C.** Dysesthesia is an abnormal sensation with or without a stimulus and is defined as an unpleasant, abnormal sense of touch and often presents as pain (may also present as an inappropriate, but not discomforting, sensation). Dysesthesia is caused by lesions of the nervous system (peripheral or central) and involves sensations (spontaneous or evoked) such as burning, wetness, itching, electric shock, and pins and needles. Dysesthesia can include sensations in any bodily tissue, including most often the mouth, scalp, skin, or legs. Paresthesia is abnormal sensation without a stimulus with a sensation of tingling, tickling, prickling, pricking, or burning of a person's skin with no apparent long-term physical effect. The manifestation of a paresthesia may be transient or chronic. The most familiar kind of paresthesia is the sensation known as "pins and needles" or of a limb "falling asleep." Neuralgia is pain sensation in the distribution of a nerve or a group of nerves (radiculopathy is pain secondary to nerve roots pathologies). Neuralgia is pain in one or more nerves caused by a change in neurological structure or function of the nerves rather than by excitation of healthy pain receptors. Neuralgia falls into two categories: central neuralgia (the cause of the pain is located in the spinal cord or brain) and peripheral neuralgia. Hyperesthesia is exaggerated response to mild stimulation or a condition that involves an abnormal increase in sensitivity to stimuli of the sense.

11. **B.** Deafferentation pain is a type of neuropathic pain that is associated with loss of sensory input from the periphery to the central nervous system, such as phantom limb pain. It is the interruption or destruction of the afferent connections of nerve cells (e.g., in animal experiments, deafferentation demonstrates the spontaneity of locomotor movement by the freeing of a motor nerve from sensory components).

12. **B.** The gasserian ganglion is formed from two roots that exit the ventral surface of the brainstem at the midpontine level, and these roots pass in a forward and lateral direction in the posterior cranial fossa across the border of the petrous bone. They enter a recess called Meckel cave, which is formed by an invagination of the surrounding dura mater into the middle cranial fossa. The dural pouch that lies just behind the ganglion is called the trigeminal cistern and contains cerebrospinal fluid. The gasserian ganglion is canoe-shaped, with the three sensory divisions—the ophthalmic (V1), the maxillary (V2), and the mandibular (V3)—exiting the anterior convex aspect of the ganglion. A small motor root joins the mandibular division as it exits the cranial cavity via the foramen ovale. The gasserian ganglion contains the cell bodies of sensory fibers of trigeminal nerve. This procedure called a gasserian ganglion block to treat facial pain is where a small amount of local anesthetic (with or without steroid) is

injected onto the part of the nerve supply to the face called the gasserian ganglion (located to the back of the face between the ear and eye socket).

13. **C.** Substance P, glutamate, aspartate, and ATP are among the major excitatory molecules responsible for pain modulation. Somatostatin, acetylcholine, and endorphin are among the major inhibitory mediators of pain.

14. **D.** Norepinephrine, adenosine, and serotonin are among the major inhibitory neurotransmitters in the pain cascade. However, calcitonin gene-related peptide is an excitatory neurotransmitter.

15. **A.** Secondary hyperalgesia is defined as an increase in pain sensitivity when a noxious stimulus is delivered to a region surrounding, but not including, the zone of injury (increased pain sensitivity outside of the area of injury or inflammation). Secondary hyperalgesia, also known as neurogenic inflammation, is associated with local redness, tissue edema, and sensitization to noxious stimuli. Local anesthetics injection or capsaicin topical application can diminish these reactions. Secondary hyperalgesia is a centrally mediated condition that may occur due to injury or disease in an area of the body. Secondary hyperalgesia is due to central neuron sensitization and requires continuous nociceptor input from the zone of primary hyperalgesia for its maintenance. Secondary hyperalgesia implies only mechanical hyperalgesia (e.g., allodynia and pin prick).

16. **D.** Certain chronic pain conditions are sympathetically maintained and will respond to sympathetic blockade, such as complex regional pain syndrome, phantom limb pain, postherpetic neuralgia, and trigeminal neuralgia. However, acute pain secondary to pelvic exenteration surgery, although very difficult to treat, is typically not mediated sympathetically and does not usually respond well to a sympathectomy.

17. **D.** One of the many reasons acute pain needs to be managed properly is its systemic effects, which include hypertension, tachycardia, and increased minute ventilation, can promote ileus and urinary retention, along with the release of catabolic hormones.

18. **C.** Piriformis syndrome is a neuromuscular disorder that occurs when the sciatic nerve is compressed or otherwise irritated by the piriformis muscle, causing pain, tingling, and numbness in the buttocks and along the path of the sciatic nerve descending down the posterior lower thigh and into the leg. The sciatic nerve can be trapped at the sciatic notch and cause impingement syndromes (buttocks and leg pain).

19. **B.** The cubital tunnel is a channel that allows the ulnar nerve to travel over the elbow and is bordered by the medial epicondyle of the humerus, the olecranon process of the ulna, and the tendinous arch joining the humeral and ulnar heads of the flexor carpi ulnaris. Cubital tunnel syndrome is a condition brought on by increased pressure on the ulnar nerve at the elbow, typically against medial epicondyle where the ulnar nerve passes. This can occur due to chronic compression of this nerve, positional or due to inappropriate cast/splint placement.

20. **D.** Myofascial pain syndromes are associated with muscle symptoms such as spasm, pain, weakness, and stiffness, and associated with autonomic dysfunction (e.g., vasoconstriction). The trigger points can spontaneously resolve, but may continue on and become latent and activated at a later time. Myofascial pain needs to be ruled out in patients with chronic lower back pain as trigger points in quadratus lumborum, and gluteus medius muscles can be the cause for it. Some systemic diseases such as connective tissue disease can cause myofascial pain. Poor posture and emotional disturbances might also instigate or contribute to myofascial pain. The diagnosis of myofascial pain is by the pain and existence of trigger points.

21. **A.** Fibromyalgia is characterized by chronic widespread pain and allodynia (a heightened and painful response to pressure). Its exact cause is unknown, but believed to involve

psychological, genetic, neurobiological, and environmental factors. Fibromyalgia symptoms are not restricted to pain. Other symptoms can include debilitating fatigue, sleep disturbances, and joint stiffness. The American College of Rheumatology diagnosis criterion indicates that the pain be at least moderate to severe in scale: Widespread Pain Index (WPI) score of 7 or higher and the Symptom Severity (SS) scale score of 5 or higher. Another category of criteria to diagnose fibromyalgia includes a WPI of 3 to 6 along with an SS scale score of 9 or higher. The other two criteria for diagnosis include chronic conditions and absence of other coexisting chronic pain disorders. Treatment includes pregabalin (Lyrica), duloxetine (Cymbalta), and milnacipran (Savella) to identify a few options.

22. **D.** Chronic lower back pain is one of the top reasons for physician office visits and also one of the greatest reasons for work absence. Lumbosacral strain, degenerative disk disease, and myofascial syndromes are the most common causes, and fibromyalgia is not typically associated with a diagnosis of lower back pain.

23. **D.** Disk herniation at L5–S1 is the most common location of vertebral disk pathology presenting as back pain (affects the S1 nerve root). Patients often have associated gluteal pain and numbness along with pain/paresthesia in the posterior thigh, posterolateral calf, lateral dorsum, and undersurface of the foot. Physical examination will also identify a diminished plantar flexion of the ankle on the affected side.

24. **B.** Disk herniation at L4–L5 is a very common location for such pathology and affects the L5 nerve root. Patients may present with pain and paresthesia anywhere along the dermatome distribution of the L5 nerve root (lateral thigh, anterolateral calf, medial dorsum of the foot, particularly between the first and second toes). The symptoms of quadriceps femoris muscle weakness would be secondary to pathology of nerve roots L2–L4.

25. **D.** Facet joints are formed by the superior and inferior processes of each vertebra. Facet syndrome is a syndrome in which the zygapophyseal joints (synovial diarthroses, from C2 to S1) cause back pain. Fifty-five percent of facet syndrome cases occur in cervical vertebrae, and 31% in the lumbar area. Facet syndrome can progress to spinal osteoarthritis, which is known as spondylosis. Back pain secondary to degenerative changes in the facet (zygapophyseal) joints is also called facet syndrome. It is characterized by near midline pain that may radiate to the gluteal region, thigh, and knee. Facet syndrome symptoms may worsen by hyperextension or lateral rotation of the back. Confirmative test is pain relief offered by intra-articular injection of local anesthetics or blockade of the posterior ramus medial nerve branch.

26. **B.** Neuropathic pain is pain caused by damage or disease that affects the somatosensory system. Neuropathic pain along with components of neuropathic pain can be associated with several chronic diseases such as diabetes, stroke, spinal cord pathology, postherpetic neuralgia, multiple sclerosis, cancer pain, or low back pain. Neuropathic pain is often described as "wax and wane" types of pain symptoms (e.g., comes and goes), burning, and electrical, as described by patients. Allodynia or hyperalgesia can often be associated with neuropathic pain.

27. **B.** Neuropathic pain can be very difficult to treat effectively and often requires multiple therapeutic modalities for treatment. These include anticonvulsants, antidepressants, antiarrhythmics, α_2-adrenergic agonists, topical agents, and analgesics (nonsteroidal anti-inflammatory drugs and opioids). Sympathetic blocks as well as spinal cord stimulation work for certain patients resistant to pharmacological interventions.

28. **D.** Complex regional pain syndrome (CRPS), formerly called reflex sympathetic dystrophy or causalgia, or reflex neurovascular dystrophy or amplified musculoskeletal pain syndrome, is a chronic systemic disease characterized by severe pain, swelling, and changes in the skin. CRPS is expected to worsen over time. Some forms of CRPS are sympathetically maintained and are therefore responsive to sympathetic blockade. CRPS type 2 is associated with documented nerve damage/injury, but not CRPS type 1. CRPS can be associated with either minor

or major surgical procedures or injuries. When the autonomic nervous system is involved, additional signs and symptoms can include sweating (sudomotor changes), color, and skin temperature changes, along with trophic changes of the skin, hair, and nails. Motor strength and range of motion of the extremity may also be affected.

29. **D.**   The general strategy in CRPS treatment is often multidisciplinary, with the use of different types of medications combined with distinct physical therapies. Physical therapy plays a central role in the multimodal treatment of CRPS. Therapy is facilitated with sympathetic blockade or intravenous regional blocks. Physical therapy typically consists of active movement without weights and desensitization therapy. If not treated in timely fashion, CRPS can result in functional disability. The incidence of a cure is about 90% with effective multimodal therapy initiated within 1 month of symptoms.

30. **B.**   Potential complications of a celiac plexus block include postural hypotension from the visceral sympathectomy and vasodilation due to the local anesthetic injection. Both the vena cava and the aorta are in close proximity and susceptible to intravascular injury/injection. Other potential complications include a pneumothorax, retroperitoneal hemorrhage, injury to the kidneys or pancreas, and sexual dysfunction. The visceral sympathetic chain is in close proximity, and blockade may result in unopposed parasympathetic activity that may lead to increased gastrointestinal motility and diarrhea.

10

Orthopedic Anesthesia

Thomas Halaszynski

1. The surgeon is performing a right total knee arthroplasty under a combined spinal–epidural anesthetic. The surgical team is providing you with information that within the next 15 minutes they plan to place bone cement (polymethylmethacrylate) to anchor the prosthesis. The most likely clinical side effect that may occur is

    A. Hypertension
    B. Increased work of breathing and hypercapnia
    C. Cardiac arrhythmias
    D. Decreased pulmonary shunt

2. Potential complications of use of a pneumatic tourniquet include all of the following, except

    A. Tourniquet pain that is relieved by performing a peripheral nerve block
    B. A compression nerve injury
    C. Development of arterial thromboembolism
    D. Pulmonary embolism

3. A 20-year-old male (status post car accident) sustained a right femur and pelvic fracture 2 days prior. In the last 24 hours, he has become progressively more short of breath, requiring 100% F_{IO_2} to maintain an oxygen saturation in the high 80s and is now becoming more confused and disoriented. Physical exam reveals petechiae on the anterior chest wall, arms, and conjunctiva along with decreased breath sounds to auscultation. The most likely diagnosis is

    A. Cognitive dysfunction
    B. Pulmonary fat embolism
    C. Undiagnosed pneumothorax
    D. Congestive heart failure

4. Incorrect statement regarding neuraxial anesthesia and deep-vein thrombosis/pulmonary embolism (DVT/PE) in orthopedic surgical procedures is

    A. Neuraxial anesthesia may reduce thromboembolic complications
    B. Neuraxial anesthesia may reduce blood loss
    C. Neuraxial anesthesia may decrease platelet reactivity
    D. Neuraxial anesthesia may increase activity of both factor VIII and von Willebrand factor

5. On postoperative day 1, an orthopedic surgeon has consulted you about his total knee arthroplasty patient who is in severe pain and has failed a regimen of patient-controlled analgesia using morphine. He is now consulting you for an epidural catheter placement for postoperative pain control, and would like to know for what time interval once-daily prophylactic low-molecular-weight heparin (LMWH) should be held prior to performing the epidural procedure:

   A. 4 hours and no absolute contraindication to placement of a catheter
   B. 6 hours and a relative contraindication to place a catheter
   C. 12 hours and no absolute contraindication to placement of a catheter
   D. 24 hours and absolute contraindication to place a catheter

6. In the anesthesia preadmission testing clinic, you are assessing a 58-year-old female with a medical history significant for hypertension, diabetes, fibromyalgia, and rheumatoid arthritis (RA). The RA is affecting the upper extremities bilaterally and the cervical spine, but her RA symptoms are well-controlled with methotrexate. She is now presenting for an elective total hip arthroplasty. The radiographs that should be ordered to rule out atlantoaxial instability are

   A. Lateral view: flexion of the cervical spine
   B. Lateral view: extension of the cervical spine
   C. No radiographs are indicated since the patient is asymptomatic
   D. Lateral view: both flexion and extension of the cervical spine

7. You were involved in a complicated left lower leg procedure (open reduced internal fixation of proximal tibia–fibula fracture repair), where the final total tourniquet time was 3 hours 15 minutes. In the postanesthesia care unit, the patient showed no signs of any peripheral nerve injury of the left lower extremity. However, on postoperative day 2, you discovered that the patient required hemodialysis secondary to rhabdomyolysis. Which of the following could be responsible for the rhabdomyolysis?

   A. Compartment syndrome
   B. Prolonged tourniquet inflation time
   C. Statin medication use that patient started 2 weeks prior
   D. All of the above

8. Concurrent administration of all of the following anticoagulants and thrombolytic therapy should be avoided when planning for neuraxial blockade, except for

   A. Fibrinolytic and thrombolytic therapy
   B. Thrombin inhibitors (desirudin, lepirudin, bivalirudin, and Argatroban)
   C. Therapeutic dosing of low-molecular-weight heparin (LMWH)
   D. Subcutaneous heparin daily dose of 10,000 U or less

9. The most correct statement regarding blood loss that may occur in a patient with a hip fracture is

   A. Intertrochanteric > base of femoral neck > subcapital
   B. Transcervical > base of femoral neck > subcapital
   C. Subtrochanteric > subcapital > transcervical
   D. Subcapital > base of femoral neck > transcervical

10. A 76-year-old female is to undergo a right femoral neck fracture repair. You perform a spinal anesthetic using 1.5 mL 0.5% bupivacaine mixed with 100 μg of preservative-free morphine. How long should the patient be monitored for postoperative apnea/hypoventilation secondary to the intrathecal morphine administration?

    A. 3 days
    B. 48 hours
    C. 12 hours
    D. 24 hours

11. A 56-year-old female with medical history significant for obesity (BMI 50), hypertension, diabetes (IDDM), tobacco abuse, and asthma is scheduled for bilateral hip replacement surgery. Preoperative laboratory results show a hematocrit (Hct) of 45%, blood urea nitrogen of 25 mg/dL, and creatinine of 1.0 mg/dL. Immediately following application of cement for the second hip, the patient became hypotension with sinus tachycardia. Arterial blood gas results reveal an Hct of 23% that responds to a crystalloid fluid bolus and blood transfusion (2 L crystalloids, 1 L albumin, and 2 U packed red blood cells). The possible cause(s) for the hypotension is/are

    A. Hypovolemia and/or low Hct
    B. Pulmonary embolism
    C. Vasodilation caused by monomer of the bone cement
    D. All of the above

12. A 68-year-old female (5'1" and 250 lb) with a medical history of chronic lower back pain and radiculopathy in the lumbar 4 to sacral 1 vertebral levels presents for anterior and posterior fusion. Her home medications include methadone 75 mg daily, oxycodone 10 mg every 3 hours as needed, a fentanyl patch (50 µg/h), and lisinopril 10 mg daily. The patient stated she has 7/10 pain daily. All of the following should be considered in the perioperative pain management regimen for this patient, except

    A. Continue with daily methadone
    B. Consider a perioperative ketamine infusion
    C. Consider transversus abdominis plane (TAP) block for the anterior abdomen
    D. Add ketorolac 30 mg every 6 hours as needed for 14 days

13. You are administering anesthesia for a cervical spine procedure, and the surgeon has indicated that she plans to monitor somatosensory-evoked potentials (SSEPs) and motor-evoked potentials (MEPs). Your anesthetic plan includes avoidance of long-acting muscle relaxants in addition to avoiding the use of

    A. 1 MAC or higher of sevoflurane as needed for maintenance anesthesia
    B. Half MAC of nitrous oxide to supplement the inhalation agent
    C. Continuous propofol infusion as anesthesia maintenance
    D. Dexmedetomidine to smooth out the anesthetic delivery

14. All of the following can be used to assist in reducing the amount of perioperative surgical blood loss in an orthopedic procedures, except

    A. Hemodilution
    B. Controlled hypotension
    C. Tranexamic acid
    D. Aprotinin

15. All of the following statements when positioning patients for spine surgery in the prone position are true, except

    A. The neck should be in neutral position (without hyperextension or hyperflexion)
    B. The eyes must be free of pressure and checked periodically
    C. The abdomen must always be supported (never permitted to hang freely)
    D. The arms are kept at less than 90 degrees of extension and flexion

16. The most incorrect statement regarding postoperative vision loss (POVL) that may occur during prone positioning in spine surgery patients is

    A. Ischemic optic neuropathy accounts for the highest incidence of POVL
    B. Ischemic optic neuropathy is associated with decreased ocular perfusion pressure
    C. Prone positioning, greater than 1 L intraoperative blood loss, and surgery lasting greater than 6 hours represent the highest risk
    D. POVL due to central retinal artery occlusion (CRAO) tends to be bilateral

17. After 180 minutes of tourniquet time during a difficult right total knee arthroplasty in a patient under sedation and intraoperative anesthesia provided by a combined spinal–epidural, the tourniquet is released and surgical closure is started. The patient may experience all the following subsequent to tourniquet release, except

   A. Hypotension and tachycardia
   B. Transient increase of end-tidal carbon dioxide
   C. Arrhythmia secondary to increased serum potassium
   D. Arrhythmia secondary to increased total serum calcium

18. The most incorrect statement regarding placement of a femoral perineural catheter for pain management during unilateral knee replacement surgery is that a femoral nerve block when compared to neuraxial blockade

   A. Provides equipotent analgesia
   B. Is associated with reduced incidence of pruritus, nausea, and vomiting
   C. Is associated with reduced incidence of urinary retention
   D. Femoral nerve block when combined with a sciatic nerve block can provide adequate analgesia for knee surgery

19. A 56-year-old female is scheduled for a right total shoulder replacement in the beach chair position. Medical history is significant for hypertension, diabetes, and a recent transient ischemic attack. The surgeon is requesting a hypotensive technique to reduce intraoperative blood loss. Where is the most optimal location to place the arterial line transducer?

   A. The level of the heart as this is the classic way of measuring
   B. The level of the sternum to measure adequate perfusion to the brain
   C. Level of the external meatus to monitor brain stem perfusion
   D. Level of shoulder to measure adequate shoulder perfusion

20. The anesthetic agent(s) that can cause adverse changes on the wave forms when monitoring somatosensory-evoked potentials (SSEPs) is/are

   A. High concentrations of inhalational agents (reduces wave form amplitude)
   B. 1 MAC of nitrous oxide (reduces wave form amplitude)
   C. Intravenous anesthesia with ketamine (exaggerates wave forms)
   D. ALL of the above

21. Which of the following surgical conditions may negatively influence changes on somatosensory-evoked potentials (SSEPs) wave forms?

   A. Spinal cord injury
   B. Ischemia induced by hypoperfusion
   C. Intraoperative bleeding
   D. All of the above

CHAPTER 10 ANSWERS

1. **C.** Placement of bone cement (bone cement implantation syndrome) can result in any combination of adverse events including hypoxia, hypotension, cardiac arrhythmias (possibly heart block or even sinus arrest), pulmonary hypertension, and decreased cardiac output.

2. **A.** Use of a compression tourniquet on upper and lower extremities can facilitate surgery and decrease blood loss, but it can result in complications and cannot be applied for prolonged periods. Use of such devices can be associated with ischemic pain that is not typically or completely relieved by performing peripheral nerve blocks of the extremity. Metabolic alterations upon tourniquet release, arterial thromboembolism, and pulmonary embolism are other potential complications.

3. **B.** A venous fat embolism will typically present itself within 72 hours following long-bone and/or pelvic fracture injuries. Such a condition may also occur following cardiopulmonary resuscitation, parental feeding with lipid infusion, and liposuction surgery. The classical triad includes dyspnea, confusion, and petechiae.

4. **D.** Advantages of neuraxial anesthesia in orthopedic surgery may include reduced incidence of DVT and PE formation, decreased platelet activity, decreased factor VIII and von Willebrand factor activity, and attenuation of stress hormone responses.

5. **C.** For patients receiving once-daily dosage of LMWH for prophylaxis, both epidural and spinal neuraxial techniques may be performed (or neuraxial catheters placed or removed) 10 to 12 hours following the previous dose of LMWH. In addition, a 4-hour time delay should occur before administering the next dose of daily prophylactic LMWH.

6. **D.** Advanced RA can affect the cervical spine such that patients may require treatment including steroids, immune therapy, and/or methotrexate. Radiographs of both flexion and extension with lateral views of the cervical spine are necessary to rule out atlantoaxial instability. If atlantoaxial instability is present, intubation should be performed with inline stabilization utilizing video or fiberoptic laryngoscopy to minimize excessive head and neck movement in order to reduce the incidence of cervical spinal cord/nerve root injury.

7. **D.** Any form of muscle damage of sufficient severity can cause rhabdomyolysis. Multiple causes can be present simultaneously in one individual. Some patients may have an underlying muscle condition, usually hereditary in nature, which may make them more prone to rhabdomyolysis. Rhabdomyolysis can be induced by several conditions including compartment syndrome, prolonged tourniquet inflation time, medications such as statins, and malignant hyperthermia. It is suggested that tourniquet times usually be kept to 2 hours or less to decrease the risk of nerve injury, ischemia, and rhabdomyolysis, which could lead to renal failure.

8. **D.** According to the American Society of Regional Anesthesia and Pain Medicine anticoagulation guidelines, medications such as antiplatelet agents (Plavix, and intravenous glycoprotein IIb/IIIa inhibitors), thrombolytics, fondaparinux, direct thrombin inhibitors, or therapeutic LMWH present an unacceptable risk for spinal and/or epidural hematoma development without sufficient time lapse between administration of such medications and neuraxial techniques. Maximum administration of subcutaneous heparin of 5,000 U bid is estimated to be safe with epidural and spinal anesthesia. Heparin administration of 5,000 U tid is not known to be accepted in clinical practice in conjunction with neuraxial blockade.

9. **A.** Blood loss in a patient secondary to a hip fracture can be significant, and some anesthesiologists plan to utilize cell savers and/or perform hypotensive techniques to minimize further blood loss. Blood loss from a hip fracture depends on the actual location of the fracture. As a general rule, intracapsular (subcapital, transcervical) fractures have been associated with less

blood loss than extracapsular (base of the femoral neck, intertrochanteric, subtrochanteric) fractures, as the capsule decreases blood loss by acting like a tourniquet. In general, blood loss from a subtrochanteric and intertrochanteric > base of femoral neck > transcervical and subcapital.

10. **D.**   Intrathecal morphine can depress ventilation and CO_2 responsiveness that can last for up to 24 hours. The first peak effect occurs about 6 to 8 hours post injection, and the second peak could happen as late as 24 hours later. The physiologic and pharmacologic mechanisms of this include vascular opioid uptake by the epidural or subarachnoid venous plexuses, rostral spread of the aqueous cerebrospinal fluid to the brainstem, and/or direct perimedullary vascular channels.

11. **D.**   Total hip arthroplasty surgery can be characterized by significant blood loss, especially in the situation of bilateral hip replacement. In acute bleeding, measuring an Hct may not accurately reflect the true value as equilibrium takes some time to show the true Hct. In addition, bone cement can cause vasodilation, which can further contribute to the low blood pressure. Cement placement has been associated with pulmonary embolism and pulmonary hypertension.

12. **D.**   Chronic pain is often a common occurrence in patients presented for spine/back surgeries. A multimodal therapeutic pain management strategy aimed at different pain cascade pathways is frequently utilized. It is a common practice to continue methadone if patients are already taking such medications and to consider starting methadone in patients with uncontrolled postoperative pain. Ketamine (GABA agonist) is effective in chronic pain patients. TAP blockade with local anesthetics can provide effective somatic pain relief of the anterior abdomen that will help in the treatment of incisional pain. Evidence supports the use of nonsteroidal anti-inflammatory drugs at low doses in spine surgeries, but higher concentrations have been associated with a rate of nonunion, so are therefore discouraged.

13. **A.**   High concentrations of potent inhalational agents (such as desflurane and sevoflurane) may increase neuromonitoring latency and decrease amplitude of the SSEP and MEP. Therefore, inhalation agents can be used for intraoperative maintenance anesthesia, but are used at less than one full MAC concentration. Intravenous (IV) anesthetics are more commonly used for maintenance of anesthesia, as they are more compatible with SSEP and MEP neuromonitoring (some expected, but tolerable changes on either latency and/or amplitude). These IV anesthetics include propofol, ketamine, etomidate, dexmedetomidine, benzodiazepines, and opioids independently and in various combinations. Opioids have the least potential to interfere SSEP and MEP neuromonitoring.

14. **D.**   Spine surgery can be associated with significant blood loss. Surgical and anesthetic techniques that have been developed to control perioperative blood loss include hemodilution, autologous blood donation preoperatively, use of cell saver, and epinephrine at wound site. Pharmacologically, antifibrinolytics such as tranexamic acid and ε-aminocaproic acid have been used with some efficacy. Tranexamic acid is a synthetic derivative of the amino acid lysine, and it is used to treat or prevent excessive blood loss during surgery and in various other medical conditions. Aprotinin has been associated with a 50% increase of cardiac side effects (myocardial infarction/congestive heart failure), increase (double) of the risk of stroke, and higher death rates (increased mortality).

15. **C.**   Prone positioning of patients needs to be carefully executed, especially during spine surgeries (prolonged procedures) and in patients who have other associated comorbidities such as rheumatoid arthritis and ankylosing spondylitis. The endotracheal tube needs to be properly secured, and eyes and nose should be padded and checked periodically to ensure that they are pressure-free. The neck and arms should be kept positioned in an anatomically neutral position. The abdomen needs to remain free to avoid increased venous pressure (assists in

reducing increased venous bleeding) and to reduce the incidence of abdominal compartment syndrome that can develop during prolonged duration of surgical intervention and aggressive fluid administration.

16. **D.** Ischemic optic neuropathy is a major cause of perioperative POVL accordingly to the vision loss registry collected by the ASA. Any increase of intraocular pressure (IOP) or decrease on mean arterial pressure (MAP) will affect ocular perfusion pressure (OPP), particularly with patients in a head-down position where edema can develop in the orbit that will increase venous pressure. OPP = MAP – IOP. CRAO accounts for a small percentage of patients who experience vision dysfunction according to the vision loss registry. CRAO may be embolic in nature or the result of direct pressure on the eyeball; therefore, it tends to be mostly unilateral.

17. **D.** Release of a tourniquet used on an extremity during surgery is often associated with the release of metabolic (acidotic) by-products from the ischemic limb that are dumped into the systemic circulation. In patients with poor preoperative functional status or those that may experience significant intraoperative blood loss, the increased systemic metabolic by-products may be enough to result in hypotension and cardiac arrhythmia that may require volume resuscitation and/or pharmacologic support. In rare instances, the hyperkalemia may need to be treated (sodium bicarbonate or calcium).

18. **D.** During unilateral knee replacement surgery, properly functioning lumbar epidural and femoral perineural catheters can provide equivalent perioperative analgesia. However, a peripheral nerve block using a femoral perineural catheter does not have several of the typical side effects that can be associated with neuraxial blockade, such as more intense sympathectomy, pruritus (when opioids are mixed with local anesthetics), nausea and vomiting, urinary retention, or orthostatic hypotension and lightheadedness. Several studies have shown that patients with regional anesthesia/analgesia (femoral catheter patients may meet discharge criterion earlier) may show earlier improved outcomes. Considering variations of surgical technique, the postoperative pain during total knee arthroplasty is located on the anterior knee that can be equally controlled by either lumbar epidural or femoral nerve block alone. For bilateral knee replacement surgery, either bilateral femoral catheters or lumbar epidural catheter may be a reasonable option.

19. **C.** Shoulder operations may be performed in either a sitting ("beach chair") or the lateral decubitus position. The beach chair position may be associated with decreases in cerebral perfusion leading to the potential for increased risk of blindness, stroke, and brain ischemia. If a controlled hypotension technique is chosen, an arterial transducer should be positioned most preferably at the level of the brain stem (i.e., external meatus of the ear).

20. **D.** Most of the currently used anesthetic agents may have some effects/negative influence on SSEP (differences may be minor or major changes). Several other perioperative variables such as hemoglobin concentration, temperature, CO_2, and arterial blood pressure may also influence the SSEP tracing.

21. **D.** There are a host of reasons causing negative SSEP-tracing changes. In addition to several anesthetic considerations (from anesthetic agent choice to techniques used), there are surgical techniques and considerations that can influence SSEP. Direct trauma, ischemia, and pressure to the spinal cord are capable of inducing acute changes on SSEP. In addition, spinal cord ischemia changes secondary to decreased blood supply, and/or vessel injury (stretching/pressure) may take as much as a half an hour to manifest itself.

11

Cardiovascular Anesthesia

Deppu Ushakumari and Ashish Sinha

1. Which of the following is responsible for the plateau phase of cardiac action potential?

   A. Slow movement of potassium out of the cell
   B. Slow movement of calcium into the cell
   C. Slow movement of calcium out of the cell
   D. Both A and C

2. A 2-year-old boy is induced with halothane-inhalation induction. The patient suddenly gets bradycardic, and you decide to administer atropine 0.4 mg intravenously. Immediately there-after, you notice that the patient is having a junctional tachycardia. Which of the following most accurately describes the sequence of events?

   A. Sinoatrial (SA) node suppression by halothane followed by anticholinergic action of atropine
   B. Atrioventricular (AV) node suppression by halothane followed by anticholinergic action of atropine
   C. SA node and AV node suppression by halothane followed by anticholinergic action of atropine
   D. SA node and AV node suppression by halothane followed by paroxysmal tachycardic action of atropine

3. Significant intravenous absorption/inadvertent intravenous injection of bupivacaine can cause profound bradycardia and sinus node arrest. Which of the following best describes the mechanism of cardiac toxicity of bupivacaine?

   A. Bupivacaine binds inactivated fast sodium channels and dissociates from them slowly
   B. Bupivacaine binds activated fast sodium channels and dissociates from them slowly
   C. Bupivacaine binds inactivated slow sodium channels and dissociates from them slowly
   D. Bupivacaine binds activated slow sodium channels and dissociates from them slowly

4. The mechanisms of depression of cardiac contractility by volatile anesthetics include all the following, except

   A. They decrease the entry of calcium into cells during depolarization
   B. They affect only L-type calcium channels
   C. They alter kinetics of calcium release
   D. They decrease the sensitivity of contractile proteins to calcium

5. The mechanism of "x" descent (descent between C and V waves) in the following right atrial tracing (Fig 11-1) is

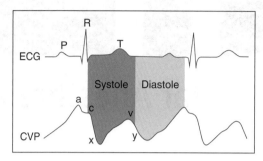

Figure 11-1.

A. Downward movement of the atrioventricular (AV) valve cusps after ventricular contraction
B. Pulling down of the atrium by ventricular contraction
C. Relaxation of atrium after atrial systole
D. Decline in atrial pressure as the AV valves open

6. A 38-year-old healthy male volunteer is undergoing cardiac function tests as part of a physiology experiment. His vital signs are HR = 62 bpm, BP = 124/74 mm Hg, respiratory rate = 12 breaths/min, SpO_2 = 100% on room air, and Hb = 14 g/dL. Which of the following is the best determination of the adequacy of his cardiac output?

A. Cardiac index 4.0 L/min/m^2
B. Cardiac output 8.1 L/min by thermodilution technique
C. Cardiac output 8.1 L/min by Fick method
D. SvO_2 of 75% from a pulmonary artery (PA) catheter

7. Which of the following patients will be affected the most from loss of atrial contribution to preload?

A. A 65-year-old patient with severe aortic regurgitation who went into recent onset atrial fibrillation
B. A 35-year-old patient with mitral-valve area of 1.0 cm^2 who went into recent onset atrial fibrillation
C. An 80-year-old patient with severe aortic stenosis who went into recent onset atrial fibrillation
D. A 55-year-old patient with acute right-ventricular myocardial infarction

8. Which of the following formulae explains the hypertrophy of heart in response to pressure or volume loads (P, intraventricular pressure; R, ventricular radius; t, wall thickness; T, circumferential stress)?

A. P = 2Tt/R
B. T = 2P/Rt
C. T = 2R/Pt
D. PT = Rt

9. Dose of heparin (U/kg) administered for cardiopulmonary bypass is (approximately)

A. 100 to 200
B. 200 to 300
C. 300 to 400
D. 400 to 500

10. The sinoatrial and the atrioventricular (AV) nodes are supplied in majority of the individuals by

    A. Left anterior descending artery
    B. Right coronary artery
    C. Circumflex artery
    D. Posterior descending artery

11. Baroreceptor reflex is ineffective for long-term blood pressure (BP) control because

    A. Renin angiotensin aldosterone system takes over the control
    B. Renal regulation of BP is more powerful
    C. Of adaptation to changes in BP over 1 to 2 days
    D. All of the above

12. Which of the following portions of myocardium has a dual blood supply?

    A. Bundle of His
    B. Atrioventricular node
    C. Posterior papillary muscle
    D. Sinoatrial node

13. Which of the following types of myocardial work needs the highest oxygen requirement?

    A. Electrical activity
    B. Volume work
    C. Pressure work
    D. Basal requirement

14. Which of the following inhalational agents causes the least coronary vasodilation?

    A. Halothane
    B. Isoflurane
    C. Desflurane
    D. Sevoflurane

15. Which of the following surgeries carries the highest cardiovascular risk?

    A. Emergency appendectomy
    B. Carotid endarterectomy
    C. Femoral–popliteal bypass surgery
    D. Inguinal hernia repair

16. A 67-year-old patient with uncontrolled hypertension presents for an elective dialysis access creation. Which of the following techniques is not suited for attenuating the hypertensive response to intubation?

    A. Administering 3 μg/kg of fentanyl intravenously
    B. Administering topical airway anesthesia
    C. Administering lidocaine 0.5 mg/kg intravenously
    D. Administering esmolol 1 mg/kg intravenously

17. The patient mentioned above develops severe hypotension immediately after intubation. Which of the following agents is most suited to bring the blood pressure back to normal values?

    A. Ephedrine
    B. Phenylephrine
    C. Epinephrine
    D. Dopamine

18. Which of the following antianginal agents has the highest coronary vasodilating potential?

   A. Nitrates
   B. Verapamil
   C. Dihydropyridines
   D. β-Blockers

19. Which of the following statements about calcium channel blockers (CCBs) is not true?

   A. CCBs potentiate both depolarizing and nondepolarizing neuromuscular blockers
   B. CCBs potentiate the circulatory effects of volatile anesthetic agents
   C. Verapamil may decrease anesthetic requirements
   D. Verapamil has no effect on cardiac contractility; it acts only on the atrioventricular (AV) node

20. Which of the following β-blockers is most suited for a patient with bronchospastic disease?

   A. Propranolol
   B. Metoprolol
   C. Acebutolol
   D. Bisoprolol

21. A 24-year-old female patient with a preoperative QTc interval of 550 ms is undergoing breast surgery under general anesthesia. Droperidol is administered to the patient for prevention of postoperative nausea, following which the patient goes into polymorphic-ventricular tachycardia. Which of the following drugs/therapies is best for the patient at this point?

   A. Amiodarone
   B. Lidocaine
   C. Pacing
   D. Diltiazem

22. Which of the following factors is not associated with severe multivessel disease during exercise electrocardiography?

   A. Sustained decrease ($\geq$10 mm Hg) in systolic blood pressure during exercise
   B. Failure to reach a maximum heart rate greater than 70% of predicted
   C. Persistence of ST-segment depression after exercising for 5 minutes or longer
   D. A 1-mm upsloping of ST segment

23. Surgical electrocautery may cause a problem with an automated implantable cardioverter defibrillator (AICD) by all the following mechanisms, except

   A. AICD interpreting a cautery current as ventricular fibrillation
   B. Inhibition of pacemaker function due to cautery artifact
   C. Increased pacing rate due to activation of a rate-responsive sensor
   D. Cautery current generating too much heat at the location of AICD and causing burns

24. Which of the following ECG leads is most sensitive to detect an anterior-wall myocardial ischemia?

   A. V5
   B. V4
   C. II
   D. V2

25. Which of the following is not true about systemic hypothermia during cardiopulmonary bypass (CPB)?

    A. Intentional hypothermia is always used following the initiation of CPB
    B. Core body temperature is usually reduced to 20 to 32°C
    C. Metabolic oxygen requirements are usually halved for every of 10°C reduction in temperature
    D. Profound hypothermia to temperatures of 15 to 18°C allows total circulatory arrest for up to 60 minutes

26. Adverse effects of hypothermia include all the following, except

    A. Platelet dysfunction
    B. Irreversible coagulopathy
    C. Potentiation of citrate toxicity
    D. Depression of myocardial contractility

27. Coronary perfusion pressure is

    A. Arterial diastolic pressure   left-ventricular end diastolic pressure
    B. Arterial diastolic pressure   left-ventricular end systolic pressure
    C. Arterial systolic pressure   left-ventricular end diastolic pressure
    D. Arterial systolic pressure   left-ventricular end systolic pressure

28. Which of the following views of transesophageal echocardiograph (TEE) is most suited to visualize blood supply of all the segments of the heart?

    A. Midesophageal fourth-chamber view
    B. Midesophageal second-chamber view
    C. Transgastric midshort axis view
    D. Midesophageal third-chamber view

29. Disadvantages of high-dose opioid induction include all the following, except

    A. Prolonged postoperative respiratory depression
    B. High incidence of recall during surgery
    C. Possible impairment of immune response
    D. Myocardial depression

30. A 66-year-old male is undergoing coronary artery bypass grafting (CABG). After the chest is opened, a progressive decline in cardiac output is noticed. The most accurate statement regarding the change is

    A. It is normal in deeply anesthetized patients
    B. Intravenous fluid administration will not help correct this change
    C. It implies imminent risk of death, and you should ask for blood to be transfused
    D. It is caused by surgeon lifting the heart, especially if it is not accompanied by a drop in blood pressure

31. Aprotinin therapy should be considered for all of the following patients, except

    A. Jehovah witnesses
    B. Redo surgeries
    C. Patients who had prior exposure to aprotinin
    D. Patients on combined clopidogrel (Plavix) and aspirin therapy

32. Which of the following statements is false regarding placement of venous cannulas for cardiopulmonary bypass (CPB)?

    A. Venous cannulas are inserted before aortic cannula placement
    B. Venous cannula insertion frequently precipitates atrial or ventricular arrhythmias
    C. Venous cannulas can impede venous return to the heart
    D. Venous cannulas can cause superior vena cava syndrome

33. Following initiation of cardiopulmonary bypass (CPB) for aortic valve replacement, you notice the mean arterial pressure (MAP) consistently above 100 mm Hg. The most appropriate next step is

    A. It is normal, and no action is needed
    B. Pump flow should be decreased to decrease the blood pressure
    C. It is usually caused by an air lock in the arterial cannula
    D. Administer midazolam to prevent awareness

34. Which of the following is not an indication of low flow rates under cardiopulmonary bypass (CPB)?

    A. SvO_2 >80%
    B. Progressive metabolic alkalosis
    C. Low urine output
    D. Hypoxemia noticed on an in-line venous oxygen saturation monitor

35. Discontinuing ventilation prematurely before full flow is achieved on cardiopulmonary bypass (CPB) causes

    A. A right-to-left shunt leading to hypoxemia
    B. Increased dead space
    C. Helps to increase venous return via the venous outflow cannula
    D. Aids the surgeon to visualize and cannulate the coronary sinus

36. Which of the following is the most sensitive to detect air bubbles at the termination of cardiopulmonary bypass (CPB)?

    A. Transesophageal echocardiography (TEE)
    B. Doppler ultrasonography
    C. Manual visualization
    D. Epiaortic echocardiography

37. Sweating during the rewarming phase of termination of cardiopulmonary bypass (CPB)

    A. Implies light anesthesia
    B. Is a hypothalamic response to perfusion with blood that is often at 39°C
    C. Necessitates cooling the operating room
    D. Can be prevented by using a forced air-warming device during the surgery

38. Use of corrected gas tensions during hypothermia

    A. Is called pH-stat management
    B. Preserves cerebral autoregulation
    C. Improves myocardial preservation
    D. Is done by adding sodium bicarbonate to the venous reservoir

39. Infusion of nitroglycerin at the termination of cardiopulmonary bypass (CPB)

    A. Dilates the coronary vessels and helps improve coronary flow
    B. Speeds the rewarming process and decreases large temperature gradients
    C. Is an old technique that produces unnecessary hemodynamic changes
    D. Improves renal blood flow

40. General guidelines for separation from cardiopulmonary bypass (CPB) include all the following, except

    A. Core body temperature of at least 34°C
    B. Stable heart rhythm or pacer rhythm
    C. Heart rate around 80 to 100 bpm
    D. Adequate ventilation with 100% O$_2$

41. Timing of inflation of an intra-aortic balloon pump (IABP) should be

    A. Just before the dicrotic notch
    B. Just after the dicrotic notch
    C. As soon as the downward slope of aortic pulse begins
    D. Synchronized with the rise of aortic pulse

42. A 68-year-old patient with an infected prosthetic aortic valve underwent a valve replacement. Post–cardiopulmonary bypass (CPB), his central venous pressure (CVP), pulmonary capillary wedge pressure (PCWP), and systemic vascular resistance (SVR) are low, while the cardiac output (CO) is high. The next step in management of this patient is

    A. Adding an inotrope
    B. Adding intra-aortic balloon pump (IABP)
    C. Adding a pulmonary vasodilator
    D. Increasing the hematocrit

43. After neutralizing heparin, which of the following is the fate of the heparin–protamine reaction product?

    A. The only product remaining will be water since it is an acid–base reaction
    B. It is removed by the reticuloendothelial system
    C. It is removed by the kidneys
    D. It is excreted unchanged via gastrointestinal (GI) tract

44. Heparin rebound after termination of cardiopulmonary bypass (CPB) is due to

    A. Redistribution of protamine to peripheral compartments
    B. Redistribution of heparin to central compartment
    C. Both A and B are true
    D. Both A and B are false; it is due to inadequate protamine dosing

45. DDAVP (desmopressin) administration can increase the activity of all the following factors, except

    A. Factor VII
    B. Factor VIII
    C. Factor XII
    D. von Willebrand factor

46. In the first few postoperative hours after an open heart surgery, the emphasis is on

    A. Monitoring for excessive postoperative bleeding
    B. Maintaining adequate urine output
    C. Trying for an early extubation
    D. Maintaining euthermia

47. Inhaled nitric oxide (NO) at 60 ppm has all of the following effects, except

    A. Drop in systemic vascular resistance (SVR)
    B. Drop in pulmonary vascular resistance (PVR)
    C. Improvement in cardiac output
    D. Better right coronary perfusion

48. Donor–recipient compatibility in cardiac transplantation is based on all, except

A. Heart size
B. ABO blood–group typing
C. Cytomegalovirus serology
D. Tissue crossmatching

49. The central venous pressure (CVP) waveform in cardiac tamponade is characterized by

A. Abolition of X descent
B. Abolition of Y descent
C. CV waveform
D. Tall C waves

50. In constrictive pericarditis,

A. Increased diastolic filling does not occur, in contrast to acute tamponade
B. The Y descent is absent in CVP waveform
C. Pulsus paradoxus is uncommon
D. Diffuse T-wave abnormalities are a rare sign

51. A 25-year-old male with a family history of sudden cardiac deaths is undergoing a laparoscopic appendectomy. Immediately after induction and intubation, you notice a heart rate of 120 bpm and blood pressure of 60/40 mm Hg, with a normal capnogram. You suspect the patient has idiopathic hypertrophic subaortic stenosis. Which of the following maneuvers is most likely to help this patient's hemodynamics?

A. Lowering the head end of the bed and administering 10 mg of ephedrine IV
B. Administering a bolus of 1 L of normal saline and esmolol 10 mg IV
C. Administering verapamil 5 mg IV immediately
D. Administering a bolus of normal saline and phenylephrine 100 µg IV

52. Pulmonary capillary wedge pressure (PCWP) does not correspond to the left-ventricular end diastolic pressure (LVEDP) in all of the following situations, except

A. Mitral stenosis
B. Tricuspid regurgitation
C. Very high positive end–expiratory pressure (PEEP)
D. Left-atrial myxoma

53. Normal mixed venous oxygen tension is _____ (mm Hg):

A. 75
B. 40
C. 45
D. 560

54. The only clinically proven method to reduce the risk of perioperative myocardial infarction (MI) and associated death is

A. Perioperative β-blocker therapy
B. Perioperative clonidine therapy
C. Both A and B
D. Use of esmolol boluses intraoperatively to keep the heart rate <80 bpm

55. Which of the following statements is false regarding perioperative myocardial infarction (MI)?

   A. Most perioperative MIs occur in the first 48 to 72 hours postoperatively
   B. A 1-minute episode of 1-mm ST-segment elevation or depression on the ECG increases the risk for cardiac events by 10-fold
   C. Perioperative risk reduction with β-blockers and clonidine is inferior to risk stratification with invasive testing, angioplasty, and coronary artery bypass grafting (CABG)
   D. Tachycardia (>105 bpm) for 5 minutes in the postoperative period can increase the risk of death by 10-fold

56. Which of the following is the most effective means of predicting a perioperative cardiac event?

   A. Echocardiography wall-motion abnormalities
   B. Echocardiography ejection fraction
   C. Dipyridamole–thallium scintigraphy
   D. Careful preoperative evaluation

57. Which of the following is most effective method of preventing the hemodynamic changes associated with intubation?

   A. Brief laryngoscopy (<15 seconds)
   B. Esmolol 1 mg/kg IV before intubation
   C. Lidocaine 2 mg/kg before intubation
   D. Deepen the anesthesia with propofol 1 mg/kg

58. Which of the following events is not likely to adversely affect hemodynamics in a patient with mitral-valve prolapse?

   A. Sympathetic stimulation
   B. Decreased systemic vascular resistance
   C. Head-up position of the patient
   D. Increased pulmonary vascular resistance

59. Anesthetic considerations in a patient with mitral regurgitation include all the following, except

   A. Avoid sudden decreases in heart rate
   B. Avoid sudden decreases in systemic vascular resistance (SVR)
   C. Minimize drug-induced myocardial depression
   D. Monitor the magnitude of the C wave of CVP as a reflection of mitral-regurgitant flow

60. Treatment of patients with prolonged QT interval include all, except

   A. β-Blockers
   B. Right stellate ganglion block
   C. Avoidance of drugs that prolong the QT interval
   D. Availability of electrical cardioversion while the patients are undergoing surgical procedures

61. Anesthetic considerations in patients with aortic stenosis include all, except

   A. Intra-arterial blood pressure monitoring
   B. Prophylactic administration of intravenous vasoconstrictor phenylephrine
   C. Avoidance of extreme bradycardia or tachycardia
   D. Avoidance of sudden increases in systemic vascular resistance (SVR)

62. Ventricular premature beats (VPCs) can be treated with lidocaine (1–2 mg/kg IV) when they

    A. Are frequent (more than six premature beats/min)
    B. Are multifocal
    C. Take place during the ascending limb of the T wave (R-on-T phenomenon)
    D. All of the above

63. Which of the following drugs needs not be avoided in the anesthetic management of a patient with Wolff–Parkinson–White (WPW) syndrome?

    A. Ketamine
    B. Pancuronium
    C. Succinylcholine
    D. Digitalis

64. Which of the following statements is false regarding management of a patient with an automated implantable cardioverter defibrillator (AICD)?

    A. The "magnet mode" is always safe
    B. The ground plate should be placed as far as possible from the pulse generator
    C. Bipolar electrocautery may be used over unipolar electrocautery to reduce interference between electrosurgical cautery and the pacemaker
    D. The magnet mode may produce asynchronous pacing at 99 bpm

65. Cardiac tamponade is characterized by

    A. Increase in diastolic filling of the ventricles
    B. Decrease in stroke volume
    C. Increase in systemic blood pressure due to increased intrapericardial pressure from accumulation of fluid in the pericardial space
    D. Systolic dysfunction, and not diastolic dysfunction, is the primary problem

66. An 81-year-old patient with a history of moderate aortic regurgitation is undergoing a coronary artery bypass grafting (CABG). The surgeon decides not to vent the left ventricle. You think this is a wrong decision, and your arguments include all the following, except

    A. Venting can be done through a drain placed from the right superior pulmonary vein into the left ventricle
    B. Venting can be done through a pulmonary venous drain
    C. Retrograde flow through the aortic valve could cause left-ventricular distension
    D. Venting done by aspirating from the antegrade cardioplegia line placed in the proximal ascending aorta will not be helpful

67. Centrifugal pumps are superior to roller pumps because of all, except

    A. They are less traumatic to blood cells
    B. They do not pump air bubbles secondary to air being less dense than blood
    C. They are afterload-dependent, and avoid the risk of line rupture with clamping of the arterial inflow circuit
    D. Roller pumps compress the fluid-filled tubing between the roller and curved metal back plate and hence avoid air

68. During cardiopulmonary bypass (CPB), the nasopharyngeal temperature is 28°C, the hematocrit is 20%, the temperature corrected $Paco_2$ is 50 mm Hg, and the uncorrected $Paco_2$ is 60 mm Hg. The most appropriate management is to

    A. Administer additional opioid
    B. Administer packed red blood cells to increase hematocrit to 25%
    C. Further decrease the patient's temperature
    D. Increase fresh-gas flow to the oxygenator

69. Two days after coronary artery bypass grafting, a 62-year-old man remains sedated, endotracheally intubated, and mechanically ventilated. Over the next 3 hours, Pao2 decreases from 90 to 70 mm Hg at an FIO_2 of 0.7, peak inspiratory pressure measured proximally in the ventilator circuit increases from 40 to 66 cm H_2O, and plateau pressure remains unchanged at 30 cm H_2O. Which of the following is the most likely case of these changes?

    A. Adult respiratory distress syndrome (ARDS)
    B. Bronchial mucus plugging
    C. Left-ventricular failure
    D. Tension pneumothorax

70. Regarding the maintenance of blood pressure during cardiopulmonary bypass (CPB), which of the following is false?

    A. Lower blood pressures may reduce cerebral blood flow and reduce emboli load to the brain, while higher pressures may improve cerebral blood flow but cause more emboli
    B. Pressures less than 40 mm Hg are avoided if possible in adults
    C. Pressures higher than 90 mm Hg are used during rewarming
    D. Pressures up to 90 mm Hg may be used in patients with cerebral vascular disease

71. During total cardiopulmonary bypass, metabolic acidosis and decreasing mixed venous oxygen saturation are noted. The most likely cause is

    A. Hypothermia
    B. Hypoperfusion
    C. Rewarming
    D. Light anesthesia

72. While monitoring coronary sinus pressure during retrograde cardioplegia,

    A. If the pressure at the distal tip of the coronary sinus catheter during cardioplegia administration at 200 mL/min is equal to central venous pressure, the catheter is not in the coronary sinus but is most likely in the pulmonary artery
    B. If the pressure is very high (>100 mm Hg), the coronary sinus catheter is in the left ventricle
    C. If the pressure in the coronary sinus catheter is 40 to 60 mm Hg during a 200-mL/min infusion, the catheter is correctly positioned
    D. If the catheter is placed too distally, delivery of cardioplegia to the left ventricle will be compromised and result in left-ventricular dysfunction

73. The electromechanically quiet heart at 22°C consumes oxygen at a rate of

    A. 2 mL/100 g/min
    B. 8 mL/100 g/min
    C. 0.3 mL/100 g/min
    D. 0.1 mL/100 g/min

74. Additional supplemental anesthetics and muscle relaxants should be administered

    A. At institution of cardiopulmonary bypass (CPB)
    B. At rewarming
    C. Both A and B
    D. In the early period after conclusion of CPB

75. The most common hemodynamic abnormality after cardiopulmonary bypass (CPB) is

    A. Low cardiac output
    B. Low systemic vascular resistance (SVR)
    C. High pulmonary vascular resistance
    D. Low heart rate

76. A 57-year-old male is undergoing coronary artery bypass grafting (left internal mammary artery to left anterior descending artery). After termination of cardiopulmonary bypass (CPB), you notice a prominent V wave in the pulmonary artery occlusion pressure (PAOP) tracing. The most likely reason for the finding is

   A. Left-ventricular dysfunction
   B. Right-ventricular dysfunction
   C. Cardiac tamponade
   D. Posterior papillary muscle dysfunction

CHAPTER 11 ANSWERS

1. **B.** The normal ventricular cell–resting membrane potential is -80 to -90 mV. Na–K ATPase bound to the membrane is responsible for concentrating K^+ intracellularly and in exchange for Na and maintaining this resting-membrane potential. Action potential (depolarization) occurs when cell membrane becomes less negative and crosses a threshold value. This depolarization raises the membrane potential of the myocardial cell, sometimes as high as $+20$ mv. The cardiac action potential is slightly different from neuronal action potential in that it has a characteristic spike and plateau appearance. The spike portion of this action potential is produced by opening of fast sodium channels along with a decreased permeability to potassium and the plateau portion (0.2–0.3 seconds) is due to opening of slower calcium channels. After depolarization, the sodium and calcium channels close and the membrane permeability to potassium is restored. This restores the resting-membrane potential to its baseline. Spontaneously depolarizing cells, responsible for the myocardial rhythm, do so primarily by intrinsic slow leakage of calcium into cells aided by leaky Na channels moving Na^+ in (Table 11-1).

Table 11-1

ACTION POTENTIAL PHASE	NAME	NET ION MOVEMENT
0	Rapid upstroke	Na^+ in (relative impermeability to K^+)
1	Early rapid repolarization	K^+ out (increased permeability to K^+ transiently)
2	Plateau (a part of repolarization)	Ca^{++} in
3	Final repolarization	K^+ out of cells
4	Resting-membrane potential	Na^+ in and K^+ out

2. **A.** Halothane and isoflurane depress SA node automaticity and make AV node refractory. By giving an anticholinergic, we stimulated the conduction system of the heart, but SA and AV nodes have been suppressed by the inhalational agent. So the next tissue in the conducting pathway (junctional pacemakers) takes over and produces junctional rhythm. While the depression of SA and AV nodes by inhalational agents is well known, the effect of inhalational agents on Purkinje fibers and ventricular myocardium is unpredictable with reports of both arrhythmia-inducing and antiarrhythmic effects. Arrhythmogenicity by inhalational agents is due to potentiation of action of catecholamines, and the direct depression of calcium channels renders some antiarrhythmic effect. Opioids depress cardiac conduction, increase AV node refractoriness, and prolong the duration of Purkinje fiber–action potential.

3. **A.** The therapeutic effects of low concentrations of lidocaine turn toxic at higher concentrations—they bind to fast Na channels and depress conduction. If we increase the concentration further, they depress the automaticity of heart by its effect on sinoatrial node. This is very different from the more potent local anesthetics like bupivacaine and ropivacaine, which cause toxicity by its effect on Purkinje fibers and ventricular muscle. Bupivacaine binds inactivated fast sodium channels and dissociates from them slowly. Its effects can be sinus bradycardia, sinus node arrest, or malignant ventricular arrhythmia.

4. **B.** All anesthetic agents can depress *cardiac contractility*. This occurs by alterations in the intracellular concentration of calcium as follows:

Inhalational agents: decreasing the entry of calcium into cells by affecting both T- and L-type calcium channels, altering the kinetics of calcium release and uptake into the sarcoplasmic reticulum, and decreasing the sensitivity of contractile proteins to calcium. These effects are more apparent with halothane than with modern inhalational agents like isoflurane, sevoflurane, and desflurane. Factors that can worsen this cardiac depression include hypocalcemia, α-adrenergic blockade, and calcium channel blockers.

Nitrous oxide: reduces the intracellular calcium concentration (dose-dependent).

Intravenous-induction agent ketamine: agent with no significant myocardial depression, except in critically ill patients with depleted catecholamines, where it acts as a direct myocardial depressant.

Local anesthetic agents: reduce calcium influx and release in a dose-dependent fashion. Bupivacaine, tetracaine, and ropivacaine cause greater depression than lidocaine and chloroprocaine.

5. **C.**   The CVP waveform consists of three positive waveforms called a, c, and v and two negative slopes called the x and y depressions.

a wave	atrial contraction
c wave	cusps bulging into the right atrium
x descent	atrial relaxation during ventricular systole
v wave	venous filling of the right atrium
y descent	atrial emptying when tricuspid valve opens

6. **D.**   Ventricular systolic function is documented most commonly as cardiac output or ejection fraction. Cardiac output is defined as the volume of blood pumped by the heart per minute. Normally, the right and left ventricles have the same output. $CO = SV \times HR$, where CO is the cardiac output, SV is the stroke volume (the volume pumped per contraction), and HR is heart rate. Variations in body size can lead to ambiguity if we just use cardiac output as a measure. This can be avoided by using cardiac index: $CI = CO/BSA$, where CI is the cardiac index and BSA is the total body surface area. BSA is usually obtained from nomograms based on height and weight. Normal CI is 2.5 to 4.2 $L/min/m^2$. As you can see, there is a wide range for CI and the patient should have a gross ventricular impairment prior to it being evident on CI. Mixed venous oxygen saturation is ideally obtained from a PA catheter. A better estimate of ventricular performance can be obtained if we subject the ventricles to some stress like exercise. This will reveal underlying inability of the heart to deliver adequate oxygen to the tissues and can be noted as a falling mixed venous oxygen saturation. Inadequate tissue perfusion relative to demand is causing the drop in mixed venous saturation. Thus, in the absence of hypoxia or severe anemia, measurement of mixed venous oxygen tension (or saturation) is the best determination of the adequacy of cardiac output.

7. **C.**   Ventricular filling is influenced by both heart rate and rhythm. Since the time spent in diastole is higher than the time spent in systole, any increase in heart rate has more effect on the diastolic filling time more than the systolic ejection time. At very high heart rates (>120 bpm) in adults, the left-ventricular filling is significantly impaired by the sheer decrease in duration of diastole. In addition, atrial contraction (kick) contributes about 20% to 30% of the ventricular filling in a normal heart. Any condition that affects the atrial contraction, like atrial fibrillation/flutter, or alters the timing of atrial kick, will negate this contribution and can have significant hemodynamic consequences in some patients. The atrial contribution to ventricular filling is more important in patients with reduced ventricular compliance who depend on active filling with atrial contraction than passive filling of the ventricle for adequate preload.

8. **A.** Afterload is the force against which ventricle is pushing the blood out. It can be denoted by the ventricular-wall tension during systole or impedance of the arterial tree. Ventricular-wall tension can be calculated by Laplace law:

Circumferential stress = intraventricular pressure × ventricular radius/2 × wall thickness

This relationship is applicable to spherical structures, but can be applied to left ventricle as well, which is a prolapsed ellipsoid. Any increase in ventricular radius as in a dilation increases the wall tension. However, any increase in thickness (hypertrophy) decreases the wall tension. This is a protective mechanism seen in patients with long-standing hypertension or aortic stenosis in an attempt to decrease the wall tension.

9. **C.** Recommended dose of heparin before initiation of cardiopulmonary bypass is 300 to 400 U/kg. The dose is given to achieve an activated clotting time of 400 to 450 seconds.

10. **B.** The SA node is supplied by the right coronary artery in 60% of individuals, and by the left anterior descending artery in 40% of the individuals. The AV node is supplied by the right coronary artery in 85% of individuals, and by the circumflex artery in 15% of individuals.

11. **C.** Baroreceptors have an important role in acute regulation of blood pressure. They are located at the bifurcation of the common carotid and in the aortic arch. These receptors sense an increase in blood pressure and enhance the vagal tone, thereby inhibiting systemic vasoconstriction. This is called the baroreceptor reflex. The afferent pathway for the baroreceptor reflex is via a branch of the glossopharyngeal nerve, sometimes called the Hering nerve. The afferent pathway for baroreceptor reflex from the aortic receptors travels along the vagus nerve. Changes in blood pressure caused by acute events like change in posture are minimized primarily by the carotid baroreceptor between mean arterial pressures of 80 and 160 mm Hg. However, readaptation to changes in acute blood pressure occurs over the course of 1 to 2 days, making this reflex ineffective for long-term blood pressure control. All volatile anesthetics depress the normal baroreceptor response, less so with isoflurane and desflurane.

12. **A.** The bundle of His is the only part of the cardiac conducting system, which has a dual blood supply derived from the posterior descending artery (PDA) and the left anterior descending (LAD) artery. Blood supply to the heart is from the right and left coronary arteries. The right coronary artery (RCA) normally supplies the right atrium, most of the right ventricle, and the inferior wall of the left ventricle. In 85% of persons, the PDA, which supplies part of the interventricular septum and inferior wall, arises from the RCA, and these people are said to have a right-dominant circulation. In the remaining 15% of persons, the PDA arises from the left coronary artery and is appropriately labeled left-dominant circulation. The left coronary artery normally supplies the left atrium and most of the interventricular septum and left ventricle. The left main coronary artery divides into the LAD artery and the circumflex (CX) artery. The LAD artery supplies the septum and anterior left-ventricular wall, and the CX artery supplies the lateral wall.

13. **C.** Autoregulatory nature of the myocardium makes the myocardial oxygen demand an important determinant of myocardial blood flow. Pressure work uses most of the oxygen, 65%, followed by basal requirements = 205, volume work = 15%, with only 1% of the supplied oxygen being used for electrical activity. The myocardium also has a very high extraction ratio. It extracts 65% of the oxygen in arterial blood, compared with 25% in most other tissues. Coronary sinus oxygen saturation is usually 30%. Hence, any drop in myocardial oxygen supply is deleterious, as it cannot compensate for reduction in flow by increasing oxygen extraction. Factors influencing the supply and demand are listed in Table 11-2.

Table 11-2

MYOCARDIAL OXYGEN SUPPLY	MYOCARDIAL OXYGEN DEMAND
Heart rate	Basal requirements
Diastolic time	Heart rate
Aortic diastolic blood pressure	Wall tension
Coronary perfusion pressure	Preload
Ventricular end diastolic pressure	Afterload
Arterial oxygen content and tension	Contractility
Hemoglobin concentration	
Coronary vessel diameter	

14. **D.** Halogenated anesthetic agents are inherent vasodilators. Their effect on coronary blood flow is variable and depends on an interplay between their effect on blood pressure, metabolic oxygen requirements of the myocardium, and their direct vasodilating properties. Although the mechanism is not clear, it may involve activation of ATP-sensitive K^+ channels and stimulation of adenosine (A_1) receptors. Halothane and isoflurane stand apart, as halothane primarily affects large coronary vessels and isoflurane affects mostly smaller vessels. Dose-dependent abolition of autoregulation may be greatest with isoflurane. Autonomically mediated vasodilation is significant for desflurane. Sevoflurane appears to lack coronary vasodilating properties.

15. **C.** According to ACC/AHA guidelines for noncardiac surgery in cardiac patients, Surgeries can be classified into high, intermediate, and low risk with high-risk surgeries having >5% risk and low-risk surgeries having <1% risk (Table 11-3).

Table 11-3 Cardiac Risk Stratification for Noncardiac Surgical Procedures.

High (reported cardiac risk often greater than 5%)
Emergent major operations, particularly in the elderly
Aortic and other major vascular surgery
Peripheral vascular surgery
Anticipated prolonged surgical procedures associated with large fluid shifts and/or blood loss
Intermediate (reported cardiac risk generally less than 5%)
Carotid endarterectomy
Head and neck surgery
Intraperitoneal and intrathoracic surgery
Orthopedic surgery
Prostate surgery
Low (reported cardiac risk generally less than 1%)
Endoscopic procedures
Superficial procedure
Cataract surgery
Breast surgery

16. **C.** Chronic hypertensive patients show wide fluctuations in blood pressure on induction (hypotension) and intubation (hypertension). Duration of laryngoscopy <15 seconds has been shown to prevent this hypertensive response to intubation. Intubation performed under deep anesthesia is also shown not to produce significant rise in blood pressure. But this comes at the price of hypotension. There are several techniques that can be used to prevent sudden spikes in blood pressure on intubation. Topical airway anesthesia, β-blockers like esmolol

0.3 to 1.5 mg/kg, short-acting opioids like fentanyl 2.5 to 5 µg/kg, intravenous preservative-free lidocaine at 1.5 mg/kg have all been shown to be effective in attenuating the hypertensive response.

17. **B.** Direct α_1 agonists like phenylephrine are preferable to indirect sympathomimetics like ephedrine to treat hypotension, following induction in patients with uncontrolled hypertension preoperatively. Catecholamines—both endogenous and exogenous—can produce exaggerated hypertensive response in these patients. We can start with small doses of phenylephrine, for example, 25 to 50 µg, provided the heart rate is not too low. If the heart rate is low, small doses of ephedrine (5–10 mg) or even epinephrine (2–5 µg) may be used. In patients who are on angiotensin-receptor blocker preoperatively, the refractory hypotension may respond only to vasopressin. Avoiding high heart rates and prolonged hypertension has been shown to decrease cardiovascular morbidity.

18. **C.** Coronary vasodilation potential of dihydropyridines (nifedipine, nicardipine, nimodipine) is much greater than those by verapamil and diltiazem. They even exceed nitrates in their vasodilatory potential. β-Blockers however have no vasodilatory action on coronary blood vessels.

19. **D.** CCBs have significant anesthetic implications. Both depolarizing and nondepolarizing neuromuscular-blocking agents are potentiated by CCBs. CCBs also potentiate the circulatory effects of volatile agents and may cause more hypotension. Both verapamil and diltiazem can potentiate cardiac depression and inhibit conduction in the AV node caused by volatile anesthetics. Verapamil may also modestly decrease anesthetic requirements. Dihydropyridine derivatives potentiate systemic vasodilation under anesthesia.

20. **C.** Cardioselectivity of agents like metoprolol is dose-dependent (β_1-receptor-specific). Even the β_1-receptor-specific agents can have some β_2-blocking action at higher doses. β-Blockers with intrinsic sympathomimetic activity, like acebutolol, provide a unique advantage in patients with bronchospastic airway disease.

21. **C.** Prolonged QT interval (QTc >0.44 second) can be caused by myocardial ischemia, drug toxicity (antiarrhythmic agents, antidepressants, or phenothiazines), electrolyte abnormalities (hypokalemia or hypomagnesemia), autonomic dysfunction, mitral-valve prolapse, or, less commonly, a congenital abnormality. Prolonged QT interval predisposes patients to ventricular arrhythmias, particularly polymorphic-ventricular tachycardia, also known as torsade de pointes or twisting points, which can lead to ventricular fibrillation. Prolonged QT interval is due to nonuniform prolongation of ventricular repolarization. This predisposes patients to reentry phenomena and results in ventricular tachycardia or fibrillation. Elective surgery should be postponed until drug toxicity and electrolyte imbalances are excluded. Polymorphic tachyarrhythmias with a long QT interval are usually treated with intravenous magnesium or by pacing. This is because they do not respond to conventional antiarrhythmics. Patients with congenital prolongation generally respond to β-adrenergic blocking agents. Left-stellate-ganglion blockade has also been tried and has some success in these patients suggesting that this may be due to an autonomic imbalance.

22. **D.** Severe multivessel disease can be detected using exercise EKG if the patient (develops)
- Cannot attain a maximum HR >70% of predicted
- Dysrhythmias at a lower HR
- Sustained fall in systolic blood pressure during exercise (>10 mm Hg)
- ST depression >2 mm, either horizontal or down sloping
- ST depression at a very low workload
- ST depression sustained even after the exercise is >5 min

23. D. Surgical electrocautery interference with AICDs and pacemaker devices are well known. The old adage of "put a magnet on it" is based on the fact that antitachycardia function in some (older) pacemakers was turned off by the application of a magnet. However, this is not true for most of the newer AICDs. Ideally, the manufacturer's representative or cardiology should be contacted to find out if the device could be reprogrammed to have the antitachycardia function off prior to the surgery. This is in addition to confirming that the pacemaker was interrogated for functionality within the last year and AICD was interrogated in the last 6 months.

Electrosurgical interference can be caused by the device interpreting the current as ventricular fibrillation and firing, interfering with its pacemaker capability, resetting of the device to backup mode. Some AICDs are programmed with a rate-responsive function, and this may be activated by a cautery device.

If there is no time to reprogram the device prior to surgery, use of a bipolar cautery, placement of electrical return pad far away from the device, using electrocautery in small bursts are some methods to decrease such an interference. In addition, all such patients should have transcutaneous pads on and a defibrillator/pacer should be available in the room. Every effort should be made to reprogram the device to its original setting prior to discharge of the patient from the postanesthesia care unit.

24. A. The sensitivity of the intraoperative/perioperative ECG in detecting ischemia is directly proportional to the number of leads monitored. V5 is the most useful lead. In order of decreasing sensitivity, V5 is followed by V4, II, V2, and V3 leads. Usually two leads are monitored simultaneously in perioperative period. Leads II and V5 are the two most commonly used leads. Lead II helps to detect arrhythmias and inferior-wall ischemia, while lead V5 is useful for detecting lateral-wall ischemia. Modified V5 lead is very useful when only one channel can be monitored (three leads applied with left-arm lead at V5 position and monitoring lead I). Posterior wall can be monitored using an esophageal lead.

25. A. It is a common practice to cool the body to a core body temperature of 20 to 32°C following CPB start. However, it is not always required. This is based on the principle that metabolic oxygen requirements can be halved with each reduction of 10°C in body temperature. This temperature is brought back to acceptable levels (where arrhythmias are lower) at the end of CPB—a phase called rewarming. Some procedures need a complete circulatory standstill—called circulatory arrest—and deep hypothermia is employed for such procedures—cooling to 15 to 18°C allows an arrest time of around 60 minutes.

26. B. The adverse effects of hypothermia are arrhythmias, platelet dysfunction, coagulopathy, decreased systolic function of myocardium, and reduction in serum-ionized calcium due to citrate toxicity.

27. A. Coronary perfusion pressure is determined by the difference between the arterial diastolic pressure and the left-ventricular end diastolic pressure. The left ventricle is perfused during diastole, while the right ventricle is perfused both during diastole and systole. An increase in heart rate reduces coronary perfusion because of a shorter diastole. Normal coronary blood flow at rest is about 250 mL/min.

28. **C.** Transgastric mid-papillary (midshort axis) view provides a snapshot of all the different blood vessels supplying the heart (Fig 11-2).

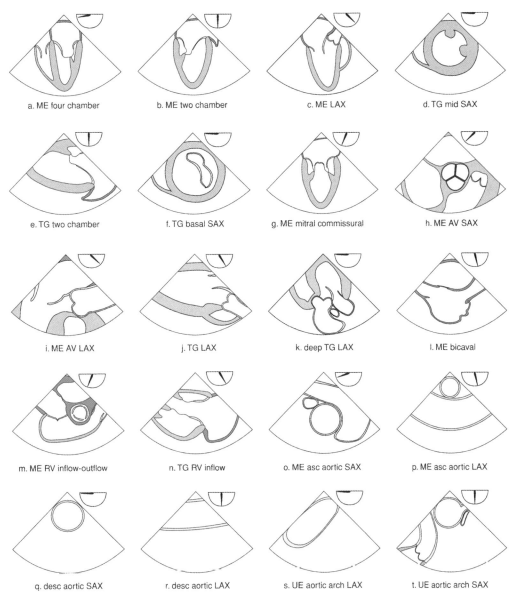

Figure 11-2. Reused with permission from Shanewise JS, Shin JJ, Vezina DP, et al. Comprehensive and abbreviated intraoperative TEE examination. In: Savage RM, Aronson S, Shernan SK, eds. *Comprehensive Textbook of Perioperative Transesophageal Echocardiography.* 2nd ed. Philadelphia, PA: Lippincott Williams & Wilkins; 2011: 86.

29. **D.** Pure high-dose opioid anesthesia (e.g., fentanyl 50–100 µg/kg or sufentanil 15–25 µg/kg) has fallen out of vogue in cardiac anesthesia practice. It was useful at a time in anesthesia when the only inhaled agents available produced unacceptable myocardial depression. The main disadvantages of high-dose opioid technique include prolonged postoperative respiratory depression (early extubation is becoming a very common trend in coronary artery bypass grafting surgeries), high incidence of patient awareness/recall, exaggerated hypertensive response to stimulation like sternotomy in a patient with good left-ventricular function, bradycardia, chest-wall rigidity, postoperative ileus, and impaired immunity.

30. A.   A progressive decline in cardiac output is sometimes seen after the chest is opened. This is attributed to the loss of negative intrathoracic pressure and decreased preload. Hence a IV fluid bolus may help. Factors potentiating such a response include deep anesthesia and preoperative angiotensin-receptor-blockade use. Another common response seen during sternal retraction and pericardiectomy is bradycardia and hypotension due to exaggerated vagal response. This is potentiated by hypoxia, β-blockers, and calcium channel blockers.

31. C.   Aprotinin, an inhibitor of serine proteases, such as plasmin, kallikrein, and trypsin, also helps to preserve platelet aggregation and adhesiveness. It has been shown to decrease blood loss and transfusion requirements and should be considered in redo surgeries, Jehovah's witnesses, recent administration of glycoprotein IIb/IIIa inhibitors (abciximab [ReoPro], eptifibatide [Integrilin], or tirofiban [Aggrastat], patients with coagulopathies, and patients with long pump runs. However, repeat exposure to aprotinin has been shown to cause allergic reactions, which may include anaphylaxis. Patients on a combination of aspirin and ADP-receptor antagonist are at high risk of bleeding and may benefit from aprotinin.

32. A.   The events occurring in sequence after heparinization are aortic cannulation followed by venous cannulation. Venous cannulation usually causes hemodynamic changes, and we have an access to provide rapid infusion through the aortic cannula if necessary. Venous cannulation also frequently precipitates arrhythmias. Premature atrial contractions and transient bursts of a supraventricular tachycardia are common. Sustained arrhythmias must be treated pharmacologically, electrically, or by immediate anticoagulation and initiation of bypass depending on the amount of hemodynamic compromise. Sometimes, stopping the surgical stimulus is all that is needed. Superior vena cava syndrome can be caused by a malpositioned venous cannulas can be interfering with venous drainage from the head and neck.

33. B.   After initiation of CPB, pump flow is gradually increased to 2 to 2.5 L/min/m^2 and MAPs are monitored. It is common to see an initial fall in BP. Initial mean systemic arterial (radial) pressures of 30 to 40 mm Hg are not unusual. Abrupt hemodilution, which reduces blood viscosity and effectively lowers systemic vascular resistance (SVR), may be responsible for this drop. The effect is partially compensated by subsequent hypothermia, which tends to raise blood viscosity again.

A disastrous scenario is a persistent and excessive decrease in MAP (<30 mm Hg); transesophageal echocardiograph evaluation is very useful in such a situation to look for unrecognized aortic dissection. If dissection is present, CPB must be temporarily stopped until the aorta is recannulated distally to prevent further extension of a dissection flap with grave consequences. Poor venous return, pump malfunction, or pressure-transducer error may all cause hypotension. Aortic cannula misdirected toward the innominate artery may be a cause for false hypertension when right radial artery is used for monitoring.

The relationship between pump flow, SVR, and mean systemic arterial blood pressure may be conceptualized as follows:

$$\text{MAP} = \text{Pump flow} \times \text{SVR}$$

With a constant SVR, MAP is proportional to pump flow. Similarly, at any given pump flow, MAP is proportional to SVR. Pump flows of 2 to 2.5 L/min/m^2 (50–60 mL/kg/min) and mean arterial pressures between 50 and 80 mm Hg are commonly used. Flow requirements are generally lower during deep hypothermia (20–25°C), as mean blood pressures as low as 30 mm Hg may still provide adequate cerebral blood flow. SVR can be increased with α agonists like phenylephrine.

High systemic arterial pressures (>150 mm Hg) are also deleterious because they promote aortic dissection or a cerebrovascular accident in addition to increasing the surgical bleeding. Hypertension is said to exist on pump when MAPs exceed 100 mm Hg, and this is treated by decreasing pump flow or deepening anesthesia using isoflurane at the oxygenator inflow gas.

Sometimes, a hypertension is refractory to these maneuvers or, if pump flow is already low, may necessitate a vasodilator like nitroprusside.

34. **B.**   Monitoring during CPB is usually done by the perfusionists. They monitor the pump flow rate, venous reservoir level, arterial inflow line pressure, blood (perfusate and venous) and myocardial temperatures, and in-line (arterial and venous) oxygen saturations. In-line pH, CO_2 tension, and oxygen-tension sensors are also available in newer bypass machines. But most machines do not provide a glucose monitor, and hypoglycemia is still a threat. Blood gas tensions and pH are confirmed by direct measurements periodically—30 minute-intervals. Inadequate tissue perfusion caused by inadequate flow rates is evidenced by low venous oxygen saturations (<70%), progressive metabolic acidosis, or low urinary output, provided there is no hypoxemia.

    During bypass, arterial inflow line pressure is almost always higher than the systemic arterial pressure recorded from a radial artery or even an aortic catheter, caused by the pressure drop across the arterial filter, the arterial tubing, and the narrow opening of the aortic cannula.

35. **A.**   Before discontinuing ventilation after initiation of CPB, it is a good practice to confirm whether full flow has been attained with the perfusionist. Discontinuing ventilation prematurely causes any remaining pulmonary blood flow to act as a right-to-left shunt, which can promote hypoxemia. The extent of hypoxemia depends on the relative ratio of remaining pulmonary blood flow to pump flow. Once the heart stops ejecting blood, ventilation can be discontinued. Following institution of full CPB, ventricular ejection may continue for a brief period of time.

36. **D.**   Epiaortic echocardiography is the most sensitive and specific technique to detect air bubbles at the termination of CPB. De-airing is facilitated by head-down position, and venting before and during initial cardiac ejection, in addition to filling up the heart with vent in place. TEE is very useful in detecting pockets of air, especially within the left ventricle. But the risk of atheromatous emboli still persists and is worse in cases where aorta was manipulated extensively, cross-clamped numerous times and in percutaneous transcatheter aortic valve replacements. Newer devices with baskets to catch such emboli have proven to be very useful.

37. **B.**   Sweating during rewarming is a hypothalamic response to perfusion with blood, which is often at 39°C. It is important to remember to administer anesthetic agents, and sometimes additional muscle relaxants, during the rewarming phase. The incidence of awareness/recall is high during rewarming because the inhalational agent delivered via the oxygenator is turned off just prior to termination of CPB to avoid residual myocardial depression.

38. **A.**   pH-stat management refers to the practice of temperature-correcting gas tensions by adding CO_2 and maintaining a "normal" CO_2 tension of 40 mm Hg and a pH of 7.40 during hypothermia. α-Stat management, on the other hand, refers to the use of uncorrected gas tensions during hypothermia. This does not require addition of CO_2 and has been shown to preserve cerebral autoregulation and improve myocardial preservation. At physiologic pH, the histidine residues of intracellular proteins play a major role in maintaining electrical neutrality. pH-stat management is commonly used in pediatric cardiac surgery, but α-stat is more commonly used in adult cardiac surgery.

39. **B.**   Rapid rewarming can release gas bubbles that were dissolved rapidly back into the blood stream. It also results in large temperature gradients between well-perfused organs and peripheral vasoconstricted tissues. The body equilibrates this gradient following separation from CPB, and patient may become hypothermic again. Methods used to speed the rewarming process include infusion of a vasodilator drug (nitroprusside or nitroglycerin) and allowing some pulsatile flow (ventricular ejection).

40. A.   Separation from CPB can be guided by a mnemonic:

A = Airway—oxygenation and ventilation with 100% oxygen

B = Blood gas—correct electrolyte abnormalities/hemoglobin

C = Coagulation—reverse heparin with protamine

D = Dysrhythmias—sinus rhythm is good; pacing needed sometimes (80–100 bpm)

E = Epinephrine—inotropes/vasopressors used as needed. Epinephrine may increase myocardial O_2 need

F = Fluids—for rapid volume resuscitation

G = Good contractility by direct visualization/transesophageal echocardiogram

H = Hypothermia is avoided; >37°C is aimed

I = Invasive monitors recalibrated

41. B.   IABP is sometimes used to facilitate weaning the patient off cardiopulmonary bypass. This provides a systolic augmentation of blood pressure in addition to improving myocardial oxygen supply during diastole. Timing and location of an IABP are critical for optimal functioning. Ideal inflation of the balloon should be just after the dicrotic notch (closure of aortic valve). Inflation while the aortic valve is still open can increase afterload, worsen aortic regurgitation and left-ventricular (LV) volume. Inflation too late in the diastolic phase will reduce diastolic augmentation and myocardial supply. Similarly, the deflation should be timed just prior to LV ejection to produce an optimal reduction in afterload. Timing is usually synchronized with EKG/arterial pulse. The location of the tip of the IABP should be just distal to the takeoff of the left-subclavian artery, usually confirmed with transesophageal echocardiograph/fluoroscopy.

42. D.   This patient has a low CVP, PCWP suggestive of low-filling pressures, indicating that he is hypovolemic. But the rest of the clinical picture of low SVR and high CO is strongly suggestive of a hyperdynamic circulatory state (vasodilated). The treatment in such a scenario will be to increase the hematocrit. If the patient had a decreased cardiac output, the treatment would be to administer volume/crystalloids. Left-heart failure (LHF) will have a high PCWP and pulmonary artery pressure. Right-heart failure (RHF) will have a high CVP and normal or low PCWP. Both LHF and RHF will have low CO.

43. B.   Protamine binds and effectively inactivates heparin because the positive charge of protamine neutralizes the negative charge of heparin. Timing of protamine administration should be determined by close communication with the surgeon. Too early administration may lead to clot formation in the cardiopulmonary bypass circuit. The electrically neutral heparin–protamine complexes are removed by the reticuloendothelial system. Protamine dosing is based on the amount of heparin initially required to produce the desired activated clotting time; protamine is then given in a ratio of 1 to 1.3 mg per 100 U of heparin. Another approach calculates the protamine dose based on the heparin dose–response curve and the estimation of heparin concentration using special monitors (Hepcon).

44. C.   The activated clotting time should return to baseline following reversal of heparin with protamine; sometimes, additional doses of protamine (25–50 mg) may be necessary. Coagulopathy often follows long bypass periods (>2 hours) and is due to multifactorial causes: surgical bleeding sites, inadequate reversal of heparin, reheparinization, thrombocytopenia, platelet dysfunction, hypothermia, preoperative coagulation defects, or newly acquired defects may be responsible. Reheparinization (heparin rebound) after apparent adequate reversal is due to a relative heparin–protamine concentration mismatch and can be caused by a redistribution either of protamine to peripheral compartments or of peripherally bound heparin to the central compartment. Hypothermia (<35°C) often exacerbates such bleeding problems.

45. A.   DDAVP, 0.3 μg/kg (intravenously over 20 minutes), can increase the activity of factors VIII and XII and the von Willebrand factor. DDAVP facilitates their release from the vascular endothelium. Hence, a second dose is usually not effective. DDAVP is very useful in reversing qualitative platelet defects, but is not recommended for routine use.

46. **A.** Immediately following cardiac surgery, the emphasis is on maintaining hemodynamic stability and monitoring for excessive perioperative bleeding. Sedation using propofol/ fentanyl/titrated doses of morphine/dexmedetomidine is used in different institutions to ensure a calm, comfortable patient. Chest-tube drainage more than 10 mL/kg/hour in the first 2 hours often raises a red flag and prompts coagulation studies and sometimes require chest reexploration. A very deadly site for postoperative monitoring is into the pericardium causing cardiac tamponade. This is usually signaled by equalization of diastolic pressures and hemodynamic compromise and needs immediate surgical intervention. After the first 2 hours, any drainage from chest tube >100 mL/hour should be closely observed.

47. **A.** NO is a potent vasodilator, which can be given as inhaled nitric oxide, which circumvents the unwanted side effect of decreased SVR and systemic blood pressure, at the same time retaining the therapeutic potential of decreasing pulmonary hypertension. Inodilators like dopamine and milrinone may help in situations with right-ventricular (RV) failure secondary to pulmonary hypertension. Vasodilators like nitroglycerin will also decrease the PVR, but they produce drop in systemic blood pressure. Inhaled prostaglandin E_1 (PGE_1) is also very specific in decreasing PVR without affecting SVR. Advanced RV failure may necessitate a RV–assist device or an intra-aortic balloon pump, which works by increasing the perfusion to the right side of the heart. Inhaled NO at 10 to 60 ppm and PGE_1 at 0.01 to 0.2 µg/kg/min are very effective pulmonary vasodilators.

48. **D.** End-stage heart disease patients have an option to get a destination ventricular-assist device therapy or get a cardiac transplantation. Their position in the transplant list is higher if they are unlikely to survive the next 6 to 12 months. Survival rates after cardiac transplantation are usually high at a 5-year survival rate of 60% to 90%. High pulmonary vascular resistance >6 to 8 Wood units (1 Wood unit = 80 dyn[middot]s/cm^5) is a predictor of right-ventricular failure, which has a high early postoperative mortality. Hence, irreversible pulmonary vascular disease is considered a contraindication to orthotopic cardiac transplantation. They still qualify for a combined heart–lung transplantation, which is allocated from a separate list. Size, ABO blood–group typing, and cytomegalovirus serology are used for donor–recipient compatibility testing. However, tissue crossmatching is generally not performed. Donor organs from patients with hepatitis B or C or HIV infection are excluded.

49. **B.** The CVP waveform is characteristic in cardiac tamponade. Cardiac tamponade is characterized by equalization of diastolic pressures throughout the heart: LAP = RAP = LVEDP = RVEDP. This produces a reduced stroke volume and high central venous pressure. The external compression on the collapsible chambers prevents emptying, and these patients compensate by having tachycardia and an increase in contractility. However, in the presence of impaired emptying, the contribution from stroke volume is very limited. This is particularly important to the anesthesiologist while inducing general anesthesia in such patients. They do not tolerate the switch from negative-pressure to positive-pressure breathing. Characteristic CVP waveform in cardiac tamponade is described as impairment of both diastolic filling and atrial emptying abolishes the *y* descent; the *x* descent (systolic-atrial filling) is normal or even accentuated. Arterial vasoconstriction (increased systemic vascular resistance) supports systemic blood pressure, whereas venoconstriction augments the venous return to the heart.

50. **C.** Constrictive pericarditis is characterized by a stiff pericardium that limits diastolic filling of the heart. Pathophysiology consists of a thickened, fibrotic, and often calcified pericardium secondary to acute or recurrent pericarditis. The adherent parietal pericardium allows the heart to fill only to a fixed volume. Filling during early diastole is typically accentuated and manifested by a prominent *y* descent on the CVP waveform. This is in contrast to cardiac tamponade, which causes a filling defect. This pathophysiology is responsible for Kussmaul

sign—paradoxical rise in venous pressure during inspiration. Chest X-ray may show some pericardial calcifications, and EKG may show atrial fibrillation, conduction blocks, low QRS voltage, and diffuse T-wave abnormalities. Clinical signs include raised jugular venous pressure, hepatomegaly, ascites, and abnormal liver function.

51. D.   The goal during management of anesthesia for patients with hypertrophic cardiomyopathy is to decrease the pressure gradient across the left-ventricular outflow obstruction. Decreases in myocardial contractility and increases in preload (ventricular volume) and afterload will decrease the magnitude of left-ventricular outflow obstruction. Intraoperative hypotension is generally treated with intravenous fluids or an α agonist such as phenylephrine. Drugs with β-agonist activity are not likely to be used to treat hypotension because any increase in cardiac contractility or heart rate could increase left-ventricular outflow obstruction. When hypertension occurs, an increased delivered concentration of isoflurane or sevoflurane can be used. Vasodilators, such as nitroprusside or nitroglycerin, should be used with caution because decreases in systemic vascular resistance can increase left-ventricular outflow obstruction.

52. B.   PCWP is an indirect measure of LVEDP, with many false positives and negatives:
    PCWP > LVEDP

- PEEP/positive-pressure ventilation
- Increased intrathoracic pressure
- Left-atrial pathology—myxoma
- Mitral-valve pathology—stenosis/regurgitation
- Pulmonary hypertension
- Chronic obstructive pulmonary disease

    LVEDP > PCWP

- LVEDP >25 mm Hg
- Premature mitral-valve closure (usually an aortic regurgitation jet causing this)
- Left-ventricular diastolic dysfunction (left-ventricular hypertrophy/ischemia)

53. B.   Mixed venous oxygen tension refers to the oxygen tension in a venous sample with blood mixed from both inferior vena cava and superior vena cava. Ideally, this sample is drawn from the tip of a pulmonary artery catheter. It is a good measure of tissue oxygen supply relative to its demand. A reduction in delivery (decreased cardiac output) or an increase in consumption (increased BMR) can both cause a reduction in PvO_2. Normal PvO_2 is about 40 mm Hg, with a saturation of 75%.

54. C.   Site of previous MI, history of coronary artery bypass grafting, site of procedure for procedures <3 hour, and type of anesthesia used (general anesthesia vs. regional) have no influence on perioperative myocardial reinfarction.

    Only three pharmacologic measures have been proven to produce a decrease in cardiovascular morbidity and mortality: β-blockers, clonidine, and statins. β-Blockers started 7 to 30 days prior to surgery and continued for 30 days postoperatively reduce the risk of cardiac morbidity (MI or cardiac death) by 90%. If started just prior to surgery and continued for 7 days, it will still confer a reduction in mortality risk by 50%. Perioperative clonidine administration reduces the 30-day and 2-year mortality risks. Statin therapy with fluvastatin for 30 days before and after surgery, in addition to β-blockade, reduces risk of MI and death by an additional 50%.

    Intraoperatively, strict hemodynamic control using an intra-arterial catheter and prompt pharmacologic intervention or fluid infusion to treat physiologic hemodynamic alterations from the normal range may decrease the risk of perioperative cardiac morbidity in high-risk patients.

55. C.   Perioperative risk-reduction therapy with medications is superior to risk stratification with invasive testing, angioplasty, and CABG. β-Blockers, clonidine, statin, and aspirin have all been used for this. A single 1-minute episode of myocardial ischemia detected by 1-mm ST-segment elevation or depression increases the risk of cardiac events 10-fold and the risk for death 2-fold. Tachycardia for 5 minutes above 120 bpm in the postoperative period can increase the risk of mortality 10 times. The incidence of perioperative myocardial reinfarction does not stabilize at 5% to 6% until 6 months after the prior myocardial infarction. Thus, elective surgery, especially thoracic and upper abdominal, or other major procedures used to be delayed for a period of 2 to 6 months after a myocardial infarction. However, recently this has reduced to 6 to 8 weeks following the ACC/AHA guidelines. Perioperative myocardial reinfarctions occur most frequently in the first 48 to 72 hours postoperatively. However, the risk of myocardial infarction remains increased for several months after surgery.

56. **D.** Careful preoperative evaluation is the most effective method of predicting a perioperative cardiac event. Risk stratification based on preoperative history and physical examination followed by some series of tests (if deemed necessary) predicts perioperative cardiac morbidity and mortality risk. Invasive testing adds little information, which can be used to produce a change in outcome. The risks of interventional procedures like angiography and an intracoronary stent or even coronary artery bypass graft (CABG) surgery adds to the already-existing risk of the proposed surgical procedure and does not reduce total risk. The combined risk of two procedures exceeds that of the original operation. The American College of Cardiology (ACC) and American Heart Association (AHA) have developed a protocol entitled ACC/AHA Guideline Perioperative Cardiovascular Evaluation for Noncardiac Surgery. The ACC/AHA guidelines have not been shown to actually reduce perioperative risk. Perioperative medical optimization of the patient with β-adrenergic blockers, clonidine, statins, and aspirin may be superior to invasive approach with angioplasty and/or CABG.

57. **A.** Deep anesthesia and brief duration of direct laryngoscopy (<15 seconds) is important in minimizing the hemodynamic changes associated with intubation. If you anticipate a longer intubation or if the patient has uncontrolled hypertension preoperatively, addition of other drugs should be considered. Lidocaine can be given IV (1.5 mg/kg IV) or topically (2 mg/kg) on the airway. Other pharmacologic options include esmolol 0.5 mg/kg and fentanyl 2 to 5 μg/kg. However, brief duration of laryngoscopy seems to be the most effective method in avoiding the sympathetic response to intubation.

58. **D.** Barlow syndrome, as it is sometimes called, refers to mitral valve. It is an abnormality of the mitral-valve structure (suspected to be myxomatous in origin) that permits prolapse of the mitral valve into the left atrium during left-ventricular systole. Any condition that increases cardiac emptying can accentuate this prolapse: (1) sympathetic nervous system stimulation, (2) decreased systemic vascular resistance, and (3) performance of surgery with patients in the head-up or sitting position all of these conditions predispose to increased cardiac emptying. Adequate preload and a sudden prolonged decrease in systemic vascular resistance must be avoided during induction of anesthesia in these patients to prevent the worsening of prolapse.

59. **D.** Anesthetic considerations in patients with regurgitant lesions:
    - Keep the heart rate high—decreases the duration of systole
    - Keep SVR high
    - Avoid decrease in myocardial contractility
    - V wave is a reflection of mitral-regurgitant flow

60. **B.** QTc >440 ms in EKG is considered a predisposing factor for ventricular dysrhythmias, syncope, and sudden death due to delayed repolarization. Common congenital syndromes associated with these conditions are Jervell and Lange-Nielsen syndrome (with deafness) and Romano Ward syndrome (no deafness). Any condition that increases the heart rate predisposes these patients to arrhythmias—avoidance of sympathetic stimulation during anesthetic induction is vital. Care should also be taken to avoid the drugs that prolong the QT interval like phenothiazines. If the patient is hemodynamically stable, these patients can be treated

with β-blockers. Unstable ventricular arrhythmias need electrical cardioversion. Left-stellate ganglion block has been shown to have some therapeutic benefit, suggesting an autonomic nervous system imbalance as possible etiology for this syndrome.

61. **D.**   Anesthetic considerations in patients with aortic stenosis:
- Maintaining a high SVR
- Optimal preload
- Avoiding extreme fluctuations in HR (60–80 bpm is ideal)
- Avoiding arrhythmias
- Rapid availability of α agonists to counter the drop in SVR with induction
- Accurate BP measurements preferably with an intra-arterial catheter

62. **D.**   VPCs are recognized on the ECG by (1) premature occurrence, (2) the absence of a P wave preceding the QRS complex, (3) a wide and often bizarre QRS complex, (4) an inverted T wave, and (5) a compensatory pause that follows the premature beat. The primary goal with VPCs should be to identify any underlying cause (myocardial ischemia, arterial hypoxemia, hypercarbia, hypertension, hypokalemia, mechanical irritation of the ventricles) if possible and correct it. VPCs can be treated with lidocaine (1 to 2 mg/kg IV) when they (1) are frequent (more than six premature beats/min), (2) are multifocal, (3) occur in salvos of three or more, or (4) take place during the ascending limb of the T wave (R-on-T phenomenon) that corresponds to the relative refractory period of the ventricle.

63. **C.**   WPW syndrome is characterized by a short PR interval (less than 120 ms), a wide QRS complex, and δ wave in EKG. The short PR interval is due to conduction along the bundle of Kent, which does not have a physiologic delay like conduction across the atrioventricular node. The composite of cardiac impulses conducted by normal and accessory pathways is the reason for δ wave and wide QRS complex. WPW is the most common preexcitation syndrome, with an incidence of approximately 0.3% of the general population. Atrial arrhythmias like paroxysmal atrial tachycardia (most frequent) and supraventricular may lead to hemodynamic collapse in patients with WPW syndrome.

Anesthetic management in the presence of a preexcitation syndrome is to avoid increase in sympathetic nervous system activity events (anxiety) or drugs (anticholinergics, ketamine, pancuronium) that might predispose to tachydysrhythmias. All cardiac antidysrhythmic drugs should be continued throughout the perioperative period.

Ketamine with its sympathomimetic property will be a poor choice for induction. Intravenous β-blockers (atenolol, metoprolol, propranolol, or esmolol) can be used to avoid tachycardia during induction of anesthesia. Histamine-releasing agents like mivacurium/atracurium are also preferably avoided. In case of a sudden onset of tachycardia, adenosine or procainamide will be a good choice to treat the arrhythmia. Digitalis and verapamil may decrease the refractory period of accessory pathways responsible for atrial fibrillation, resulting in an increase in ventricular response rate during this dysrhythmia and should be avoided.

64. **A.**   The magnet mode of many implanted devices, especially the newer AICDs, is now programmable and does not always default to asynchronous pacing. Hence, it should not be considered "safe." The specific magnet mode for a patient's device should be identified by interrogation prior to surgical procedures as some magnet modes change with device state or are programmable. Electrosurgical cautery is interpreted as spontaneous cardiac activity by the artificial cardiac pacemaker when the ground plate for electrocautery is placed too near the pulse generator or with use of a unipolar cautery. For this reason, the electrical return plate (wrongly called ground plate) should be placed as far as possible from the pulse generator. Other techniques to improve safety include using a bipolar cautery, and placement of external pads prior to the beginning of the case.

Magnet mode for many pacemakers (not AICDs) is asynchronous at 99 bpm. However, in some devices, the magnet mode shifts to asynchronous at 50 bpm at the end of battery life. Asynchronous pacing at such a low heart rate with the sensing function off may lead to R-on-T phenomenon if the patient has a spontaneous heart rate above 50 bpm.

65. B.   Cardiac tamponade is characterized by (1) decreases in diastolic filling of the ventricles, (2) decreases in stroke volume, and (3) decreases in systemic blood pressure due to increased intrapericardial pressure from accumulation of fluid in the pericardial space. Inadequate ventricular filling leads to a decreased stroke volume, which in turn results in activation of the sympathetic nervous system (tachycardia, vasoconstriction) in attempts to maintain the cardiac output. These patients need to be kept "full and fast" as the right-sided filling occurs only when central venous pressure exceeds the right-ventricular end diastolic pressure.

66. D.   If the aortic valve is not competent, the regurgitant flow from the aorta will keep distending the left ventricle, impairing perfusion and myocardial preservation. This can be avoided (1) by a drain placed from the right superior pulmonary vein into the left ventricle, (2) by aspirating from the antegrade cardioplegia line placed in the proximal ascending aorta, or (3) via a pulmonary venous drain. The goal is to keep the ventricle from overdistention when it is not pumping. Venting of blood returning via the Thebesian or bronchial veins may also be necessary.

67. D.   The bypass pump serves to pump the oxygenated blood back to the arterial side of the patient. They are of two types: centrifugal and roller pump. The centrifugal pump has three disks rotating at 3,000 to 4,000 rpm that use blood viscosity to pump blood. Centrifugal pumps are less traumatic to blood cells, do not pump air bubbles secondary to air being less dense than blood, and are afterload-dependent, avoiding the risk of line rupture with clamping of the arterial inflow circuit. Roller pumps generate flow by compression of fluid-filled tubing between the roller and curved metal back plate and can pump air. Because of their mechanism, they can cause tube rupture with arterial inflow clamping. The flow is determined by a dial on the cardiopulmonary bypass machine, and usual flows for normothermia or mild hypothermia aim for a cardiac index between 2 and 4 $L/min/m^2$.

68. D.   In the clinical scenario described, the patient has an increased CO_2 in the blood (irrespective of temperature correction).
$Paco_2$ is a balance of CO_2 production and removal. If removal exceeds production, $Paco_2$ decreases. If production exceeds removal, $Paco_2$ increases. The resulting $Paco_2$ is expressed by the alveolar CO_2 equation:

$$Paco_2 = k. VCO_2/VA$$

In the equation, k is a constant (0.863) that corrects units, VCO_2 is carbon dioxide production, and VA is alveolar ventilation. Since the patient is on cardiopulmonary bypass, increasing the fresh-gas flow to the oxygenator will wash out more CO_2. None of the other options has any role in CO_2 production or elimination during cardiopulmonary bypass.

69. B.   This patient has a drop in Pao_2 from 90 to 70 mm Hg despite having a Fio_2 of 70. Along with the relative hypoxemia, he also developed an increase in peak inspiratory pressure with no change in plateau pressure. The lack of change in plateau pressure rules out any intrinsic change in the lung compliance. Both ARDS and left-ventricular failure (pulmonary edema) will result in a change in lung compliance. The clinical scenario described can result from both tension pneumothorax and bronchial mucous plugging. But the fact that it occurred after 2 days of mechanical ventilation and without any change in the hemodynamic status makes bronchial mucous plugging the most likely cause.

70. C.   The drop in mean arterial pressure at the beginning of CPB is caused by a sharp decrease in systemic vascular resistance caused by the drop in hematocrit caused by the priming solution on pump. This drop in blood pressure along with decreased hematocrit may cause a drop in tissue oxygen delivery. This is very important for tissues with high oxygen consumption like myocardium and brain. Use of α agonists to keep the mean arterial pressure may aid the cerebral perfusion. The correct blood pressure during bypass is often decided based on the patient's coexisting conditions, carotid stenosis, etc. Lower pressures may reduce cerebral blood flow and emboli load to the brain. Higher pressures may improve cerebral blood flow and reduce watershed infarction but higher pressures come from higher flows and more emboli per unit time. Pressures less than 40 mm Hg are avoided if possible in adults. Pressures higher than 60 mm Hg are used during rewarming. Pressures up to 80 to 90 mm Hg may be used in patients with cerebral vascular disease.

71. **B.** A mixed venous PO_2 lower than 30 mm Hg associated with metabolic acidosis suggests inadequate tissue perfusion. Temperature correction of $Paco_2$ and pH is probably not necessary. Urine output may serve as a guide to the adequacy of renal perfusion, with an output of 0.5 to 1 mL/kg/hr, indicating adequate renal perfusion.

72. **C.** Monitoring of coronary sinus pressures during retrograde administration is used to assess proper catheter placement. The anatomical location of coronary sinus ostia makes it very difficult for proper visualization by the surgeon. A properly placed coronary sinus catheter will have pressure of 40 to 60 mm Hg during a 200-mL/min infusion. If the pressure at the distal tip of the coronary sinus catheter during cardioplegia administration at 200 mL/min is equal to central venous pressure, the catheter is not in the coronary sinus but is most likely in the right atrium or in the superior vena cava. Being up against a wall produces a very high (>100 mm Hg) pressure. Positioning of the coronary sinus catheter should be checked with transesophageal echocardiography and manual feel by the surgeon. If the catheter is too deep, cardioplegia to the right ventricle will be compromised, resulting in poor right-ventricular protection.

73. **C.** At 30°C, the heart muscle consumes oxygen at a rate of 8 to 10 mL/100 g/min, provided it is normally contracting. Oxygen consumption in the fibrillating ventricle at 22°C is 2 mL/100 g/min. The electromechanically quiet heart at 22°C consumes oxygen at a rate of 0.3 mL/100 g/min.

74. **A.** The extra volume of crystalloid used in priming the CPB circuit may produce a sudden dilution of circulating drug concentrations. This creates a high chance of patient recall/movement. Supplemental anesthetics, such as benzodiazepines or opioids, and an additional dose of nondepolarizing muscle relaxant, may be administered prophylactically. Volatile anesthetics delivered using vaporizers incorporated into the CPB circuit have largely negated this problem along with the use of BIS monitors. The effect of hemodilution on drug concentrations is likely to be offset by a decreased need for drugs during hypothermia. On the contrary, anesthetic requirements seem to be minimal if the patient was adequately rearmed at the conclusion of CPB. Therefore, additional anesthesia is not routinely required during rewarming at the termination of CPB.

75. **B.** Low SVR is a very common hemodynamic abnormality after CPB. This makes weaning from CPB very difficult. SVR is usually calculated using the formula mean arterial pressure (mm Hg) − central venous pressure (mm Hg)/pump flow (L/mi) × 80.

    SVR should be between 1,200 and 1,400 prior to CPB separation. The units of SVR are dyn s/cm⁵. SVR can be normalized with a vasoconstrictor prior to weaning from CPB. By this, we are attempting to match the vascular input impedance to the cardiac output impedance and optimizing energy transfer.

76. **D.** Acute mitral regurgitation (MR) post–CPB is often noticed as a prominent V wave in PAOP tracing. If there is a transesophageal echocardiograph (TEE) in place, we may be able to see a wide MR jet, with observation of an echogenic mass attached to the mitral valve or when a mobile mass is seen to prolapse into the left atrium during systole and to move back into the left ventricle during diastole. The posterior papillary muscle, along with the posterior wall, is entirely perfused either by the right coronary artery (RCA) or by the third obtuse marginal branch, usually by a single artery unlike the anterior, which derives its blood supply from two arteries. It is usually a complication of acute mitral infarction but maybe seen at the end of CPB due to inadequate myocardial protection (warm blood in the adjacent descending aorta providing inadequate protection) during CPB or air entry into the RCA. Acute MR due to volume overload from excessive fluid administration is usually a central MR as evidenced in TEE with a distended ventricle and can be managed by decreasing the preload.

12

Thoracic Anesthesia

Deppu Ushakumari and Ashish Sinha

1. Which of the following is not a characteristic feature of asthma?

   A. Chronic inflammatory changes in the submucosa of the airways
   B. Airway hyper responsiveness
   C. Reversible expiratory airflow obstruction
   D. Elastase deficiency in the airways

2. A 55-year-old male presented to you with a pulmonary function test report, which shows an increase of FEV_1 percent predicted of more than 12%, and an increase in FEV_1 of greater than 0.2 L in response to bronchodilators. Which characteristic of his respiratory illness is depicted here?

   A. Bronchial asthma—acute bronchodilator responsiveness
   B. Chronic obstructive pulmonary disease (COPD)—variability in airflow obstruction
   C. COPD—acute bronchodilator responsiveness
   D. All the above are correct

3. Which of the following techniques is associated with a lower complication rate related to bronchospasm in the asthmatic population?

   A. Regional anesthesia
   B. General anesthesia—laryngeal mask airway (LMA)
   C. General anesthesia—endotracheal tube (ETT)
   D. Combined general and neuraxial anesthesia

4. A 22-year-old patient with a history of moderate persistent asthma on medium-dose inhaled corticosteroids and long-acting inhaled β-agonist presents for an emergency appendectomy. On clinical examination, he is actively wheezing, but maintaining an oxygen saturation of 99% on room air. Which of the following statements about this clinical scenario is most appropriate?

   A. Presence of wheezing on physical examination indicates that he is having a severe attack of asthma
   B. Volatile anesthetics cause bronchodilation through catecholamine-independent mechanisms
   C. Increased airway resistance that occurs intraoperatively is usually due to acute exacerbation of asthma
   D. A laryngeal mask airway (LMA) is more stimulating to the airway than an endotracheal tube, and should be avoided in asthmatics

5. During the above case, the end-tidal sevoflurane concentration reads 3.5, but the anesthesia ventilator is alarming because of high peak airway pressures. Which of the following is the most likely cause?

   A. Acute bronchospasm
   B. Anaphylactic reaction to intravenous muscle relaxant that you just administered
   C. Mechanical causes of obstruction
   D. Inadequate depth of anesthesia

6. At the end of the above case, the surgeon requests you to extubate the patient fully awake because he found extensive intestinal adhesions and is afraid of retained gastric contents in the stomach. Which of the following will be your most likely plan of action?

   A. Insert an orogastric tube, empty the stomach as much as you can, and proceed with a deep extubation to avoid bronchospasm
   B. Administer intravenous lidocaine to decrease the likelihood of airway stimulation and wait till the patient is fully awake before extubation
   C. Shut off the inhalational agent and use intravenous propofol to avoid transitioning through a rocky stage-2 wake up
   D. Transition to a laryngeal mask airway (LMA) under sevoflurane anesthesia and let the patient wake up with an LMA

7. Which of the following is true regarding administering general anesthesia to a chronic obstructive pulmonary disease (COPD) patient?

   A. Nitrous oxide + opioid technique is ideal
   B. Use large tidal volumes
   C. Use lower breathing rates to permit more exhalation time
   D. Correct the hypercapnia intraoperatively to help extubate early

8. Anesthetic considerations for a patient with severe pulmonary hypertension include all the following, except

   A. Right heart catheterization is the gold standard for diagnosis
   B. Mortality in pregnant patients undergoing vaginal delivery is very small as opposed to cesarean section
   C. Minimize tachycardia, hypoxemia, and hypercapnia during anesthetic management
   D. Cardiac output from a failing right ventricle depends on filling pressure from venous return and pulmonary pressure

9. Which of the following is not a part of the "STOP BANG" screening questionnaire for obstructive sleep apnea (OSA)?

   A. Snoring
   B. Observed apnea
   C. Exercise tolerance
   D. High blood pressure

10. Risk factors associated with increased perioperative morbidity and mortality in thoracic surgery patients include all the following, except

   A. Extent of lung resection
   B. Age older than 70 years
   C. Experience of the operating surgeon
   D. Male sex

11. The following is not necessarily a part of prethoracotomy respiratory assessment

   A. Pulmonary capillary wedge pressure >18 mm Hg
   B. Predicted postoperative FEV_1 >40%
   C. VO_2 max >15 mL/kg/min
   D. Predicted postoperative diffusing capacity for carbon monoxide (DLCO) >40%

12. Which of the following is one of the benefits regarding cessation of smoking 12 to 24 hours prior to surgery?

   A. Shift of oxyhemoglobin dissociation curve to the right
   B. Improvement in mucociliary transport
   C. Decrease in sputum production
   D. Improved small-airway function

13. In surgical cases requiring lung isolation

   A. Measurement of tracheal width from a posteroanterior chest radiograph is of no use in selecting the size of a double-lumen tube (DLT)
   B. More frequent use of left-sided DLT is based on the anatomy of tracheobronchial tree
   C. Uniform ventilation to all lobes is most likely achieved by a right-sided DLT because it has a ventilation slot in the bronchial tube
   D. Fiber–optic confirmation of correct DLT placement is not required if you have good clinical confirmation

14. A 59-year-old lady is intubated with a 37 left-sided double-lumen tube (DLT) for wedge resection of left lower lobe nodule. After intubation, you inflate the bronchial cuff and ventilate the left lung through the bronchial lumen without any difficulty. Then you proceed to inflate the tracheal cuff and ventilate through the tracheal lumen. You notice a very high resistance to air flow. Which of the following events is most *unlikely* with the said clinical picture?

   A. Left DLT too deep with the tracheal outlet into the left main-stem bronchus
   B. Left DLT displaced with the bronchial cuff herniated at carina
   C. Left DLT entered the right bronchus with the tracheal outlet in the right main stem
   D. DLT too far out with the bronchial lumen sitting just above the carina

15. What would you do if you have the following situation with a bronchial blocker for left lung surgery?

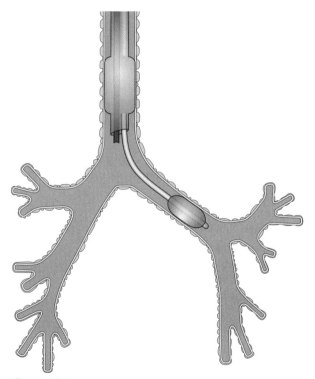

Figure 12-1.

   A. Appropriate positioning for this surgery
   B. Withdraw the bronchial blocker a couple of centimeters
   C. Insert the bronchial blocker a few centimeters farther down
   D. Remove the bronchial blocker and reinsert it into the left side

16. In which of the following situations is applying continuous positive-airway pressure (CPAP) to the nondependent lung most ideal for improving oxygenation?

    A. Bronchopleural fistula
    B. Open lobectomy
    C. Massive pulmonary hemorrhage
    D. Sleeve resection

17. Which of the following statements is false regarding ventilation/perfusion relationship in a lateral decubitus position during spontaneous ventilation?

    A. The ventilation/perfusion matching is preserved
    B. Contraction of dependent hemi diaphragm is more efficient
    C. Dependent lung is on a more favorable part of the compliance curve
    D. The lower lung receives less ventilation and more perfusion than the upper lung

18. In an open pneumothorax, the major effect of mediastinal shift is to

    A. Decrease the contribution of dependent lung to the tidal volume
    B. Move air to and fro between the dependent and the nondependent lung
    C. Decrease the perfusion to the dependent lung
    D. Compress the big veins and decrease cardiac preload

19. Factors known to inhibit hypoxic pulmonary vasoconstriction (HPV) and thus worsen the alveolar–arterial oxygen gradient include all of the following, except

    A. Hypocapnia
    B. Nitroglycerin
    C. Hypercapnia
    D. Pulmonary infection

20. A 64-year-old female is undergoing a left video-assisted thoracoscopy for a suspicious pulmonary nodule. Immediately after positioning the patient laterally, which of the following alarms indicates a malposition of the double-lumen tube (DLT)?

    A. High CO_2 alarm
    B. Low O_2 alarm
    C. Low tidal volume alarm
    D. Unable to drive bellows alarm

21. A bronchial blocker is useful in all of the following clinical situations, except

    A. Patient to be left intubated post operatively
    B. Anatomical abnormality precluding the placement of a double-lumen tube (DLT)
    C. Tamponading bronchial bleeding in adult patients
    D. To attain better collapse of the nondependent lung

22. Which of the following statements about lung resection surgery is false?

    A. Mortality rate for pneumonectomy is 5% to 7%
    B. Mortality rate for lobectomy is 2% to 3%
    C. Mortality is higher for left-sided pneumonectomy
    D. Most postoperative deaths result from cardiac issues

23. Regarding lung resection surgery, which of the following statements is false?

    A. Perioperative arrhythmias are common
    B. Supraventricular tachycardias (SVTs) are thought to result from surgical manipulation or distension of the right atrium
    C. Incidence of arrhythmia decreases with age due to the ageing of cardiac conduction system
    D. Postoperative hypoxemia and acidosis due to atelectasis and shallow breathing are common

24. Which of the following has the least effect on hypoxic pulmonary vasoconstriction (HPV)?

    A. Nitrous oxide
    B. Desflurane   end tidal 5.5%
    C. Sevoflurane   end tidal 2.5%
    D. Isoflurane   end tidal 1.5%

25. Which of the following statements is not true regarding "lower lung syndrome"?

    A. It is caused by excessive fluid administration in a lateral decubitus position
    B. It increases intrapulmonary shunting
    C. It is gravity-dependent transudation of fluid into the dependent lung
    D. It is due to volutrauma caused during one-lung ventilation

26. The first step recommended to improve oxygenation if a patient is exhibiting drop in oxygen saturation during one-lung ventilation is

    A. Apply continuous positive-airway pressure (CPAP) to the collapsed lung
    B. Apply positive end–expiratory pressure (PEEP) to the dependent lung
    C. Periodic inflation of the collapsed lung
    D. Continuous inflation of oxygen into collapsed lung

27. During apneic oxygenation,

    A. Adequate oxygenation can be maintained only for short periods of time
    B. Arterial PCO_2 rises 3 to 4 mm Hg in the first minute
    C. Arterial PCO_2 rises 1 to 2 mm Hg each subsequent minute after the first minute
    D. Progressive respiratory acidosis limits the use of this technique to 10 to 20 minutes in most patients

28. A 68-year-old male patient with a lung nodule underwent a right upper lobectomy. On post-operative day 4, the patient develops a sudden large air leak from the chest tube associated with increasing pneumothorax and partial lung collapse. The most likely cause is

    A. Bronchopleural fistula on the right from necrosis of suture line
    B. Bronchopleural fistula on the right from inadequate surgical closure of the bronchial stump
    C. Atelectasis causing shifting of the mediastinum to the left
    D. A normal finding

29. An 80-year-old female underwent a left lower lobectomy. In the ICU on postoperative day 2, she develops hemoptysis. The vital signs are stable, but on the chest X-ray a homogenous density is seen in the left lower lung area. After subsequent bronchoscopy, the left upper lobar orifice is closed. The most likely diagnosis is

    A. Acute herniation of the heart into the left lower lobe area
    B. It is a normal finding and the homogenous opacity is due to accumulation of fluid in the left lower lobe area
    C. Torsion of the left upper lobe as the left upper lobe expanded to occupy the left hemithorax
    D. Reexpansion edema of the left upper lobe

30. A 45-year-old recent immigrant from Vietnam is admitted to the emergency department with massive hemoptysis (>600 mL in the last 24 hours). You are called to evaluate the patient for a possible bronchial artery embolization or a rigid bronchoscopy. In your discussion with the patient, which of the following statements is not appropriate about his clinical condition?

    A. Operative mortality exceeds 20%
    B. It can be done as a semi-elective procedure, and there is no need to do it emergently
    C. The most common cause of death is asphyxia secondary to blood in the airway
    D. Medical management has a lower mortality rate than operative management

31. An 81-year-old chronic smoker, with a history of 60 pack year smoking, is admitted with progressive dyspnea and a huge right-sided pulmonary cyst. The cyst is compressing her remaining right lung, and she is brought to the OR for an emergency pulmonary cystectomy. Which of the following is right regarding anesthetic management of this patient?

A. The greatest risk of rupture of the cavity is during preoxygenation just prior to induction

B. These cavities allow to and fro movement of air and have a very low chance to progressively enlarge

C. Maintenance of spontaneous ventilation is desirable until a double-lumen tube (DLT) is in place

D. Assisted ventilation is not necessary immediately after induction and can be harmful

32. A 66-year-old patient with a history of severe tracheal stenosis is presenting for a tracheal resection. The most *unlikely* clinical finding is

A. Progressive dyspnea

B. Wheezing evident on exertion

C. Dyspnea worse on sitting up and leaning forward

D. Patient may have a history of blunt/penetrating tracheal trauma

33. In the anesthetic management of the above patient, which of the following statements is correct?

A. Flow–volume loops aid the clinician in evaluating the severity of the lesion

B. Right radial artery blood pressure monitoring is preferred over the left side for lower tracheal resection

C. Slow-inhalation induction is not advisable and a rapid-sequence induction should be used

D. Early extubation is not advisable at the end of the procedure for risk of rupturing the suture lines

34. Complications associated with mediastinoscopy include all the following, except

A. Vagally mediated reflex bradycardia

B. Cerebral ischemia

C. Pneumothorax

D. Thoracic duct injury

35. Anesthetic considerations for bronchoalveolar lavage include all the following, except

A. It is performed for patients who make excess quantities of surfactant and fail to clear it

B. It is performed under general anesthesia with lung isolation

C. It is usually performed in the supine position

D. It involves positioning the patient in a lateral position to aid active suctioning of the lavage fluid

36. Considerations for lung transplantation include all the following, except

A. Cor pulmonale does not necessarily require combined heart–lung transplantation

B. Patients with diminished left-ventricular function can be transplanted as long as they have normal right-ventricular function

C. Patients with Eisenmenger syndrome require combined heart–lung transplantation

D. Organ selection is based on size and ABO compatibility

37. After a double-lung transplantation

A. Loss of lymphatic drainage predisposes to pulmonary edema

B. Respiratory pattern changes to a slow deep respiration

C. Cough reflex is abolished above the carina

D. Hypoxic pulmonary vasoconstriction is abolished

38. Anesthetic considerations for esophageal surgery include

    A. Very low risk of pulmonary aspiration

    B. Mandatory pulmonary artery catheter monitoring

    C. Diaphragmatic retractors interfering with cardiac function

    D. Always performed with a double-lumen tube (DLT)

39. Lung-volume-reduction surgery (LVRS)

    A. Has been demonstrated to have very good efficacy by the National Emphysema Treatment Trial (NETT)

    B. Necessitates limiting of peak inspiratory pressure to 30 cm H_2O following intubation

    C. A prolonged inspiratory time is recommended for facilitating exposure of the surgical segments

    D. Patients have a better outcome if kept intubated at the end of the surgery

40. Which of the following flow–volume loops will be expected in a child with variable extrathoracic obstruction?

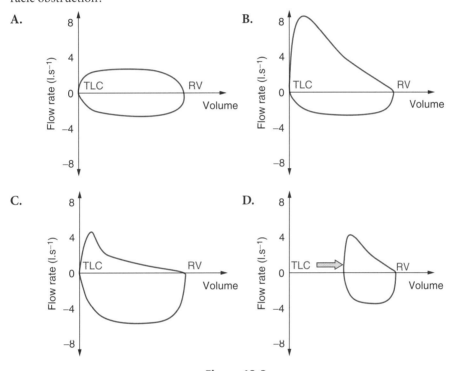

Figure 12-2.

41. A 12-year-old boy with suspected lymphoma presents to you for a lymph node biopsy. When you go to visit the patient, you notice that he has venous engorgement and edema of the head, neck, and arms. He refuses to lie down, and is tachycardiac and tachypneic. The preferred management for this boy would be

    A. Safest thing will be to secure the airway immediately by using rapid-sequence induction

    B. Preferably biopsy the lymph node under local anesthesia so that the patient can be sent for radiotherapy immediately after a tissue diagnosis

    C. Empiric treatment with steroids and surgery under general anesthesia only after the airway compromise is alleviated

    D. Get a chest X-ray and rule out mediastinal compression prior to any active management

CHAPTER 12 ANSWERS

1. **D.** Asthma is a type of reactive airway disease characterized by hyperresponsive airways, reversible expiratory airflow obstruction, and chronic inflammation. Sudden bronchospasm in response to external/internal stimuli and response to bronchodilators like β_2-agonists are important distinguishing features of asthma. Elastase deficiency in the airways is a feature of emphysema.

2. **A.** Response to a bronchodilator drug resulting in relief of airway obstruction is highly suggestive of bronchial asthma. A more than 12% increase in predicted FEV_1 and an absolute increase in FEV_1 of more than 0.2 L suggest acute bronchodilator responsiveness and variability in airflow obstruction. The reversibility of this magnitude is almost always indicative of bronchial asthma. COPD patients do respond to bronchodilators but not to the same extent. Early stages of asthma are diagnosed by decreased mid expiratory flow rates (effort independent) and decreased FEV_1 and by its reversibility.

3. **A.** In a severely asthmatic patient, regional anesthesia is superior to general anesthesia with an LMA, which is better than general anesthesia with ETT. The choice of anesthetic technique is often influenced by the severity of asthma, history of previous intubations for asthma, dependence on inhaled bronchodilators, and patient preference. The goal in any such circumstance is to decrease airway manipulation and stimulation. If a general anesthetic technique is pursued, inhaled bronchodilator therapy immediately prior to induction, use of non–histamine-releasing drugs, airway manipulation only after deep anesthetic plane, and use of intravenous lidocaine prior to intubation have all been proven to be useful.

4. **B.** History and physical examination can suggest presence of severe asthma if the patient has had repeated intubations for asthma. Even though high-pitched, musical wheezes are characteristic of asthma, they are not specific and they have no correlation with the severity of obstruction. Spirometry is the only objective method to quantify the severity of obstruction. Sudden severe bronchospasm can present as high airway pressures with absence of breath sounds and very high resistance to mechanical ventilation. Mechanical causes of obstruction such as a kinked endotracheal tube or a mucous plug can also present a similar clinical picture and are more common. If bronchospasm is suspected, anesthesia should be augmented with an intravenous anesthetic such as propofol. General anesthesia through a LMA is less stimulating to the airway than through an endotracheal tube. Volatile anesthetics are potent bronchodilators, and they act through catecholamine-independent mechanisms. They are rarely used as second-line agents in cases of bronchospasm refractory to medical therapy.

5. **C.** Acute bronchospasm causes expiratory wheezing, increased peak inspiratory pressure or decreased tidal volume (depending on the mode of ventilation), and a characteristic upslope of the capnogram. Any airway stimulation can cause severe reflex bronchoconstriction and bronchospasm in severely asthmatic patients with hyperactive airways. Mechanical causes of obstruction such as a kinked endotracheal tube or a mucous plug can also present a similar clinical picture and are more common. When troubleshooting such a scenario, an intravenous anesthetic agent is very helpful to deepen the plane of anesthesia as the delivery of inhaled anesthetic agents may not be effective.

6. **B.** A patient who has adequate return of neuromuscular function and has a regular spontaneous breathing pattern with adequate tidal volumes can be considered a candidate for deep extubation. After clearing out the secretions from the oropharynx and the endotracheal tube, extubation is performed under a deep plane of anesthesia and ventilation continued by a mask/LMA. Careful patient selection is very important, and it should not be considered in those at increased risk for aspiration of gastric content and if the necessary airway

management skills are not immediately available. When extubation is delayed for reasons of patient safety, (presence of gastric contents in a case with acute appendicitis), intravenous administration of lidocaine (1.5–2 mg/kg bolus) may decrease the likelihood of airway irritation and bronchospasm. Thus, extubation can be performed after the patient is awake and following commands if airway irritation can be avoided.

7. **C.**   Balanced anesthesia using an inhaled anesthetic and opioid is a safe choice for anesthesia for a COPD patient. Use of nitrous oxide (N_2O) is normally safe but not strictly necessary. The ability of N_2O to diffuse into closed air spaces may lead to the enlargement of an emphysematous bulla or a pneumothorax and possibly rupture. Air trapping and development of auto positive end–expiratory pressure can be decreased by providing a prolonged expiratory time. This can be done by using a normal tidal volume and a slow respiratory rate and an I:E ratio of $\geq$1:3. Care should be taken to avoid hyperventilation and creation of a respiratory alkalosis as these patients tolerate marked hypercapnia secondary to hypoventilation. However, high $Paco_2$ levels will increase pulmonary artery pressure, which may be poorly tolerated in patients with a compromised right-ventricular function and cor pulmonale. Bronchodilation using inhaled β_2-agonists and pulmonary toilet through blind suctioning or fiberoptic bronchoscopy may facilitate safe extubation of the trachea.

8. **B.**   Pulmonary hypertension is defined as an increase in mean pulmonary artery pressure above 25 mm Hg at rest or 30 mm Hg with exercise in the presence or absence of an elevated pulmonary capillary wedge pressure. Right-sided heart catheterization is the gold standard for diagnosing and quantifying the degree of pulmonary hypertension. Care should be taken to avoid all the factors that increase pulmonary vascular resistance in a patient with severe pulmonary hypertension presenting for surgery. This includes avoiding hypoxia, hypercarbia, hypothermia, light anesthesia, pain, dysrhythmias, and maintaining adequate cardiac output. Progressive right-ventricular dilation and hypertrophy in response to an increased afterload generated by chronic pulmonary hypertension will eventually lead to right-ventricular systolic dysfunction, inadequate left-ventricular filling, and eventually biventricular failure. The interventricular septal bulge decreases left-ventricular cavity filling, further worsening the left-ventricular failure. Cardiac output from a failing right ventricle depends on the filling pressure from venous return and pulmonary pressure. Pulmonary hypertension in pregnant patients has a high mortality rate up to 50% for vaginal delivery and even higher for cesarean delivery.

9. **C.**   Snoring, daytime sleepiness, hypertension, obesity, and a family history of OSA are risk factors for OSA. There is a high risk for OSA if >3 yes to the below questions.

S (snore) Have you been told that you snore?
T (tired) Are you often tired during the day?
O (obstruction) Do you know if you stop breathing or has anyone witnessed you stop breathing while you are asleep?
P (pressure) Do you have high blood pressure or on medication to control high blood pressure?
B (BMI) Is your body mass index greater than 28?
A (age) Are you 50 years old or older?
N (neck) Are you a male with a neck circumference greater than 17 inches, or a female with a neck circumference greater than 16 inches.
G (gender) Are you a male?

10. **D.**   The extent of lung resection (pneumonectomy > lobectomy > wedge resection), age older than 70 years, and inexperience of the operating surgeon are risk factors associated with increased perioperative morbidity and mortality rates. In patients with anatomically resectable lung cancer, pulmonary function tests—$ppoFEV_1$, lung perfusion scanning, and exercise testing to measure maximum oxygen consumption (VO_2max)—may predict postoperative pulmonary function and outcome.

11. **A.**   The prethoracotomy respiratory assessment has been labeled as a three-legged stool that incorporates assessment of respiratory mechanics, cardiopulmonary reserve, and lung parenchymal function. The following findings are considered favorable: respiratory mechanics assessment demonstrates ppoFEV$_1$ >40%, MVV, RV/TLC, and FVC; the cardiopulmonary reserve measurements show VO$_2$ max >15 mL/kg/min, 6-minute walk test, exercise Spo$_2$ <4%, stair climb >2 flights, and assessment of lung parenchymal function shows ppoDLCO >40%, Pao$_2$ >60, Paco$_2$ <45 mm Hg. The choices B, C, and D are the most valid tests out of the "three-legged stool."

12. **A.**   Any patient presenting for elective surgeries with a history of smoking should be advised smoking cessation regardless of the time available prior to surgery. Smoking can affect the pulmonary system in multiple ways—increase in airway irritability and secretions, decreased mucociliary transport, and increased incidence of postoperative pulmonary complications. Patients are more receptive toward interventions immediately prior to surgery and this provides a good teachable moment. Prolonged abstinence (8–12 weeks) is required to improve mucociliary transport and small-airway function and decrease sputum production. The incidence of postoperative pulmonary complications decreases with abstinence from cigarette smoking for more than 8 weeks in patients undergoing coronary artery bypass surgery, and more than 4 weeks in patients undergoing pulmonary surgery. However, even 12 to 24 hours of cessation may be beneficial because it decreases the level of carboxyhemoglobin and it shifts the oxyhemoglobin dissociation curve to the right.

13. **B.**   The angle between the right main bronchus and trachea is 25 degrees at the level of carina, but the left main bronchus takes off at an acute angle of 45 degrees. Thus, right main bronchus is shorter, wider, and more in line with the trachea. There is a good correlation between tracheal and bronchial width (bronchial diameter is predicted to be 0.68 of tracheal diameter).

    The right upper lobe bronchus takes off at an acute angle from the point of origin of the right primary bronchus and is easily occluded if the ventilation port on the right-sided DLT is not aligned properly. Because of these reasons, a left-sided DLT is most commonly used. Uniform ventilation to all lobes can be achieved more easily with a left-sided DLT than a right-sided one. Measurement of tracheal width from a posteroanterior chest roentgenogram can help select the size of a left-sided DLT. In addition to physical examination, fiberoptic assessment should be done to confirm proper position of a left-sided DLT because the malposition incidence if confirmed with auscultation alone is considered to be 20% to 48%.

14. **C.**   There is no single predictor that can accurately predict the appropriate size of a DLT. But a general guideline is a woman shorter than 160 cm should be intubated with a 35-Fr tube, a woman taller than 160 cm should be intubated with a 37-Fr tube, and a man shorter than 170 cm should be intubated with a 39-Fr tube, and a man taller than 170 cm should be intubated with a 41-Fr tube. This tube size of 37 Fr may be too big for this lady. When we inflated the bronchial cuff and attempted ventilation, the unoccluded outflow tract of the bronchial lumen made it easy to ventilate. However, after inflating the tracheal cuff (with the bronchial cuff already inflated), failure to ventilate suggests that something is occluding the tracheal lumen (the bronchial cuff in this situation). The presence of breath sounds only on the right side with both the cuffs inflated suggests that the bronchial lumen is patent and ventilating the right side. The ventilated gas coming out of tracheal lumen is being trapped between the tracheal and the bronchial balloons. This finding can be confirmed with fiberoptic bronchoscopy, and the tube needs to be repositioned with bronchial cuff in the left main-stem bronchus. If with the same clinical picture, you are hearing breath sounds only on the left side with both the cuffs inflated, it could be that the DLT is too far into the left bronchus with the tracheal lumen opening into the left main stem. It is also possible that the bronchial cuff is barely into the left main stem with a herniated bronchial cuff preventing the inflation of right-sided lung via the tracheal lumen.

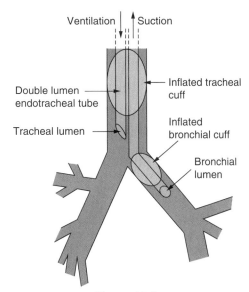

Figure 12-3.

15. B. Figure 12-4A is a bronchial blocker for a left-sided lung surgery placed deeply into the left main-stem bronchus. Figure 12-4B is a bronchial blocker advanced too far into the right main stem, and the balloon of the bronchial blocker is occluding the right upper lobe takeoff. For both situations, the bronchial blocker should be withdrawn a couple of centimeters to a level just below the carina.

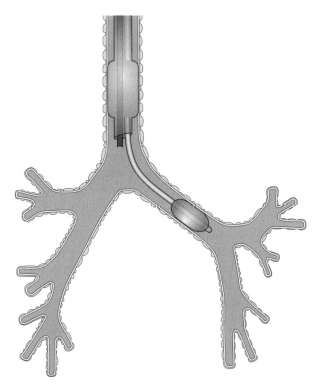

A Blocker positioned deeply into
left main-stem bronchus

Figure 12-4.

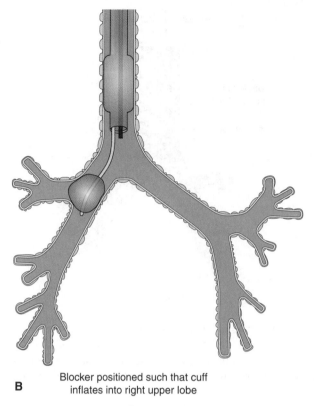

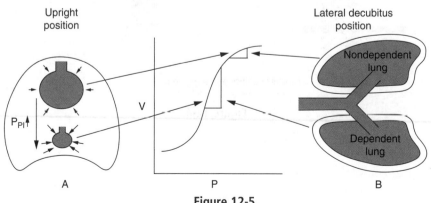

B   Blocker positioned such that cuff
     inflates into right upper lobe

Figure 12-4.

16. **B.** Difficulties with oxygenation are fairly common during one-lung ventilation. If the SpO$_2$ is below acceptable range, various techniques that can be tried to improve the oxygenation include increasing FiO$_2$ to 1, intermittent two-lung ventilation, applying positive end–expiratory pressure (PEEP) to the dependent lung. However, the most effective method is the application of 5 to 10 cm H$_2$O CPAP to the nondependent lung. This should be done prior to application of PEEP to the dependent lung. This low level of CPAP results in minimal lung inflation and generally does not interfere with surgery. A slow inflation of 2 L/min of oxygen into the nonventilated lung for 2 seconds and repeated every 10 seconds for 5 minutes or until the saturation rises to 98% has been shown to improve oxygenation during one-lung ventilation. CPAP applied to the operative lung may be disadvantageous in some cases like thoracoscopy, bronchopleural fistula, sleeve resection, or massive pulmonary hemorrhage.

17. **D.** During spontaneous ventilation in lateral decubitus position, ventilation/perfusion matching is preserved because the lower lung receives more perfusion due to gravity and more ventilation due to better contraction of the dependent hemidiaphragm. The dependent hemidiaphragm gets a better displacement from a higher position in the chest. The dependent lung has a better compliance as well—this improves ventilation.

Figure 12-5.

18. **A.** Inspiration in a lateral position during spontaneous ventilation causes more negative pleural pressure on the dependent side of the open pneumothorax. The relatively higher pressure on the nondependent side causes a downward shift of the mediastinum during inspiration. The reverse happens on expiration, and the mediastinum shifts upward. This results in an ineffective respiratory exchange, but the major effect is by decreasing the contribution of the dependent lung to the tidal volume.

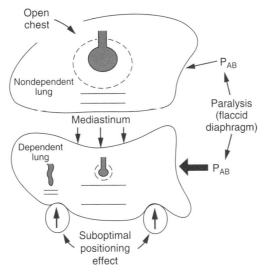

Figure 12-6.

19. **C.** HPV is a protective mechanism by which body shunts away blood from a nonventilated lung. It plays a significant role in maintaining oxygenation during one-lung ventilation. Factors inhibiting HPV include infection, pulmonary hyper/hypotension, low $Paco_2$, changes in Svo_2 (mixed venous oxygen saturation), and pharmacological agents like vasodilators—nitroglycerin and nitroprusside, β-agonists, calcium channel blockers, and inhalational anesthetic agents.

20. **C.** Left-sided DLTs are most commonly used in clinical practice. Any change in position of the patient after the DLTs have been placed includes a risk of malpositioning of the DLT. Low exhaled tidal volumes and poor lung compliance are the most common initial indicators. Left-sided DLT may be malpositioned back into the trachea, into the right main-stem bronchus, or too far into the left primary bronchus. If it is in the trachea, the inflated bronchial cuff is preventing any ventilated gas from going past it. If it is in the right side or pushed too far into the left bronchus, the bronchial cuff may be obstructing the left upper or left lower lobe bronchus. These two situations can be immediately relieved by deflating the bronchial cuff.

21. **D.** DLTs are considered to be the best lung isolation device currently in use. In certain situations, placement of a DLT is difficult and bronchial blockers are used for lung isolation. They are similar to Fogarty catheters and are single-lumen devices with an inflatable balloon at the tip. They are passed through a single-lumen endotracheal tube under fiberoptic guidance and the balloon is inflated within the bronchus of the operative side. The cuff of the bronchial blocker is a high-pressure–low-volume cuff. The single narrow lumen within the blocker allows the lung to deflate (though slowly) and can be used for suctioning or insufflating oxygen (below). The biggest problem is caused by the small size of the channel, which impairs exhalation. However, in patients with a history of difficult intubation bronchial blockers circumvent the need to reintubate a patient prior to transferring out of the operating room.

22. **C.** The mortality rate for pneumonectomy is about 5% to 7%, compared with 2% to 3% for a lobectomy. Mortality is higher for right-sided pneumonectomy than for left-sided pneumonectomy. This is attributed to the greater loss of lung tissue. Lung cancer resection surgeries involve finding the right balance between resecting enough lung tissue to obtain a tumor-free margin, at the same time leaving enough for residual postoperative pulmonary function.

Wedge resections for peripheral lesions, lobectomy for bigger tumors, pneumonectomy for tumors involving the main bronchus, sleeve resections for patients with proximal lesions, and limited pulmonary reserve are among the various choices the surgeons can make.

23. **C.**   The incidence of arrhythmias increases with age and with the amount of pulmonary resection. Perioperative arrhythmias are fairly common after thoracic surgery—atrial fibrillations/SVTs and PVCs are all seen and are thought to be a result of the surgical manipulation of the heart and distension of the right atrium as a result of decreased pulmonary vascular bed. Pulmonary complications after surgery can be decreased by preoperative incentive spirometry, bronchodilator therapy, and good pulmonary hygiene.

24. **B.**   Halogenated agents generally have minimal effects on HPV in doses <1 minimum alveolar concentration (MAC). Balanced anesthetic technique using a combination of inhaled anesthetic agents and intravenous opioids is beneficial. Inhalational agents allow delivery of 100% oxygen, are potent bronchodilators, and can be easily titrated to desired concentration and opioids have minimal hemodynamic effects as well as providing analgesia. They complement each other very well. However, use of long-acting opioids should be limited during surgery to prevent excessive postoperative respiratory depression. The only choice with <1MAC is B.

25. **D.**   Anesthetic management of pulmonary resections includes very tight fluid management. Most of the time restrictive fluid management strategy facilitated by use of blood/colloids is entertained. Lower lung syndrome refers to gravity-dependent transudation of fluid into the dependent lung, which decreases effective oxygenation, increases ventilation–perfusion mismatch, shunting, and promotes hypoxemia. This transudation is worsened by excessive administration of intravenous crystalloids. On the nondependent side, reexpansion of the collapsed lung can result in pulmonary edema due to alteration in the pressures on either side of the Starling equation.

26. **A.**   Hypoxemia is fairly common after institution of one-lung ventilation in the lateral position. Various interventions can be tried when it happens—some have better efficacy than the others. These include periodic reinflation of the collapsed lung with oxygen, which interferes with surgery; early ligation or clamping of the ipsilateral pulmonary artery—seldom used but can be tried in pneumonectomies; and CPAP (5–10 cm H_2O) to the collapsed lung causing partial reexpansion of the lung and may interfere with surgery. The mechanism of action of CPAP application is supposed to oxygenation as well as displacement of blood from the pulmonary vasculature into the dependent lung. Other less efficacious methods that can be tried include PEEP (5–10 cm H_2O) to the ventilated lung, oxygen insufflation to collapsed lung (diffusion respiration), and change in dependent lung minute ventilation (Vt 5 mL/kg is usually recommended but can be increased). Application of CPAP to the collapsed lung should be done before instituting PEEP to the ventilated lung, as the effect of PEEP depends on where the lung falls on the PEEP–PVR curve. Persistent hypoxemia requires immediate return to two-lung ventilation.

27. **D.**   Apneic oxygenation refers to insufflation of 100% oxygen at a rate greater than the oxygen consumption (>250 mL/min) while the ventilation is stopped. Progressive respiratory acidosis limits the use of this technique to 10 to 20 minutes in most patients. Oxygenation can be maintained in patients with normal DLCO for more than this time interval. During apneic oxygenation, arterial PCO_2 rises 6 mm Hg in the first minute followed by 3 to 4 mm Hg every subsequent minute.

28. **A.**   Bronchopleural fistula refers to a communication between the bronchial and pleural spaces. It presents as a sudden large air leak from the chest tube that may be associated with an increasing pneumothorax and partial lung collapse. Inadequate surgical closure of the bronchial stump usually presents itself with a bronchopleural fistula in the first 24 to 72 hours. Necrosis of the suture line (bronchial/parenchymal) caused by ischemia or infection usually

presents after 72 hours. This is a rare complication, but small air leaks are fairly common after segmental or lobar resection due to collateral ventilation from small channels at the sites of incomplete fissures. They are usually smaller in volume, will not cause significant impairment of ventilation, and will close by itself after a few days—after which chest tubes can be discontinued.

29. **C.**   This is the classical picture of torsion of a lung lobe as it expands to fill up the space left by resection of the other lobe. This is because the torsion results in occlusion of the pulmonary vein, which drains blood flow to that part of the lung and presents clinically as hemoptysis and radiographically as an enlarging homogenous density. This can be confirmed by visualizing a closed lobar orifice on bronchoscopy. On the other hand, an acute herniation of the heart into the operative hemithorax is associated with hemodynamic changes and a shift in the cardiac shadow on chest X-ray. This is caused by a large pressure difference between the two hemithoraces. Herniation to the right causes severe hypotension and an elevated central venous pressure due to torsion of the vena cava. Herniation to the left causes compression of the heart at the atrioventricular groove, resulting in hypotension, ischemia, and infarction.

30. **D.**   With the given history, the massive hemoptysis (defined as >500–600 mL of blood loss in 24 hours) is most likely infectious in origin with tuberculosis being a strong possibility. The other causes of massive hemoptysis include bronchiectasis, aspergillomas, neoplasms, foreign body in the trachea, and trauma. A potentially lethal hemoptysis with severe hemodynamic compromise necessitates emergency surgery. Bronchial artery embolization may be attempted if the patient is hemodynamically stable. Whenever possible, surgery is carried out in a semi-elective way, but the operative mortality is still high, >20%. However, medical management is associated with a much higher mortality, >50%. The most common cause of death is asphyxia secondary to blood in the airway.

31. **C.**   Pulmonary cysts or bullae are large cavitary lesions that behave as if they have a one-way valve, gets progressively large and may compress the remaining lung tissue. They may also rupture producing a tension pneumothorax. They can be congenital or acquired as a result of emphysema. They are usually scheduled for lung resection surgeries when they cause recurrent pneumothorax or progressive dyspnea. Positive-pressure ventilation results in further expansion of such cavities and increased risk of rupture along with impaired oxygenation from the affected lung. Maintenance of spontaneous ventilation (negative inspiratory pressure) is recommended until the affected lung is isolated using a DLT or until a chest tune is placed. Inhalational agents can be used to facilitate this, but the large dead space caused by the presence of huge cyst may result in progressive hypercarbia. Assisted ventilation is helpful in such circumstances. Care should be taken to avoid complete positive-pressure ventilation.

32. **C.**   Tracheal stenosis is narrowing of the airway as a result of tracheal mucosal damage followed by scarring. It can also be caused by tumors—squamous or adenoid cystic carcinoma. The inciting factors for the mucosal damage include trauma or prolonged endotracheal intubation. These patients present with progressive dyspnea, hemoptysis, and stridor on exertion. The dyspnea is characteristically worse on lying down and is made better by sitting up and leaning forward.

33. **A.**   Anesthetic considerations for tracheal resection include invasive monitoring, use of anticholinergics to prevent increased secretions, slow inhalational induction maintaining spontaneous ventilation, airway stimulation after attaining a deep plane of anesthesia, return of spontaneous ventilation, and early extubation. The left radial artery is preferred for lower tracheal resections because of the potential for compression of the innominate artery. A nonirritating inhalational agent like sevoflurane in 100% oxygen can be used along with short-acting opioids like remifentanil. Care should be taken to decrease the FIO_2 to below 0.3 if the surgeon is using laser to resect the scar tissue. After opening the stenosed segment, the surgeon can insert a sterile endotracheal tube into the segment of trachea below the lesion and patient can be ventilated through that. There will be a brief period of apnea as the surgeon is

anastomosing the anterior part of trachea after resection. Once the anastomosis is complete, the initial endotracheal tube can be readvanced below the lesion. The neck is kept flexed in the postoperative period to minimize tension on the tracheal suture line. Heliox offers a method to avoid turbulence due to its lower density. Flow–volume loops confirm the location of the obstruction and aid the clinician in evaluating the severity of the lesion.

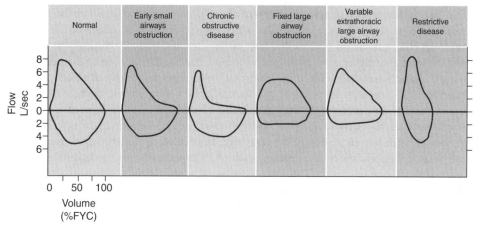

Figure 12-7.

34. D. Mediastinoscopy involves operating on an area covered with blood vessels and nerves. The complications include reflex bradycardia due to vagal stimulation, bleeding from damage to the great vessels, pneumothorax, air embolism, post-op hoarseness due to recurrent laryngeal nerve injury, and phrenic nerve injury. A false drop in blood pressure may be observed due to compression of the innominate artery if the arterial line is placed on the right arm. A spontaneously breathing patient with head end elevated is also at risk for a pneumothorax that presents postoperatively.

35. D. Pulmonary alveolar proteinosis is a condition in which patients produce excessive quantities of surfactant and fail to clear it, producing bilateral lung involvement and recurrent pneumonias. Bronchoalveolar lavage is performed in these patients for severe hypoxemia or worsening dyspnea. They undergo sequential lung lavages interspaced by a few days with the worse lung getting lavage first. It is an absolute indication for lung isolation. If both lungs are lavaged during the same procedure, it significantly impairs effective oxygenation.

Lung isolation for unilateral bronchoalveolar lavage is obtained by a double-lumen tube under general anesthesia. Proper positioning of the tube by bronchoscopy is essential prior to the lavage to prevent contamination of the opposite lung. A water-tight seal with the cuffs is also essential prior to the lavage. The procedure is normally done in the supine position; lavaging a dependent lung in a lateral position helps to minimize soiling of the nondependent lung, but the ventilation–perfusion mismatch caused by ventilating a nondependent lung which is not perfused is severe and makes this clinically impossible. Warm normal saline is infused into the lung to be treated and is drained by gravity; treatment continues until the fluid returning is clear (about 10–20 L). Patient can be extubated after carefully suctioning out both the lungs or the double-lumen tube is replaced by a single-lumen tube at the end of the procedure.

36. B. Right-ventricular failure caused by increase in right-sided afterload (increased pulmonary artery resistance) may recover after isolated lung transplantation, and they do not require combined heart–lung transplantation. Such is not the case in patients with Eisenmenger syndrome who require combined heart–lung transplantation. However, normal left-ventricular function and absence of significant coronary artery disease or other serious health problems is ensured before lung transplantation, as the wait list of patients for the organs are long. Respiratory failure caused by cystic fibrosis, bullous emphysema, or vascular diseases are usually bilateral and necessitate a double-lung transplant. It can be done using cardiopulmonary bypass or sequentially using one-lung ventilation depending on the pulmonary artery pressures and the ventricular function. Single-lung transplantation is being increasingly performed for patients with chronic obstructive pulmonary disease. Organ selection is based on size, ABO compatibility, and cytomegalovirus serology matching.

37. **A.** A newly transplanted lung lacks the neural innervation, lymphatic drainage, and bronchial circulation, which were present in the explanted lung. Central respiratory pattern generated by centers in the brain stem is unaffected. Hypoxic pulmonary vasoconstriction, mediated locally is also unaffected. However, loss of lymphatic drainage increases extravascular lung water and predisposes the transplanted lung to pulmonary edema. Fluid restriction is fairly common after lung transplantation to prevent this from happening. Although some patients develop bronchial hyperreactivity, cough reflex is abolished below the carina. These patients usually get postoperative bronchoscopy to assess bronchial suture line, as they are prone for ischemic breakdown in the absence of bronchial circulation.

38. **C.** Anesthetic considerations in patients with esophageal disease include the risk of pulmonary aspiration, use of a DLT, invasive monitoring, intravenous access sufficient for rapid fluid resuscitation, maintaining normothermia, and use of transcutaneous pads for defibrillation if needed. The esophageal disease process predisposes them to aspiration due to obstruction, altered motility, or abnormal sphincter function. The risk of aspiration continues into the postoperative period. Even though a DLT (Double lumen tube) facilitates surgical exposure, it is not always required. Invasive monitoring with arterial line and central venous pressure monitoring help guide hemodynamic management. However, a PAC (Pulmonary artery catheter) is used only for patients with significant cardiac disease. Substernal and diaphragmatic retractors used during the transhiatal approach to esophagectomy can interfere with cardiac function. Surgeons hand can interfere with cardiac filling while bluntly dissecting the esophagus from the posterior mediastinum. Since the vagus runs very close to the esophagus, marked vagal stimulation can result in profound bradycardia or even cardiac arrest—transcutaneous pads helps in these situations. Hypothermia increases coagulopathy and increases cardiac arrhythmias and should be avoided. The potential for rapid massive blood loss is significant as the surgery is near the major blood vessels.

39. **B.** There has been a recent resurgence in LVRS, even though NETT, a trial of usual medical therapy versus usual medical therapy plus LVRS, suggested lack of efficacy of LVRS. Anesthetic considerations for LVRS include watching out for pneumothorax caused by a ruptured bleb, use of double-lumen tubes to allow selective ventilation and to facilitate surgery, using a lower F_{IO_2} to a goal SpO_2 of 90%, limiting the degree of positive-pressure ventilation (<30 cm H_2O peak inspiratory pressure), prolonging the expiratory time, and early extubation. Total IV anesthesia techniques using propofol and remifentanil or inhalational agents like desflurane with short-acting neuromuscular blocking agents help facilitate early extubation. If the patient cannot be extubated at the conclusion of the procedure, the double-lumen tube is exchanged for a single-lumen tube to decrease airway resistance.

40. **B.** Equal pressure point refers to the point in the airway where intraluminal pressure and extraluminal pressure (pleural) are the same. This is normally beyond the 11th to 13th generation of bronchioles where cartilaginous support is absent. This is the point where dynamic airway compression can occur—this refers to the phenomenon in which collapsible membranous portion of the airway gets compressed by the extraluminal pressure generated by a forced expiration. It is facilitated by the large pressure drop across the airways causing a higher gradient between extra and intraluminal pressures. Obstructive airway diseases predispose the patients to dynamic airway compression. Elastase deficiency in emphysema causes decreased elastic support in smaller airways. The bronchoconstriction and inflammation of asthma predisposes to reversal of transmural gradients. Such patients usually adapt by pursed-lip breathing and terminating the expiration early before functional residual capacity falls below closing capacity (auto PEEP). However, the increase in lung volume and slowing of expiration caused by such a maneuver helps to stent the airway open. The increase in lung volume

increases the intraluminal pressure and dilates the airways, and the slow expiration reduces the decrease in pressure from the alveoli to the mouth because lower driving pressures are sufficient for lesser flows. This shifts the equal pressure point to the noncollapsible larger airways or to the mouth.

41. C.   Any lesion causing a compression of the superior vena cava (SVC) and impedes blood return from head and neck can cause venous engorgement and edema of the head, neck, and arms. This is usually produced by a mediastinal tumor causing compression of the mediastinal structures including the SVC. It can also be caused by an occlusive thrombus in the SVC. Among the mediastinal neoplasms, lymphomas are the most common causes for SVC syndrome. But other mediastinal tumors like germ-cell tumors or pulmonary lesions with secondary lymphadenopathy may also be responsible. These cases are very difficult as induction of anesthesia in a supine position causes severe airway obstruction and cardiovascular collapse. The airway obstruction is due to direct mechanical compression as well as mucosal edema. Attempts should be made to decrease the size of the mass and the degree of mediastinal compression should be made prior to elective surgery. This includes radiation therapy, chemotherapy, and steroids. An empiric treatment with steroids may be attempted prior to a tissue diagnosis in this 12-year old. A preoperative echocardiogram can quantify the degree of compromise in cardiac function, presence of a thrombus, or dynamic inflow obstruction in the presence of pericardial fluid. A CT scan/MRI will help diagnose the presence of tracheomalacia/erosion and the level of the lesion. If induction of general anesthesia is required in the presence of SVC syndrome, awake fiberoptic intubation is the preferred method and inhalational anesthetics can be used to attain a deep plane of anesthesia in a spontaneously breathing patient after intubation. A rigid bronchoscope and ability to go on cardiopulmonary bypass are other precautionary measures that can be taken.

13

Neuroanesthesia

Dipty Mangla and Ashish Sinha

1. Total normal cerebral blood flow (CBF) is

   A. 25 mL/100 g/min
   B. 50 mL/100 g/min
   C. 100 mL/100 g/min
   D. 150 mL/100 g/min

2. The factor associated with maximum increase in intracranial pressure (ICP) is

   A. Increased central venous pressure to 14 mm Hg
   B. Hypercarbia with $Paco_2$ of 50 mm Hg
   C. Ventilation with positive end–expiratory pressure (PEEP) of 5 cm H_2O
   D. Bucking and coughing on endotracheal tube

3. Cerebral perfusion pressure (CPP) (mm Hg) in a patient with intracranial pressure (ICP) of 12 mm Hg, central venous pressure (CVP) of 15 mm Hg, and mean arterial pressure (MAP) of 70 mm Hg will be

   A. 58
   B. 55
   C. 52
   D. 48

4. Treatment of a patient with mannitol can lead to all the following, except

   A. Oliguria
   B. Hypotension
   C. Hypervolemia
   D. Hypokalemia

5. A patient is undergoing craniotomy for subdural hematoma. During the procedure, the surgeon requests lowering the intracranial pressure. All the following can be used, except

   A. Mannitol
   B. Hyperventilation
   C. Steroids
   D. Furosemide

6. The desired level of $Paco_2$ in a neurosurgical patient is

   A. 30 to 35 mm Hg
   B. 25 to 30 mm Hg
   C. 20 to 25 mm Hg
   D. 15 to 25 mm Hg

7. An absolute contraindication for electroconvulsive therapy (ECT) is

   A. Hypertension
   B. Pheochromocytoma
   C. Aortic aneurysm
   D. Stroke

8. Signs of air embolism in a patient include all, except

   A. Hypertension
   B. Heart murmur
   C. Arrhythmia
   D. Decreased $EtCO_2$

9. A 65-year-old male is undergoing surgery for medulloblastoma in the posterior fossa of brain. Approximately 1 hour into surgery you notice arrhythmias on the monitors. The next step will be

   A. Inform the surgeon
   B. Give β-blockers
   C. Administer lidocaine
   D. Give 100% oxygen

10. Nitrous oxide should be avoided in patients with

   A. Subdural hematoma
   B. Brain tumor
   C. Closed head injury
   D. Pneumocephalus

11. The following fluid should be avoided in a patient undergoing craniotomy

   A. Lactated Ringerés
   B. Normal saline
   C. Dextrose 5%—normal saline
   D. Hetastarch

12. Most sensitive method to detect air embolism is

   A. Transesophageal echocardiogram (TEE)
   B. Decreased end-tidal carbon dioxide
   C. Increased end-tidal nitrogen
   D. Mill wheel murmur

13. Best measure to reduce cerebral oxygen consumption includes

   A. Administration of barbiturates
   B. Hyperventilation
   C. Administration of opioids
   D. Institution of hypothermia

14. All of the following decrease cerebral blood flow (CBF), except

   A. Etomidate
   B. Propofol
   C. Thiopental
   D. Ketamine

15. In a patient undergoing craniotomy, the transducer of arterial line should be zeroed at the

    A. Level of hypothalamus
    B. Level of heart
    C. Level of external auditory meatus
    D. Level of atmosphere

16. Jugular venous oxygen saturation

    A. Estimates oxygen extraction
    B. Is unaffected by systemic hypoxia
    C. Involves placement of catheter through inferior vena cava
    D. Monitors global oxygenation of both cerebral hemispheres

17. The effect of ischemia on somatosensory-evoked potentials (SSEPs) is

    A. Decreased latency, decreased amplitude
    B. Increased latency, increased amplitude
    C. Decreased latency, increased amplitude
    D. Increased latency, decreased amplitude

18. A patient with spinal injury, sustained 3 hours ago, comes to the OR for exploratory laparotomy. Anesthetic management of the patient includes which of the following?

    A. Rapid-sequence induction with succinylcholine
    B. Hypothermia for better neurologic outcome
    C. Managing autonomic hyperreflexia
    D. Avoiding corticosteroids

19. The electrophysiological monitor most resistant to anesthetic agents is

    A. Somatosensory-evoked potentials
    B. Motor-evoked potentials
    C. Brain-stem auditory-evoked potentials
    D. Electroencephalography

20. The most reliable monitor for neurologic monitoring in a patient undergoing carotid endarterectomy is

    A. Electroencephalogram
    B. Jugular venous oxygen saturation
    C. Awake neurologic exam
    D. Stump pressure

21. Anesthetic management of a patient with multiple sclerosis (MS) includes

    A. Avoiding hypothermia
    B. Avoiding hyperthermia
    C. Spinal anesthesia is safe
    D. Use of succinylcholine can result in hypokalemia

22. All the following are true for Guillain–Barré syndrome (GBS), except

    A. Respiratory paralysis is frequent complication
    B. Presence of labile autonomic nervous system
    C. Ascending motor paralysis
    D. Exaggerated reflexes

23. True statement about autonomic hyperreflexia is

   A. Lesions below T10 is responsible for the reflex
   B. It can be treated with deep general anesthetic
   C. It is associated with vasoconstriction above the site of injury
   D. It can be provoked by thermal stimulation

24. A 16-year-old patient with acute lysergic acid diethylamide (LSD) intoxication and head injury comes to emergency room. All the following can be used in anesthetic management, except

   A. Propofol
   B. Succinylcholine
   C. Ketamine
   D. Phenylephrine

25. A 25-year-old patient with severe depression is undergoing an electroconvulsive therapy (ECT). The duration of seizure can be increased by

   A. Hypoventilating the patient
   B. Hyperventilating the patient
   C. Administering succinylcholine
   D. Administering rocuronium

26. All of the following are contraindications of electroconvulsive therapy (ECT), except

   A. Pacemaker
   B. Recent stroke
   C. Raised intracranial pressure
   D. Severe osteoporosis

27. True statement regarding cerebral physiology is

   A. Normal cerebral metabolic oxygen consumption is 5 mL/100g/min
   B. Normal Intracranial pressure (ICP) is approximately 15 mm Hg
   C. Normal cerebral blood flow (CBF) is 50 mL/100g/min
   D. Cerebral autoregulation is strictly maintained at blood pressures between 60 and 150 mm Hg in all patients

28. True statement about cerebrospinal fluid (CSF) is

   A. It is formed in the third ventricle
   B. It is absorbed in arachnoid granulations present in fourth ventricle
   C. Total volume of CSF is about 150 mL
   D. Major mechanism of formation is by passive diffusion of ions

29. A precordial Doppler can detect a minimal of ___ mL of intracardiac air:

   A. 0.1
   B. 0.25
   C. 0.5
   D. 1

30. The only inhalational anesthetic that can cause an isoelectric EEG among the following is

   A. Isoflurane
   B. Halothane
   C. Enflurane
   D. Nitrous oxide

31. Intraoperative anesthetic management of a patient undergoing cerebral aneurysm repair includes all, except

    A. Maintenance of hypotension
    B. Mannitol for facilitating surgical exposure
    C. Maintaining mild hypothermia
    D. Patient remaining intubated for 24 hours postoperatively

32. Which of the following types of neuromonitoring can be done in a patient undergoing transsphenoidal resection of a pituitary tumor?

    A. EEG
    B. Motor-evoked potentials
    C. Visual-evoked potentials
    D. Auditory-evoked potentials

33. The drug of choice for treating nausea and vomiting in a patient with parkinsonism would be

    A. Ondansetron
    B. Promethazine
    C. Droperidol
    D. Metoclopramide

34. All the following anesthetic agents can cause seizurelike activity on the electroencephalogram (EEG), except

    A. Ketamine
    B. Etomidate
    C. Enflurane
    D. Thiopental

35. The neuromuscular blocking agent relatively contraindicated in a patient with raised intracranial pressure (ICP) is

    A. Rocuronium
    B. Vecuronium
    C. Atracurium
    D. Cisatracurium

36. The afferent input for somatosensory-evoked potentials is carried by which spinal cord tract

    A. Corticospinal
    B. Dorsal columns
    C. Spinothalamic
    D. Spinocerebellar

37. You are called to evaluate a 50-year-old patient for brain death. All the following are criteria for brain death, except

    A. Apnea for 10 minutes
    B. Absence of corneal reflex
    C. Presence of spinal reflexes
    D. Decerebrate posturing

38. A 30-year-old male is found unresponsive outside a supermarket. The emergency response team finds him in ventricular fibrillation. After 10 minutes of CPR, the emergency response team is successful in reviving the patient. In the emergency room, it is decided to cool the patient to 34°C from 37°C. By this measure, the cerebral metabolic demand will decrease by

    A. 12%
    B. 18%
    C. 24%
    D. 30%

39. All the following are relative contraindications to a sitting craniotomy, except

    A. Right-to-left cardiac shunt
    B. Patent foramen ovale
    C. Ventriculoatrial shunt
    D. Ventriculoperitoneal shunt

40. An 80-year-old female comes to the ER with closed distal radial fracture. On further questioning, she gives a history of stroke about 2 weeks ago. How long should one wait before it can be assumed that her risk of perioperative stroke is same as a healthy 80-year-old?

    A. 6 days
    B. 6 weeks
    C. 6 months
    D. 6 years

41. A 28-year-old male is being treated in the ICU for raised intracranial pressure (ICP). All the following measures can aid in decreasing ICP *quickly*, except

    A. Corticosteroids
    B. Hyperventilation to $Paco_2$ of 30 mm Hg
    C. Mannitol
    D. Head elevation to 30 degrees

42. Which of the following agents will have the least effect on somatosensory-evoked potentials (SSEPs)?

    A. Vecuronium
    B. Propofol
    C. Fentanyl
    D. Nitrous oxide

43. Signs and symptoms of raised intracranial hypertension include all the following, except

    A. Hypertension
    B. Tachycardia
    C. Bradycardia
    D. Irregular respiration

44. Etomidate in a dose of 0.2 mg/kg can lead to all the following, except

    A. Abolish ventilatory response to carbon dioxide
    B. Increase amplitude and latency of somatosensory-evoked potentials (SSEPs)
    C. Decrease cerebral metabolic oxygen demand
    D. Decrease cerebral blood flow (CBF)

45. The most important factor governing cerebral blood flow (CBF) is

    A. Cerebral metabolic oxygen demand
    B. $Paco_2$
    C. pH
    D. Cerebral perfusion pressure

46. The following graph depicts the relationship between cerebral perfusion and

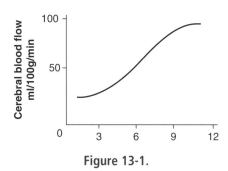

Figure 13-1.

    A. $Paco_2$
    B. Pao_2
    C. Mean arterial pressure
    D. Cerebrospinal fluid pH

47. The following graph depicts the relationship between cerebral perfusion and

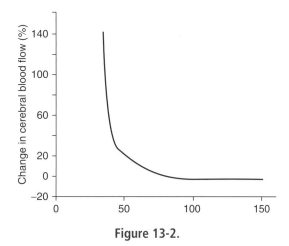

Figure 13-2.

    A. $Paco_2$
    B. Pao_2
    C. Mean arterial pressure
    D. Cerebrospinal fluid pH

48. A 45-year-old male is seen in the preadmission testing for pituitary adenoma resection surgery. All the following would be expected if this adenoma was causing acromegaly, except

    A. Hypotension
    B. Obstructive sleep apnea
    C. Difficult airway
    D. Hyperglycemia

49. The fastest measure to decrease intracranial pressure (ICP) in a patient is

    A. Mannitol
    B. Dexamethasone
    C. Furosemide
    D. Hyperventilation

50. Therapy for cerebral vasospasm includes

    A. Hypertension, hypervolemia, hemodilution
    B. Normotension, euvolemia, hypocarbia
    C. Hypotension, hypovolemia, hypocarbia
    D. Hypertension, hypervolemia, hypocarbia

CHAPTER 13 ANSWERS

1. **B.** Normal total CBF is about 50 mL/100 g/min. CBF below 20 mL/100 g/min is associated with cerebral ischemia. CBF is modulated by various factors, which include $Paco_2$, Pao_2, blood pressure, intracranial pressure, etc.

2. **D.** Intracranial pressure is supratentorial CSF pressure measured in the lateral ventricles or cerebral cortex. Normal ICP is 10 mm Hg or less. Between $Paco_2$ values of 20 and 80 mm Hg, CBF increases by 1 mL/100 g/min and cerebral blood volume increases by 0.05 mL/110g/min per mm Hg increase in $Paco_2$. Increase in CVP and adding PEEP will minimally increase ICP by affecting venous return. Coughing and bucking can cause a much higher increase in ICP (acute increase) than any of the above factors.

3. **B.** CPP = MAP − ICP or CVP, whichever is higher.
    Thus, CPP = 70 − 15 = 55 mm Hg.

4. **A.** Mannitol, a six-carbon sugar, is the most commonly used diuretic in neuroanesthesia practice. It is an osmotic diuretic and undergoes little or no reabsorption. It also improves renal blood flow. Side effects include an initial increase in circulatory volume, which can cause pulmonary edema. Diuresis attributed to mannitol can lead to hypovolemia and hypokalemia.

5. **C.** Treatment of intracranial hypertension includes hyperventilation to $Paco_2$ of 25 to 30 mm Hg, improving CSF drainage by elevating the head by 30 degrees or surgical placement of CSF drain, using an osmotic diuretic (mannitol), hypertonic saline, decompression craniectomy, barbiturates, and corticosteroids. The latter have been used to decrease cerebral edema, and take a few hours to have effect, but routine use of corticosteroids in managing intracranial hypertension is not recommended.

6. **B.** $Paco_2$ is the most potent physiologic determinant of cerebral blood flow. Maximal reductions in ICP can be achieved by decreasing $Paco_2$ to 25 to 28 mm Hg, and the reduction in ICP lasts up to 24 to 36 hours.

7. **B.** ECT is commonly used for treatment of refractory major depression. It involves using electricity to shock one or both cerebral hemispheres to induce a seizure lasting 30 to 60 seconds. Contraindications to ECT include pheochromocytoma, recent myocardial infarction (<3 months), recent stroke (<1 month), intracranial mass or increased ICP, angina, poorly controlled heart failure, significant pulmonary disease, bone fractures, severe osteoporosis, pregnancy, glaucoma, and retinal detachment.

8. **A.** Clinical signs of venous air embolism include a decrease in end-tidal CO_2, a decrease in arterial oxygen saturation, sudden hypotension, mill wheel murmur, and even sudden circulatory arrest. Presence of a patent foramen ovale, which has an incidence of 20% in adults, can lead to paradoxical air embolism, with the potential of causing coronary ischemia or a stroke.

9. **A.** For posterior fossa tumor resection, the patient is frequently placed in the sitting or prone position. Monitoring of the patient includes arterial blood pressure line, a central venous catheter (for access, pressure monitoring, aspiration of any air—if required), and a precordial Doppler to detect intracardiac air (venous air embolism). Operations on posterior fossa tumors can injure vital brain-stem respiratory and circulatory nuclei, resulting in hemodynamic fluctuations or depression of ventilation. The surgeon should be informed at the first sign of cardiac arrhythmias.

10. **D.** Nitrous oxide can diffuse into closed air spaces, which may be of significant clinical consequences. The blood/gas coefficient of nitrous oxide is 0.47, whereas that of nitrogen

is 0.015. This means that nitrous oxide is about 33 times more diffusible than nitrogen. As a result, at any given partial pressure, far more nitrous oxide can be carried into a closed gas space than nitrogen removed. Thus, nitrous oxide can quickly expand closed gas spaces, such as middle ear or a pneumothorax.

11. **C.**   In a patient undergoing craniotomy, intravenous fluid replacement should be performed by using glucose-free isotonic crystalloid or colloid solutions. Hyperglycemia is known to worsen ischemic brain injury.

12. **A.**   The most sensitive intraoperative monitor for detecting venous air embolism is TEE. The second best monitor is precordial Doppler sonography, which can detect as little as 0.25 mL of air. Changes in end-tidal respiratory gas concentrations, such as nitrogen and carbon dioxide, and changes in pulmonary artery pressures are less sensitive. Hypotension and mill wheel murmur are late manifestations of venous air embolism.

13. **D.**   Hypothermia is one of the most effective methods for protecting the brain against ischemia. Hypothermia decreases both basal and electrical metabolic requirements throughout the brain, unlike intravenous anesthetic agents or hyperventilation.

14. **D.**   Propofol, barbiturates, and etomidate produce dose-dependent decreases in cerebral metabolic rate and CBF. Ketamine is the only induction agent that dilates the cerebral vasculature and thus increases CBF (50% to 60%).

15. **C.**   In a seated patient, the arterial pressure in the brain differs significantly from left ventricular pressure. Cerebral perfusion pressure is determined by setting the transducer to zero at the level of the ear, which approximates the circle of Willis.

16. **D.**   Jugular venous bulb oximetry involves placing a sampling catheter in the internal jugular vein (IJV). The normal range for mixed venous oxygen saturation at IJV is 50% to 75%. It gives an estimate of balance between oxygen supply and demand of the brain, and measures global cerebral oxygenation (not focal).

17. **D.**   SSEPs reflect the integrity of neuronal pathway from the peripheral nerves through the spinal cord (dorsal columns) to the brain. SSEPs are electrical manifestations of the central nervous system response to external stimulation. Intraoperative changes in amplitude or latency or complete loss of waveforms are indicators of compromised sensory pathway integrity. SSEP amplitude loss greater than 50% or a latency increase greater than 10% is considered significant.

18. **A.**   In the early management of acute spinal injury patients, particular emphasis should be placed on preventing further spinal damage, which may occur during patient movement, airway manipulation, and positioning. High-dose corticosteroids are often administered to help improve neurological outcome. The head and neck should be stabilized using manual inline stabilization, and awake fiberoptic intubation should be considered in high cervical injuries. Patients with high cord transections may have impaired airway reflexes, hypotension, and bradycardia and may be prone to hypothermia in view of generalized vasodilation. Succinylcholine can be used safely in first 24 hours following spinal injury.

19. **C.**   Somatosensory- and motor-evoked potential monitoring is commonly used to detect ischemia of spinal cord in spine surgeries. Brain-stem auditory–evoked responses monitor ischemia during posterior fossa surgeries. Inhalational agents in general increase the latency and decrease the amplitude of evoked potentials (if used at more than 0.5–0.75 MAC). The effect of inhalational anesthetics on evoked potentials in decreasing order is visual > motor > somatosensory > brain-stem auditory.

20. **C.** Awake neurological status is the most reliable method to detect cerebral ischemia. In patients undergoing carotid endarterectomy under local anesthesia and mild sedation, global and focal neurological status can be continuously assessed. In patients undergoing carotid endarterectomy under general anesthetic indirect methods to detect cerebral ischemia can be used. These include EEG monitoring, transcranial Doppler, arteriography, and measurement of blood flow using xenon.

21. **B.** MS is characterized by progressive demyelination in the brain and spinal cord. Stress, anesthesia, and surgery can have detrimental effects on the course of the disease. Elective surgery should be avoided in acute relapse of MS. Regarding the effect of anesthetic technique on MS, spinal anesthesia can exacerbate MS symptoms, epidural anesthesia usually does not affect MS, succinylcholine should be avoided to prevent hyperkalemia, and hyperthermia should be avoided as an increase in temperature may block nerve conduction. Advanced MS may be associated with autonomic dysfunction.

22. **D.** GBS affects about 2/100,000 people. It is characterized by a sudden onset ascending motor paralysis, areflexia, and paresthesias. Bulbar involvement with respiratory failure is a frequent complication. Succinylcholine should be avoided in these patients, as it can cause hyperkalemia. Regional anesthesia may make GBS worse. Anesthetic management may be complicated by liability of the autonomic nervous system (hypotension or hypertension).

23. **B.** Autonomic hyperreflexia is seen in patients with spinal cord injury at or above T6. It is characterized by acute generalized sympathetic hyperactivity in response to a triggering stimulus. The triggering stimulus can be any stimulus occurring below the level of the lesion, and is most commonly a distension of hollow viscera (bowel or bladder). Clinical signs include severe hypertension, bradycardia, arrhythmias, profuse sweating, vasodilation above the level of lesion, and pallor and vasoconstriction below the level of lesion. Antihypertensives may have to be utilized to treat the hypertension. Spinal anesthesia (not preferred because of technical difficulty and unpredictable level) or deep general anesthesia has been used in preventing autonomic hyperreflexia.

24. **C.** LSD is a hallucinogen and causes CNS excitation, sensory distortion, delusions, hallucinations, and euphoria. Autonomic effects, mediated via the hypothalamus, include tachycardia, hypertension, mydriasis, piloerection, salivation, lacrimation, and vomiting. In view of hypertension and tachycardia that can be caused by LSD, ketamine should be avoided.

25. **B.** Propofol when used for induction in patients undergoing ECT can increase the seizure threshold and decrease the duration of the seizure. Hyperventilation and administration of caffeine or etomidate can increase seizure duration. Muscle relaxants do not affect the threshold or duration of the seizure.

26. **A.** Contraindications to ECT include recent myocardial infarction (<3 months), a recent stroke (<1 month), an intracranial mass and raised intracranial pressure, angina, poorly controlled congestive heart failure, significant pulmonary disease, bone fractures, severe osteoporosis, pregnancy, glaucoma, and retinal detachment.

27. **C.** The cerebral metabolic rate is reflected by oxygen consumption, which is about 3 to 3.8 mL/100 g/min. Total CBF averages 50 mL/100 g/min. In normal individuals, CBF remains nearly constant between mean arterial pressures of about 60 and 160 mm Hg. The cerebral autoregulation curve is shifted to right in patients with chronic arterial hypertension. ICP by convention means supratentorial CSF pressure measured in the lateral ventricles or over the cerebral cortex, and the normal CSF pressure is 10 mm Hg or less.

28. **C.** CSF is formed by the choroid plexuses of cerebral lateral ventricles. In adults, normal CSF production is about 20 mL/hour with a total volume of 150 mL. The CSF is absorbed in arachnoid granulations over cerebral hemispheres. CSF formation involves active secretion of sodium in the choroid plexuses, and not passive diffusion.

29. **B.** A precordial Doppler can detect as little as 0.25 mL of intracardiac air. A precordial Doppler is the next best sensitive indicator to detect intracardiac air after a transesophageal echocardiogram.

30. **A.** Isoflurane can produce an isoelectric EEG at 2 to 2.5 MAC, while enflurane typically produces a spike and wave pattern at 2 to 3 MAC. Seizure activity may be seen on EEG with 3% enflurane in a hypocapnic patient. Halothane causes slowing of EEG activity with increasing concentration until 4 MAC, after which it produces uniform activity. Increasing sevoflurane concentration from 2 to 5 MAC changes the cortical EEG pattern from a high-amplitude slow wave to burst suppression to an isoelectric EEG interspersed with spikes.

31. **D.** Intraoperative management of cerebral aneurysms should include availability of blood, avoidance of hypertension during induction, central venous pressure and arterial blood pressure monitoring, mannitol after the dura is opened to help surgical exposure, elective hypotension as it decreases transmural pressure across the aneurysm (avoiding rupture), administration of thiopental and mild hypothermia for cerebral protection, and awake extubation depending on neurological status.

32. **C.** The transsphenoidal or bifrontal craniotomy approach may be used to gain access to pituitary gland. The former (transsphenoidal approach) has several advantages including elimination of frontal lobe retraction, microsurgical removal of small adenomas, reduced blood loss, and shorter hospital stay. Patients are intubated endotracheally (oral), and oropharyngeal packing is done to prevent bleeding into the esophagus. Additionally, epinephrine or cocaine may be injected submucosally to reduce bleeding. The cavernous sinus forms the lateral border of the sella turcica and includes the internal carotid artery, venous structures, and cranial nerves III, IV, V, and VI. Therefore, visual-evoked potentials may be monitored in the OR for early detection of visual pathway damage.

33. **A.** Parkinson disease is a movement disorder that affects individuals 50 to 70 years of age. It is caused by progressive loss of dopamine in the nigrostriatum. Patients have bradykinesia, postural instability, rigidity, facial masking, and a resting pill-rolling tremor. Antidopaminergic activity associated with butyrophenones, phenothiazines, and metoclopramide can worsen symptoms and thus these should be avoided.

34. **D.** Ketamine, etomidate, and enflurane can cause seizurelike activity on the EEG. Thiopental increases the threshold and decreases the duration of seizure activity.

35. **C.** In a patient with increased intracranial pressure, a nondepolarizing muscle relaxant is commonly used to facilitate controlled ventilation and tracheal intubation. Rocuronium and vecuronium are commonly used as they provide the greatest hemodynamic stability. Succinylcholine and atracurium (due to associated histamine release) may increase ICP, particularly if intubation is attempted before deep general anesthesia. Hyperventilation prior to intubation is utilized to decrease the ICP.

36. **B.** Somatosensory-evoked potentials are transmitted through the following pathway:

    peripheral stimulus → peripheral nerve → dorsal root ganglia → first-order fibers in the ipsilateral posterior column to dorsal column nuclei → second-order fibers crossing to the opposite side → medial lemniscus to the thalamus → third-order fibers continuing to the frontoparietal sensory-motor cortex.

37. **D.** Brain death is irreversible cessation of all brain activity. Generally accepted clinical criteria for brain death include presence of coma, absence of motor activity, absence of brain-stem reflexes (papillary, corneal, vestibule–ocular, and gag/cough), absence of ventilatory effort ($Paco_2$ >60 mm Hg), exclusion of hypothermia or effect of sedatives, isoelectric EEG, and absence of cerebral perfusion by angiography.

38. B.   Cerebral metabolic rate decreases by 6% per degree Celsius decrease in body temperature below 37°C. Hence, a 3°C drop in temperature will decrease the cerebral metabolic rate by 18%.

39. D.   The incidence of venous air embolism in sitting craniotomies is about 20% to 40%. The presence of right-to-left shunt can cause paradoxical air embolism. Air embolism can have catastrophic consequences, such as coronary ischemia and stroke. Thus, sitting position should be avoided in patients with a right-to-left shunt, patent foramen ovale, or ventriculoatrial shunt.

40. B.   Regional blood flow and metabolic rate are normal after 2 weeks following a stroke. Alterations in CO_2 responsiveness and blood–brain barrier abnormalities require more than 4 weeks to be corrected. Thus, most clinicians postpone elective surgery for at least 6 weeks following stroke.

41. A.   Definitive treatment of intracranial hypertension is ideally directed at the underlying cause. Treatment modalities include fluid restriction, head elevation, osmotic agents and loop diuretics, moderate hyperventilation (up to 24–36 hours), avoidance of hypotension, hypoxia and hypercarbia, and corticosteroids. The latter is used to decrease cerebral edema in patients with known intracranial tumors, and take a few hours to take effect.

42. A.   Inhalational volatile anesthetics produce an increase in latency and decrease in amplitude of evoked potentials. Nitrous oxide produces a decrease in amplitude with no change in latency. Propofol decreases amplitude and an increase in latency of SSEPs. Muscle relaxants have no effect on SSEPs. Narcotics cause dose-dependent decrease in amplitude and increase in latency.

43. B.   Increased intracranial pressure (ICP) can lead to altered mental status, intractable vomiting, and focal or global neurological deficits. Clinical signs include hypertension, bradycardia, irregular respiration, and pupillary changes (papilledema may be seen on fundoscopy). Cushing triad consists of raised ICP, hypertension, and bradycardia.

44. A.   Etomidate decreases cerebral metabolic rate, CBF, leading to a decrease in intracranial pressure. It enhances SSEP. It is a sedative hypnotic but lacks analgesic properties. Ventilation is affected to a lesser extent with etomidate when compared to barbiturates or benzodiazepines. Induction doses usually do not result in apnea.

45. A.   Increased metabolic activity leads to an increase in CBF. Regional CBF parallels metabolic activity and can vary from 10 to 300 mL/100 g/min. For example, motor activity of a limb is associated with a rapid increase in regional blood flow of the corresponding motor cortex.

46. A. CO_2 gas tension has the greatest influence on cerebral blood flow (CBF). Between a $Paco_2$ of 20 and 80 mm Hg, CBF changes approximately 1 to 2 mL/100 g/min per mm Hg in $Paco_2$.

47. B.   Marked changes in Pao_2 affect cerebral blood flow (CBF), although minimally. Hyperoxia is associated with only minimal decreases in CBF. On the other hand, hypoxemia ($Pao_2 < 50$ mm Hg) greatly increases CBF.

48. A.   The acromegalic patient suffers from general overgrowth of skeletal, soft, and connective tissues. This results in coarse facial features and enlarged hands and feet. Patients may also have a difficult airway because of overgrowth of soft tissues of upper airway, enlargement of tongue and epiglottis, overgrowth of mandible with increased distance from lips to vocal cords, and glottic and subglottic narrowing. These changes may also lead to obstructive sleep apnea. Patients also are prone to hyperglycemia, hypertension, congestive heart failure, increased lung volumes, increased ventilation–perfusion mismatch, peripheral neuropathy, skeletal muscle weakness, osteoarthritis, and osteoporosis.

49. D. The quickest way to reduce ICP in a patient is hyperventilation, often to a $Paco_2$ of 25 mm Hg. Reduced $Paco_2$ (hypocarbia) causes cerebral vasoconstriction leading to a reduction in cerebral blood flow and cerebral blood volume. However, hyperventilation is only used as a temporizing measure only in periods of acute raised ICP.

50. A. Cerebral vasospasm occurs in about one-third of patients surviving the initial aneurysmal rupture, and carries a high degree of morbidity and mortality. The degree of vasospasm depends on the degree of initial subarachnoid hemorrhage. Vasospasm usually develops 3 to 14 days postsubarachnoid hemorrhage results in narrowing of cerebral blood vessels and decreased blood flow distally. This may lead to an ischemic deficit and cerebral infarction, if left untreated. Therapies for cerebral vasospasm include "triple-H therapy" (hypertension/hypervolemia/hemodilution), balloon angioplasty, and intra-arterial nicardipine and other vasodilators.

14

Gastrointestinal, Liver, and Renal Diseases

Thoha Pham

1. A 38-year-old woman with a history of diverticulosis is scheduled for an exploratory laparotomy for lysis of adhesions. Which of the following is the best way of maintaining core body temperature during the initial hour of general endotracheal anesthetic?

   A. Providing warm and humidified inspired gases
   B. Increasing ambient temperature
   C. Administration of warm intravenous fluids
   D. Use of warm irrigating fluids

2. Each of the following would be expected in an otherwise-healthy 125-kg (BMI 40 kg/m^2) man undergoing open cholecystectomy, except

   A. Decreased functional residual capacity
   B. Increased intra-abdominal pressure and risk of reflux
   C. Increased metabolism of volatile anesthetics
   D. Decreased metabolism of atracurium

3. Which of the following has a dual effect of increasing gastric pH, and decreasing the gastric volume to minimize risks associated with aspiration?

   A. Prochlorperazine
   B. Ranitidine
   C. Ondansetron
   D. Metoclopramide

4. This finding is indicative of microatelectasis on the second postoperative day after major abdominal surgery:

   A. Hypercarbia
   B. Hypoxemia
   C. Diffuse wheezing
   D. Tactile fremitus

5. A morbidly obese 60-year-old man with a 65-pack year history of tobacco smoking is awake after an uncomplicated general anesthetic with sevoflurane for routine endoscopy and colonoscopy screening. After 45 minutes in the recovery room (PACU), while breathing 6 L/min of oxygen via nasal cannula, his pulse oximetry drops to 88%. His rest of the vital signs are stable, and the lungs are clear to auscultation. The most effective management at this point is

   A. Coughing with deep breathing
   B. Reintubation of the trachea
   C. Intravenous administration of doxapram
   D. Continuous positive-airway pressure

6. During rapid-sequence induction of anesthesia for emergent laparotomy to explore multiple stab wounds, a 45-year-old man vomits a large quantity of undigested food particles. During intubation of the trachea, food particles are noted near the cords. After instituting ventilation with 100% oxygen, the most appropriate next step in this patient's management is

   A. Place patient in Trendelenburg position
   B. Ventilate with positive end–expiratory pressure of 15 cm H_2O
   C. Administer corticosteroids
   D. Administer antibiotics

7. A 71-year-old female develops a severe case of diarrhea with multiple loose bowel movements since awakening this morning. When she arrives preoperatively for her surgery, an arterial blood gas (ABG) is obtained. The most likely finding would be

   A. $pH = 7.30$, $Paco_2 = 50$, $Pao_2 = 60$, $HCO_3^- = 24$
   B. $pH = 7.35$, $Paco_2 = 32$, $Pao_2 = 85$, $HCO_3^- = 18$
   C. $pH = 7.45$, $Paco_2 = 30$, $Pao_2 = 80$, $HCO_3^- = 28$
   D. $pH = 7.40$, $Paco_2 = 45$, $Pao_2 = 85$, $HCO_3^- = 15$

8. A 65-year-old patient is noted to have excessive bleeding during a colectomy with an activated clotting time (ACT) of 200 seconds. The most unlikely reason for this oozing is

   A. Undiagnosed factor VII deficiency
   B. Prior administration of heparin 5,000 U subcutaneously
   C. Preoperative ingestion of aspirin and ibuprofen
   D. Dilutional thrombocytopenia

9. During laparotomy, a patient has required infusion of 4 L of lactated Ringer's and 4 U of packed red blood cells (pRBCs). As the fifth unit of pRBCs begins infusing, patient has sudden onset of tachycardia and hypotension. Within a few minutes, Foley bag reveals dark urine. The most likely cause of unexplained oozing is

   A. Hemolytic transfusion reaction
   B. Leukoagglutinin reaction
   C. Dilutional thrombocytopenia
   D. Dilutional coagulopathy

Questions 10 to 12

A 26-year-old male patient with a history of severe ulcerative colitis, unresponsive to conservative measures, presents for elective open total abdominal colectomy with end ileostomy. He has been unable to eat for the last 2 weeks and was started on total parenteral nutrition (TPN) several days prior.

10. Intraoperative effect that should be expected and monitored for is

    A. Dilutional anemia
    B. Hyperglycemia
    C. Sepsis
    D. Hyperphosphatemia

11. At the conclusion of the surgery, the patient fails to regain consciousness. The metabolic complication of TPN (Table 14-1) that is likely is

Table 14-1 Metabolic Complications of TPN.

Glucose (hypoglycemia, hyperosmolar nonketotic coma)
Protein (hyperammonemia)
Hypercalcemia
Hypophosphatemia
Essential fatty acid deficiency
Vitamin toxicity

- **A.** Azotemia
- **B.** Hyperkalemia
- **C.** Hyperosmolar ketotic hyperglycemia
- **D.** Hyperosmolar nonketotic hyperglycemia

12. Consider that the patient opens his eyes and is extubated in the operating room. However, 15 minutes after arriving to the recovery room (PACU) he is unable to maintain adequate ventilation and oxygenation. Physical exam reveals profound global weakness with absent reflexes. The specific electrolyte abnormality that should be evaluated considering his TPN requirement is

- **A.** Potassium
- **B.** Phosphate
- **C.** Sodium
- **D.** Glucose

13. Each of the following statements about the preoperative management of an adrenal pheochromocytoma is true, except

- **A.** Adequate blockade can be assessed by in-house blood pressures <160/90 mm Hg for 24 hours prior to surgery
- **B.** β-Blockers should be administered only in conjunction with adequate α-blockade
- **C.** Administration of α-blocker can decrease operative mortality
- **D.** Nasal congestion is a sign of inadequate α-adrenergic block

14. A 40-year-old man undergoing an open resection of a pheochromocytoma under isoflurane general endotracheal anesthesia suddenly develops tachycardia, hypertension, and multifactorial ventricular ectopy. Each of the following could be considered an appropriate treatment option, except

- **A.** Switching from isoflurane to sevoflurane
- **B.** Intravenous vasodilator
- **C.** Intravenous α-blocker
- **D.** Intravenous lidocaine

15. An otherwise-healthy 38-year-old female patient is undergoing repair of a large ventral hernia under intrathecal anesthesia. A T2 sensory level is obtained with hyperbaric bupivacaine prior to incision. A false statement concerning this situation includes

- **A.** Effective cough is preserved
- **B.** The cardioaccelerator nerves are blocked
- **C.** Examination of the biceps reveals full strength bilaterally
- **D.** Bupivacaine binds to the intracellular portion of sodium channels

16. A patient with cholestasis presents for preoperative evaluation with laboratory findings revealing normal aspartate aminotransferase (serum glutamic–oxaloacetic transaminase) and prothrombin time but with a markedly elevated alkaline phosphatase. He will need a muscle relaxant for upcoming colon surgery. Which of the following anesthetic scenarios should be considered?

   A. Prolonged duration of vecuronium action
   B. Increase intubating dose of atracurium
   C. Prolonged duration of succinylcholine action
   D. Shortened duration of pancuronium action

17. An alcoholic 62-year-old male patient is noted to have jaundice one day after a laparoscopic cholecystectomy under halothane/fentanyl general endotracheal anesthesia. Bilirubin and alkaline phosphatase are elevated, but alanine aminotransferase (serum glutamic–pyruvic transaminase [SGPT]) and aspartate aminotransferase (serum glutamic–oxaloacetic transaminase [SGOT]) are within normal ranges. Of note, all values were within normal limits in this patient preoperatively. The most likely cause of his jaundice is

   A. Idiopathic halothane hepatic injury
   B. Worsening of underlying chronic liver dysfunction
   C. Posthepatic biliary obstruction
   D. Intravenous acetaminophen administration

18. An initial bolus of pancuronium was administered to a patient with end-stage liver disease with associated ascites for general anesthesia. Appropriate anesthetic considerations include all of the following, except

   A. Increased sympathomimetic activity due to vagolysis
   B. Intense histamine release immediately after administration
   C. Larger volume of distribution requiring initial larger doses
   D. Longer duration of action requiring smaller maintenance doses

19. A chronic alcoholic patient with liver cirrhosis is likely to demonstrate all of the following during administration of anesthesia, except

   A. A high minimum alveolar concentration (MAC) for desflurane
   B. Opioid hyperalgesia
   C. Resistance to the hypnotic effects of thiopental
   D. Resistance to the analgesic effects of opiates

20. A woman with long-standing alcoholic cirrhosis (Child-Turcotte-Pugh B) presents to the emergency room for chronic shortness of breath and abdominal pain. A review of her lab findings reveal a hematocrit concentration of 36% (hemoglobin 12.4 g/dL) with an arterial blood gas revealing a PaO_2 of 65 mm Hg breathing a FIO_2 of 0.5 via face mask. Her vitals are a blood pressure of 135/60 mm Hg and a heart rate of 88 bpm. The most likely cause of her hypoxemia is

   A. Intrahepatic arteriovenous shunts
   B. Intrapulmonary arteriovenous shunts
   C. Anemia
   D. Decreased cardiac output

21. Which of the following cardiovascular abnormalities is *least* likely to be present in a patient with end-stage alcoholic cirrhosis

   A. Resting tachycardia
   B. Widened pulse pressure
   C. Increased peripheral vascular resistance
   D. Increased cardiac output

Questions 22 to 23

A 120-kg diabetic male is scheduled for emergent pinning of his mandible after a motor vehicle accident. His wife reports that he snores loudly every night with occurrences of breathing cessation. Medical history is also significant for hypertension controlled with a diuretic. On physical examination, he has a large tongue and a wide neck with inadequate mouth opening revealing a Mallampati grade 4 view. His BMI is 38 kg/m^2 with a neck circumference of 44 cm.

22. Arterial blood gas (ABG) finding that would confirm Pickwickian syndrome is

   A. pH = 7.44, $Paco_2$ = 44, Pao_2 = 90, HCO_3 = 24
   B. pH = 7.35, $Paco_2$ = 44, Pao_2 = 65, HCO_3 = 26
   C. pH = 7.42, $Paco_2$ = 36, Pao_2 = 80, HCO_3 = 22
   D. pH = 7.37, $Paco_2$ = 55, Pao_2 = 67, HCO_3 = 28

23. The dose of thiopental required for rapid-sequence induction would be *increased*, as compared with what would be required at his ideal body weight, because of changes in

   A. Decreased basal metabolic rate
   B. Increased blood volume
   C. Increased muscle mass
   D. Decreased liver metabolism

24. A patient with chronic liver disease is scheduled for a laparoscopic abdominal operation. The risk of mortality during surgery for this patient is assessed using

   A. Mayo end-stage liver disease
   B. Child-Turcotte-Pugh score
   C. Ranson criteria
   D. Alvarado score

25. The variable *not* used to calculate an MELD (model for end-stage liver disease) score to prioritize patients for liver transplantation is

   A. Creatinine
   B. INR (international normalized ratio)
   C. Bilirubin
   D. Albumin

Questions 26 to 28

A 30-year-old male patient without preoperative renal dysfunction is undergoing a primary orthotopic liver transplant (OLT) for failure due to inherited α_1-antitrypsin deficiency.

26. During cross-clamping of the suprahepatic inferior vena cava (IVC), the most accurate effect created by use of venovenous bypass (VVB) is that it

   A. Induces urinary retention
   B. Prevents metabolic acidosis
   C. Requires heparinization
   D. Supports cardiac output

27. Immediately before unclamping and reperfusion of the transplanted liver, sodium bicarbonate and calcium chloride are administered intravenously to *counteract*

   A. Coagulopathy
   B. Decreased cardiac output
   C. Increased systemic vascular resistance
   D. Hypertension

28. At the end of the case as the drapes are taken down, diffuse microvascular bleeding is noted in this patient who required 15 U of blood during his intraoperative course. Platelet count is 40,000/mm^3, prothrombin time is 18 seconds, activated partial thromboplastin time (PTT) is 54 seconds, D-dimer is 2,000 ng/mL, and serum fibrinogen concentration is 40 mg/dL. The most likely cause of bleeding is

A. Disseminated intravascular coagulation (DIC)
B. Abnormal platelet function
C. Depressed levels of factor VIII
D. Citrate toxicity

29. A patient presents for preoperative evaluation for upcoming surgery. He has a history of liver transplantation 2 years ago, otherwise feeling well. Which of the following is most likely to be present during preoperative evaluation?

A. Elevated serum creatinine concentration
B. Hypoalbuminemia
C. Prolonged partial thromboplastin time
D. Hypocalcemia

30. Following a gastric bypass procedure, a 130-kg woman is extubated and breathing spontaneously in the recovery room (PACU). She is breathing at a rate of 24 breaths/min on 10 L/min of oxygen via nasal cannula, and is complaining of continued subjective dyspnea. Arterial blood gas analysis shows Pao_2 = 95 mm Hg, $Paco_2$ = 44 mm Hg, and pH = 7.37. The parameter most closely related to her increased alveolar–arterial oxygen-tension gradient is

A. Decreased minute volume
B. Decreased functional residual volume
C. Decreased expiratory reserve volume
D. Decreased respiratory drive

31. During laparoscopic cholecystectomy, the risk of failure to visualize contrast material entering the duodenum during intraoperative cholangiogram is highest with the administration of

A. Buprenorphine
B. Nalbuphine
C. Morphine
D. Naloxone

32. Drugs that can decrease or reduce opioid-induced biliary spasm include all of the following, except

A. Diltiazem
B. Atropine
C. Metoclopramide
D. Glucagon

33. Each of the following is associated with delayed gastric emptying, except

A. Diabetes mellitus
B. Celiac plexus block
C. Vagotomy
D. μ-Receptor agonism

Questions 34 to 39

A 33-year-old otherwise-healthy female suffering from moderately severe abdominal pain of unclear etiology is set to undergo an exploratory laparoscopy. The abdominal cavity is insufflated using carbon dioxide (CO_2).

34. All of the following are correct statements regarding pathophysiologic changes associated with creation of the pneumoperitoneum, except

    A. Increased risk of reflux and aspiration
    B. Decreased venous return
    C. Decreased systemic vascular resistance (SVR)
    D. Increased intrathoracic pressures

35. Inherent risks of abdominal laparoscopy include

    A. Renal failure
    B. Bronchospasm
    C. Gas emboli
    D. Hypothermia

36. The patient is placed in a steep Trendelenburg position. Her oxygen saturation begins to gradually decline over the course of several minutes while being ventilated with 100% oxygen ($F_{IO_2} = 1.0$). The initial step in the management of her hypoxemia is

    A. Add positive end–expiratory pressure (PEEP)
    B. Intravenous bolus of 500 mL saline
    C. Reposition the patient
    D. Switch to pressure support ventilation

37. The exploratory surgery progresses slowly. Over the next 3 hours, her $EtCO_2$ begins to gradually rise, requiring increasing minute ventilation. All of the following contribute to the degree of systemic CO_2 absorption, except

    A. Solubility of the gas
    B. Intra-abdominal pressures (IAP)
    C. Duration of surgery
    D. Blood pressure

38. Each of the following is hemodynamic change associated with hypercarbia, except

    A. Arrhythmias
    B. Bradycardia
    C. High cardiac output
    D. Low systemic vascular resistance (SVR)

39. The surgery continues on with a request to increase the pneumoperitoneum to 30 mm Hg to improve the surgical view. All of the following are appropriate in the differential diagnosis for hypotension during laparoscopy, except

    A. Compression of the inferior vena cava
    B. Increase cardiac afterload
    C. Too small blood pressure cuff
    D. CO_2 embolism

40. This physical exam finding is *inappropriately* paired with the possible nerve injury resulting from ill positioning during surgery:

    A. Inability to evert the foot   common peroneal nerve
    B. Inability to stand on toes   sciatic nerve
    C. Difficulty climbing stairs   femoral nerve injury
    D. Foot drop   saphenous nerve injury

41. A 50-year-old male patient is to undergo an open nephrectomy for renal carcinoma. The patient requests an epidural for perioperative pain management, as he is strongly intolerant to μ-agonist opiate therapy with nausea and vomiting. After a T2 sensory level is obtained, the patient is induced with propofol 200 mg and rocuronium 70 mg, followed by tracheal intubation. The expected response to intubation in this patient includes

A. Hypertension
B. Tachycardia
C. Tachypnea
D. Mydriasis

42. A 24-year-old female status postrecent living-related renal transplant requires chronic immunosuppression with cyclosporine and steroids to combat organ rejection. She now presents for right-knee arthroscopic anterior cruciate ligament repair and mentions significant history of postoperative nausea and vomiting (PONV). The most appropriate next step in planning her anesthetic management is

A. Proceed with total IV anesthesia (TIVA), avoiding inhaled anesthetics
B. Avoid regional anesthesia
C. Liberally infuse intravenous fluids
D. Use metoclopramide to decrease gastric secretions

Questions 43 to 45

A 70-year-old 70-kg male with benign prostatic hypertrophy and difficulty with urination presents for a transurethral resection of his 65-g prostate (TURP). His other pertinent history includes hypertension and hyperlipidemia, both well controlled. He has a remote history of a lumbar spinal fusion with no current lumbar symptomatology. The patient requests a general anesthetic for the procedure and refuses spinal anesthesia.

43. Assuming the use of a hypotonic irrigant, these factors will contribute to the amount of fluid absorbed by the patient, except

A. Venous pressure
B. Hydrostatic pressure of the irrigation infusion
C. Lithotomy position
D. Size of prostate

44. In the recovery room, he complains of bothersome localized suprapubic pain and is requesting pain medicine. He denies pain or discomfort anywhere else. His review of systems is negative for fevers or chills. The relatively common complication of this procedure that should be ruled out at this time is

A. Hyponatremia
B. Glycine toxicity
C. Extraperitoneal perforation
D. Transient bacteremia

45. The patient is administered hydromorphone intravenously, and 20 minutes later is feeling well with minimal pain complaints. At this time, his postoperative laboratories have returned, revealing a serum sodium value of 130 mEq/L. The most appropriate next step in the management of his hyponatremia is

A. Hypertonic saline infusion
B. Fluid restriction
C. Demeclocycline administration
D. Insulin and glucose administration

46. Effects of furosemide administration in the perioperative period include

    A. Hypernatremia
    B. Decreased risk for acute tubular necrosis
    C. Metabolic alkalosis
    D. Hyperkalemia

Questions 47 to 51

A 38-year-old woman is set to undergo extracorporeal shock wave lithotripsy to disintegrate a painful stone trapped in her upper ureter. The patient is requesting an epidural anesthetic and is choosing to be otherwise awake and cooperative with her positioning and procedure.

47. The step of the epidural placement that should be *avoided* in this patient is

    A. Loss of resistance to air
    B. Loss of resistance to hanging drop
    C. Test dose injection
    D. Bolus dose of local anesthetics

48. Once the epidural is adequately placed and the patient is immersed sitting in the water tank, the physiologic change that should be expected is

    A. Decreased central venous pressure
    B. Increased vital capacity
    C. Increased functional residual capacity
    D. Lower extremity peripheral pooling

49. Extracorporeal shock wave lithotripsy therapy proceeds with the shock wave synchronized with what ECG phase of the cardiac cycle?

    A. The P wave
    B. The Q wave
    C. The R wave
    D. The S wave

50. Which of the following statements would be considered *false* with regard to extracorporeal shock wave lithotripsy (ESWL)?

    A. Delivery of the shock wave is timed to coincide with the ventricular refractory phase
    B. Neuraxial anesthesia up to T2 sensory level is adequate
    C. If able to control ventilation, use high tidal volumes and low respiratory rate
    D. Removal of the patient from the bath water can be accompanied by a decrease in the blood pressure

51. All of the following are contraindications to immersion extracorporeal shock wave lithotripsy, except

    A. Harrington rod implants
    B. Abdominally placed rate-responsive cardiac pacemaker
    C. Positive pregnancy test
    D. Large calcified abdominal aortic aneurysm

52. Which of the following is considered the most sensitive indicator of impending traumatic renal failure?

    A. Decreased creatinine clearance
    B. Decreased central venous pressure
    C. Decreased fractional excretion of sodium
    D. Increased urine osmolality

53. A 26-year-old male patient with Alport syndrome requires hemodialysis (every third day) and presents for an arteriovenous fistula creation. His last dialysis treatment was yesterday. Patient requests general anesthesia for this procedure. Which of the following drugs will have a prolonged duration of action?

   A. Fentanyl
   B. Neostigmine
   C. Atracurium
   D. Methadone

54. Each of the following is associated with acute tubular necrosis, except

   A. Hyaline casts
   B. Urine specific gravity <1.010
   C. Muddy casts
   D. Fractional excretion of sodium of 4%

Questions 55 to 56

A 75-year-old patient who is awaiting urgent laparotomy has had oliguria for the past 12 hours since the onset of his acute abdominal pain last night. His medical history includes well-controlled hypertension. Vital signs include a BP of 120/65 mm Hg and a HR of 72 bpm. His laboratory findings reveal

   Urine osmolality: 550 mOsm/L
   Urine specific gravity: 1.020
   Urine sodium concentration: 15 mmol/L
   Fractional excretion of sodium: 0.5%
   Ratio of urine-to-plasma urea concentration: 10

55. The most appropriate treatment of his oliguria is

   A. Fluid restriction
   B. Fluid challenge
   C. Renal ultrasound
   D. Foley placement

56. Fluid resuscitation is done with 4 L of normal saline. The potential acid–base abnormality that can occur is

   A. Hyperchloremic acidosis
   B. Metabolic alkalosis
   C. Hyperkalemic acidosis
   D. Respiratory alkalosis

57. A 67-year-old patient with chronic renal failure presents for hip arthroscopy to address and treat his labral tears and associated hip pain. The best option for opioid therapy in this patient is

   A. Meperidine
   B. Codeine
   C. Dextropropoxyphene
   D. Fentanyl

CHAPTER 14 ANSWERS

1. **B.**   The initial reduction in core temperature during general anesthesia is caused by redistribution of heat from the core to the periphery, which can be attenuated by increasing ambient temperature to minimize the gradient.

2. **D.**   Perioperative morbidity related to obesity is associated with changes in respiratory (e.g., difficult airway, decreased functional residual capacity), cardiovascular (e.g., increased cardiac output), and gastrointestinal (e.g., gastroesophageal reflex disease, increased abdominal pressure) systems that will impact the delivery of anesthesia. Given that metabolism of inhalational agents is increased over normal weight patients, higher minimum alveolar concentrations may be required. Atracurium (including cis-atracurium) is metabolized via Hofmann degradation and is unaffected by the obese state.

3. **B.**   Aspiration of acidic gastric juices poses a potential threat during induction and intubation. H_2-blockers (e.g., cimetidine, ranitidine) can decrease gastric volume and raise pH to a level that should be protective from fatal aspiration. Metoclopramide promotes gastrointestinal motility without directly affecting pH itself. $5\text{-}HT_3$ (serotonin) receptor antagonism (e.g., ondansetron) and D_2 (dopamine) antagonism (e.g., prochlorperazine) are useful antiemetics, with no effect on gastric pH or volume.

4. **B.**   Atelectasis likely occurs in all patients who undergo general anesthesia, in particular those postabdominal surgeries. Changes of microatelectasis develop routinely and do not significantly delay discharge for most patients despite the relative state of hypoxia (decreased Pao_2). Deep breathing, use of an incentive spirometer, early mobilization, and adequate pain control are all measures used to expand lung volumes and promote improved oxygenation.

5. **A.**   Postsurgical atelectasis is treated by physiotherapy, focusing on deep breathing while encouraging coughing. An incentive spirometer is often used to promote full expansion of the lungs. Ambulation is also highly encouraged to improve lung inflation. These measures are considered first-line options for his presumed microatelectasis. In the smoker, coughing will also clear the airways of mucous to improve aeration. Doxapram stimulates chemoreceptors in the carotid bodies, which in turn stimulates the respiratory center in the brain stem to increase tidal volume and respiratory rate.

6. **A.**   Initial management involves the recognition of a possible aspiration event when there are visible gastric contents in the oropharynx. Once diagnosis is suspected, the patient should be placed in Trendelenburg position to limit pulmonary contamination, followed by suctioning of the oropharynx. Empirical antibiotic therapy is strongly discouraged unless it is apparent that the patient has developed a subsequent pneumonia. Corticosteroids should not be given prophylactically, as there is no evidence to support this practice.

7. **B.**   Gastrointestinal secretions, including diarrhea and intestinal fistulas, are rich in bicarbonate and, therefore, losses will cause a metabolic acidosis. However, respiratory compensation for metabolic processes will occur almost immediately by increasing ventilation to blow off CO_2 to reduce the acidosis, effecting change in as quick as 15 to 30 minutes. Therefore, one would expect ABG findings of a metabolic acidosis with full respiratory compensation.

8. **A.**   The ACT enables one to monitor the anticoagulant effect of unfractionated heparin. ACT prolongation can also indicate coagulation-factor deficiency, severe thrombocytopenia, or severe platelet dysfunction. The ACT is sensitive to a deficiency or dysfunction of all the clotting

factors (except factor VII)—indicating problems with the intrinsic or common pathways. Factor level must be less than 5% of normal to prolong the ACT.

9. A. An acute hemolytic transfusion reaction is associated with hemolysis of transfused blood, usually related to ABO incompatibility with associated hemoglobinuria. Pulmonary leukoagglutinin reaction is related to the presence of antileukocyte antibodies in donor plasma leading to transfusion-related acute lung injury.

10. B. Malnourished surgical patients are at greater risk for postoperative morbidity and mortality compared to a well-nourished patient undergoing similar operations for similar indications. However, providing TPN to the malnourished patient in the perioperative period carries its own inherent risks, such as greater risk of infection, hyperglycemia, and electrolyte abnormalities.

11. D. For those on TPN, the anesthesiologist must monitor blood glucose levels meticulously to avoid hypo- or hyperglycemia. Hyperosmolar, nonketotic, hyperglycemic coma has been reported in patients who fail to regain consciousness after anesthesia.

12. B. Ensuring the presence of normal serum phosphate levels in the patient receiving TPN is essential, as hypophosphatemia has been associated with acute respiratory failure due to profound areflexic muscle weakness.

13. D. The most critical element to safe perioperative care of the pheochromocytoma patient is adequate preoperative blockade against the effects of the circulating catecholamines. The main goals of preoperative blockade are to normalize blood pressure and heart rate, restore volume depletion, and prevent surgery-induced catecholamine storm. A sign of adequate α-blockade is the development of nasal congestion due to smooth-muscle relaxation of nasal mucosal arterioles.

14. A. Switching from isoflurane to sevoflurane is not an appropriate method to treat the catecholamine storm, which can occur during direct surgical manipulation of the tumor. An α-blocker, vasodilator, and lidocaine are appropriate options to counter the effects of catecholamine storm.

15. A. Sympathetic preganglionic fibers originate in the intermediolateral cell column of the spinal cord from T1 to L2. Cardiac innervation is principally via sympathetic fibers from T1 to T4. As such, high thoracic blockade up to T2 will block the cardioaccelerator nerves, leading to bradycardia and hypotension. The respiratory system is usually unaffected, as diaphragmatic breathing alone can maintain relatively normal arterial blood gases. However, patients may feel unable to breath and are often unable to cough effectively.

16. A. The pharmacokinetics of many nondepolarizing muscle relaxants in the presence of cholestasis and obstructive jaundice may be altered. The prolonged duration of action likely results from both inhibition of hepatic uptake by the accumulated bile salts and a general deterioration of liver transport function. Succinylcholine, atracurium, and cis-atracurium have theoretical advantages because their elimination occurs via plasma cholinesterases and Hofmann degradation, respectively, mostly independent of renal or hepatic function.

17. C. Postoperative liver dysfunction is common, but is generally mild and asymptomatic (Table 14-2). Mild transient increases in serum levels of liver enzymes (SGOT/SGPT) are often seen within hours of surgery, but rarely persist >2 days. Subclinical hepatocellular injury can occur in up to 50% of those receiving an inhaled anesthetic with halothane. Though volatile anesthetics are often implicated as the cause of postoperative jaundice, there are many other causes to consider. A surgical cause is likely if the operation involved the liver or biliary tract. Drugs, including antibiotics, and other metabolic or infectious causes must also be ruled out.

Table 14-2 Postoperative Liver Dysfunction—Causes and Differentiation.

	PREHEPATIC	**INTRAHEPATIC**	**POSTHEPATIC**
Etiology	Hemolysis Hematoma reabsorption Bilirubin overload	Severe arterial hypoxemia Cirrhosis Congestive heart failure Sepsis Viruses Drug-induced	Stones Sepsis Cancer
Bilirubin	↑ (unconjugated)	↑ (conjugated)	↑ (conjugated)
Aminotransferases	Unchanged	↑↑	Unchanged
Alkaline phosphatase	Unchanged	Unchanged	↑↑
Prothrombin time	Unchanged	↑	Unchanged
Albumin	Unchanged	↓	Unchanged

18. **B.**   Chronic liver disease may interfere with the metabolism of drugs due to decreased number of functional hepatocytes or decreased hepatic blood flow that typically accompanies cirrhosis of the liver. Prolonged elimination half-life times for morphine, diazepam, lidocaine, pancuronium, and, to a lesser degree, vecuronium have been demonstrated in this population. Cirrhotic patients will require a larger initial dose of pancuronium due to increased volume of distribution for this hydrophilic agent with smaller maintenance doses for prolonged duration of action. Pancuronium has slight vagolytic activity resulting in increased heart rate and cardiac output. Mivacurium and atracurium are associated with histamine release.

19. **B.**   Certain physiologic and pathologic states may alter MAC of inhaled anesthetics. MAC is higher in infants and lower in the elderly. Also, MAC increases with hyperthermia, alcoholism, and thyrotoxicosis. Furthermore, hypothermia, hypotension, and pregnancy seem to decrease MAC, while duration of anesthesia, gender, height, and weight seem to have little effect on MAC. Those with chronic liver disease are also at increased risk of arterial–venous shunting.

20. **B.**   Those with chronic liver disease are at increased risk of arterial–venous shunting. The presence of intrapulmonary shunting will result in hypoxemia.

21. **C.**   Cirrhosis is typically associated with several cardiovascular abnormalities including a hyperdynamic circulation characterized by increased cardiac output and decreased peripheral resistance. Other cardiovascular changes include a resting tachycardia, warm peripheries, a bounding pulse, and a widened pulse pressure.

22. **D.**   Obesity hypoventilation syndrome (aka Pickwickian syndrome) is a state in which the severely overweight patient fails to breathe rapidly or deeply enough, resulting in hypoxia and hypercarbia. If Pickwickian syndrome is suspected, the most important initial test is the demonstration of elevated carbon dioxide in the blood. This requires either an ABG or a measurement of bicarbonate levels in venous blood. Expected ABG findings would reveal a chronic, compensated respiratory acidosis.

23. **B.**   Redistribution of thiopental to inactive tissue sites rather than metabolism is the most important determinant of early awakening following a single intravenous injection.

24. **B.**   The Child-Turcotte-Pugh score is used to predict mortality during surgery in patients with chronic liver disease, namely, cirrhosis. The Mayo or model for end-stage liver disease was initially developed to predict death within 3 months of surgery in patients who had undergone a transjugular intrahepatic portosystemic shunt procedure and was subsequently found to be useful in determining prognosis and prioritizing patients for liver transplant. Alvarado score is used for appendicitis, while the Ranson criteria assess pancreatitis.

25. **D.**   The MELD score is a formulaic calculation utilizing three variables: creatinine, INR, and bilirubin. For dialysis-dependent patients, the creatinine score is automatically set to 4 mg/dL despite true serum levels.

$$\text{MELD score} = 10 \times [0.957 \times \log e \,(\text{creatinine}) + \log e \,(\text{bilirubin}) + 1.12 \times \log e \,(\text{INR})] + 6.43$$

26. **D.**   Standard technique of OLT causes changes in hemodynamics during the anhepatic phase because of cross-clamping of the suprahepatic IVC. Interruption of the IVC and portal vein flow causes a decrease in preload, cardiac output, and arterial blood pressure. VVB has been used to achieve hemodynamic stability by avoiding venous congestion, promoting venous return with decrease incidence of renal dysfunction.

27. **B.**   Postreperfusion syndrome is the most common hemodynamic derangement in liver transplantation, manifesting mainly as decreased heart rate, mean arterial pressure, and systemic vascular resistances. Ventricular function, both right and left, has been shown to be normal during reperfusion, in which case the visceral and liver vasodilation that occurs would be the main cause of arterial hypotension. Prophylaxis with atropine prevents bradycardia but not hypotension. Administration of calcium chloride and sodium bicarbonate together with hyperventilation mitigates the symptoms related to the reduced cardiac output.

28. **A.**   Coagulopathy following massive transfusion is a consequence of posttraumatic and surgical hemorrhage. Bleeding following massive transfusion can occur due to hypothermia, dilutional coagulopathy, platelet dysfunction, fibrinolysis, or hypofibrinogenemia. Transfusion of 15 to 20 U of blood products causes dilutional thrombocytopenia contributing to the bleeding. Excessive fibrinolysis and low fibrinogen are further causes of bleeding in these patients. The hemostatic signatures of DIC are low platelets, low fibrinogen, prolonged prothrombin, prolonged PTT, elevated D-dimers, and low antithrombin.

29. **A.**   Long-standing insufficient liver function is believed to cause changes in the circulation that changes vessel tone and blood flow in the kidneys. The likely presence of renal insufficiency is a consequence of these changes in blood flow, rather than direct damage to the kidney itself.

30. **C.**   Dyspnea is a common complaint in individuals with class II or III obesity, especially following a general anesthetic. As such, individuals present with a pronounced reduction in expiratory reserve volume and an increase in the alveolar–arterial oxygen gradient.

31. **C.**   µ-Receptor agonism may contribute to sphincter of Oddi spasm, preventing passage of contrast with full µ-agonist more likely to contribute versus partial µ-agonists (e.g., buprenorphine) and agonist–antagonist (e.g., nalbuphine). Naloxone, as a µ-antagonist would alleviate any opioid-induced spasm.

32. **C.**   A variety of agents that can produce smooth-muscle relaxation have been used. Nitrates and calcium channel blockers have been the most extensively studied. Anticholinergics, including atropine and glucagon, are additional agents that can provide sphincter of Oddi relaxation. Metoclopramide is a promotility agent that enhances sphincter smooth-muscle contraction.

33. **B.**   Sympathetic celiac plexus blockade leaves parasympathetic fibers unopposed with associated increased gastrointestinal motility and possible diarrhea.

34. **C.**   Abdominal laparoscopy requires insufflation of the abdominal cavity, most commonly using CO_2, to create a pneumoperitoneum. Increase in intra-abdominal pressures will place the patient at a greater risk of reflux and aspiration; thus, general anesthesia with an

endotracheal tube is required. High pressures in the abdominal cavity can also compress both small and large blood vessels, hampering venous return to the heart. Intrathoracic pressures are also increased, associated with diaphragm elevation, compromising cardiac output further. Increase in SVR occurs during pneumoperitoneum, reflected as an increase in afterload for left-sided heart chambers.

35. **C.** Abdominal laparoscopy, though relatively safe, is associated with a few inherent dangers including gaseous embolism, potential inability to control bleeding, an increase in CO_2 partial pressures and changes in arterial blood pressure and heart rate. CO_2 absorption from the peritoneal cavity can result in a state of acidosis as $Paco_2$ rises.

36. **A.** The supine position under general anesthesia results in a decrease in functional residual capacity (FRC). Pneumoperitoneum and the Trendelenburg position shifts the diaphragm cephalad, further decreasing FRC. If FRC becomes less than closing capacity, airway collapse, atelectasis, and ventilation/perfusion mismatch can further compromise respiratory function. The judicious use of PEEP can be helpful to mitigate end-expiratory alveolar collapse; however, too much PEEP can contribute to deterioration in right-sided cardiac performance.

37. **D.** Systemic absorption of gas from pneumoperitoneum is determined by factors including solubility of the gas, IAP, and duration of surgery. Therefore, CO_2 laparoscopy may produce hypercarbia, particularly during long surgeries under high IAP unless minute ventilation is increased. In those with severely compromised cardiopulmonary function and restricted CO_2 clearance, severe hypercarbia can occur despite aggressive hyperventilation.

38. **B.** Hypercarbia causes hemodynamic changes by its direct action on the cardiovascular system and indirect actions through the sympathetic nervous system. Manifestations while under general anesthesia include tachycardia, arrhythmias, high cardiac output, increased arterial blood pressure, and low SVR with flushed skin.

39. **C.** The effects of pneumoperitoneum include compression of the inferior vena cava resulting in poor venous return and low preload. Systemic vascular resistance increases proportionately when the intra-abdominal pressure is elevated, providing a larger afterload against which the left ventricle must function. During insufflation, a gas embolus can occur, entering the venous system to create an "air lock" with mechanical obstruction of the right-side chambers. A blood pressure cuff that is too small for the arm will result in erroneously high blood pressure readings.

40. **D.** The saphenous nerve is the largest and longest branch of the femoral nerve that supplies sensory innervation to the medial aspect of the lower leg. Movement of the foot is unaffected.

41. **D.** High thoracic epidural blockade up to T2 blocks the cardiac accelerators, providing adequate sympathectomy to prevent hypertension and tachycardia. Sympathetic outflow to the pupil travels via the intermediolateral cell column at the C8 to T2 cord level and remains intact; thus, the sympathetic surge can still result in mydriasis.

42. **A.** Transplant recipients are always under various regimens of immunosuppression to prevent organ rejection. Clinically significant reductions in serum levels of these medications can be caused by dilution with massive fluid resuscitation perioperatively, as well as with cardiopulmonary bypass. Many immunosuppressants are metabolized in the liver via the cytochrome P450 system such that drugs administered during anesthesia (or perioperatively) may affect blood levels including increased concentrations with cimetidine and metoclopramide and decreased levels with octreotide. Regional anesthesia and/or TIVA are reasonable options to minimize PONV in this patient.

43. C.   Normally, about 20 mL/min of irrigation fluid is absorbed (1–1.5 L for a normal case with resection time about 45–60 minutes), which increases as the duration of the surgery increases. In clinical practice, it is almost impossible to accurately assess the volume absorbed. The amount of fluid absorbed depends on several other factors as well, including the hydrostatic pressure of the irrigation infusion (determined by the height of the bag), venous pressure (more fluid absorbed if patient is hypotensive), the size of the prostate to be resected (associated with longer time required), blood loss (implies a large number of open veins), and surgical skills of the surgeon (efficiency with time management and hemostasis).

44. C.   Another relatively common complication of TURP is perforation of the bladder. Perforations usually occur during difficult resections and are often made by the cutting loop or knife electrode. The tip of the resectoscope can also cause injury, as well as overdistention of the bladder with irrigation fluid. Most perforations are extraperitoneal, and in the awake patient, they result in pain in the periumbilical, inguinal, or suprapubic regions; additionally, the urologist may note the irregular return of irrigating fluid. Less often, the perforation is through the wall of the bladder and thus intraperitoneal. In such cases, pain may be generalized, in the upper abdomen, or referred from the diaphragm to the shoulder. Bacteremia is usually asymptomatic and easily treated with commonly used antibiotic combinations that are effective against gram-positive and gram-negative bacteria.

45. B.   For normovolemic, asymptomatic hyponatremic patients, free water restriction is generally the treatment of choice. There is no role for hypertonic saline in these patients. The volume of restriction should be based on the patient's renal diluting capacity. If patient is unable to adhere to fluid restrictions, consider use of a loop diuretic (e.g., furosemide) to increase free water excretion in the kidneys. Demeclocycline is a tetracycline antibiotic that has a secondary effect of reducing the responsiveness of the collecting tubule cells to antidiuretic hormone, thus improving free water loss.

46. C.   As with many diuretics, furosemide can cause dehydration and electrolyte imbalance, including loss of potassium, calcium, sodium, and magnesium. Excessive use of furosemide will most likely lead to a metabolic alkalosis due to hypochloremia and hypokalemia.

47. A.   With epidural anesthesia, consider avoiding the use of loss of resistance to air for identifying the epidural space, as air will provide an interface and cause dissipation of shock wave energy resulting in local tissue injury. Animal experiments have shown epidural tissue damage following injection of air followed by exposure to shock waves.

48. D.   Water immersion produces significant changes in the cardiovascular and respiratory systems. Cardiovascular changes include an increase in central blood volume, with an increase in central venous and pulmonary artery pressures, which are directly correlated with the depth of immersion. The sitting position, together with either general or epidural anesthesia, would tend to cause peripheral pooling and decreased venous return. Respiratory changes with immersion up to the clavicles are significant: functional residual capacity and vital capacity are reduced by 20% to 30%; pulmonary blood flow has been shown to increase; and tight abdominal straps and the hydrostatic pressure of water on the thorax impart a characteristic of shallow, rapid breathing pattern.

49. C.   Shock wave–induced cardiac arrhythmias occur in up to 10% to 14% of patients undergoing lithotripsy despite the fact that shock waves are purposefully synchronized with the patient's ECG and are delivered in the refractory period of the cardiac cycle (R wave).

50. C.   An advantage of providing a general anesthetic for ESWL is that ventilatory parameters can be controlled using high frequency and low volumes to decrease stone movement with respiration.

51. A. Contraindications for lithotripsy include the following: pregnancy, a large aortic aneurysm, certain bleeding conditions, and certain skeletal deformities that prevent accurate focus of shock waves. Patients with abdominally placed cardiac pacemakers should notify their doctor. Rate-responsive pacemakers that are implanted in the abdomen may be damaged during lithotripsy. Orthopedic prostheses, including hip prostheses and even Harrington rods, are generally not a problem as long as they can be kept out of the blast path.

52. A. Creatinine clearance test evaluates how efficiently the kidneys clear creatinine from the blood. Creatinine, a waste product of muscle energy metabolism, is produced at a constant rate that is proportional to the muscle mass of the individual. Because the body does not recycle it, all of the creatinine filtered by the kidneys in a given amount of time is excreted in the urine, making creatinine clearance a very specific measurement of kidney function.

53. B. Succinylcholine, atracurium, and cis-atracurium have theoretical advantages because their elimination occurs via plasma cholinesterases and Hofmann degradation, respectively, mostly independent of renal or hepatic function. Fentanyl and methadone are also considered relatively safe in renal failure as they have no active metabolites. Methadone has limited plasma accumulation in renal failure as it is primarily eliminated in the feces. In terms of reversal agents, renal excretion accounts for approximately 50% of the clearance of neostigmine and approximately 75% of elimination of edrophonium and pyridostigmine. Renal failure allows some protection against residual neuromuscular blockade because renal elimination half times of anticholinesterase drugs is prolonged.

54. A. Acute tubular necrosis is classified as a "renal" (e.g., not prerenal or postrenal) cause of acute kidney injury. Diagnosis is made by a fractional excretion of sodium >3%, greater than expected urine sodium concentration with low osmolality and presence of muddy casts on urinalysis. A sensitive indicator of tubular function is sodium handling because the ability of an injured tubule to reabsorb sodium is impaired, whereas an intact tubule can maintain this resorptive capacity. If the patient has tubular damage for any reason, the urinary sodium will be greater than expected. Keep in mind that the use of diuretics, however, can complicate the interpretation of these results. Low urine flow, concentrated urine, or an acidic environment can contribute to the formation of hyaline casts, pointing to hypovolemia and prerenal failure (Table 14-3).

Table 14-3 Differentiation between Prerenal and Intrinsic Renal Failure.

PARAMETER	PRERENAL FAILURE	ACUTE TUBULAR NECROSIS
Urine Na+ (meq/L)	<20	>40
Urine osmolality (mOsm/kg)	>500	<350
FENa %	<1	>2
Urea %	<35	>35
Urine specific gravity	>1,020	<1,010
Urine:plasma urea ratio	>10:1	<7:1

55. B. Urinalysis reveals a prerenal state. Treatment focuses on correcting the cause of the prerenal acute renal failure, most often with a fluid challenge. Depending on the cause, the condition often reverses itself within a couple of days after normal blood flow to the kidneys has been restored. But if it is not reversed or treated successfully and quickly, prerenal acute renal failure can cause tissue death in the kidneys and lead to intrinsic (intrarenal) acute renal failure.

56. A. Hyperchloremic acidosis is a well-recognized entity as a consequence of large volume administration of some intravenous fluids. Normal saline (0.9% sodium chloride solution) and colloids suspended in normal saline are often infused because they are easily available, and are isotonic with plasma. When a patient is given normal saline (a hyperchloremic solution), chloride levels can significantly increase. It is the chloride anion that is the ultimate cause of the acidosis. Consider this equation: sodium chloride combines with water: $NaCl + H_2O \rightarrow HCl + NaOH$. The strong acid (HCl) and the strong base (NaOH) should cancel each other out, with no effect on pH. However, because the normal concentrations of Na^+ and Cl^- in the serum are 140 and 100, respectively, adding normal saline (154 mEq Na and 154 mEq Cl) causes the chloride to increase proportionately more than the sodium. This increase in chloride tips the acid–base balance toward HCl, thereby causing a metabolic acidosis.

57. D.   Chronic pain is common in chronic kidney disease and most will rate their pain as moderate to severe. The absorption, metabolism, and renal clearance of opioids are complex in renal failure. However, with the appropriate selection and titration of opioids, patients with renal failure can achieve analgesia with minimal risk of adverse effects. Meperidine is not recommended in renal failure due to accumulation of normeperidine, which may cause seizures. Morphine is not recommended for chronic use in renal insufficiency due to the rapid accumulation of its active nondialyzable metabolite (morphine-6-glucuronide). Codeine has been reported to cause profound renal toxicity, which can be delayed and may occur after trivial doses. Dextropropoxyphene is associated with central nervous system and cardiac toxicity and is not recommended for use in patients with renal failure. On the other hand, fentanyl is considered relatively safe in renal failure, as it has no active metabolites.

CHAPTER 15

Endocrine Diseases

Jean Kwo and Edward Bittner

1. Type 1 diabetes mellitus

   A. Is characterized by a relative lack of insulin plus resistance to endogenous insulin
   B. Always requires insulin
   C. Affects 95% of patients with diabetes
   D. Can be controlled with diet, weight loss, and oral hypoglycemic agents

2. Preoperative assessment of patients with diabetes mellitus should include

   A. An assessment of functional status
   B. 24-Hour creatinine clearance
   C. Pulmonary function testing
   D. Cancellation of the surgical case if $HbA_{1c} > 10\%$

3. Preferred anesthetic agent in a patient with hyperthyroidism includes

   A. Desflurane
   B. Ketamine
   C. Sevoflurane
   D. Meperidine

4. Multiple endocrine neoplasia (MEN) I syndrome includes

   A. Pheochromocytoma, medullary thyroid carcinoma, parathyroid hyperplasia
   B. Pancreas tumors, medullary thyroid carcinoma, pituitary adenoma
   C. Pheochromocytoma, medullary thyroid carcinoma, mucosal neuromas
   D. Pancreas tumors, pituitary adenoma, parathyroid hyperplasia

5. Laboratory findings in primary hypothyroidism are

   A. Low TSH, elevated T3, elevated T4
   B. Low TSH, low T3, low T4
   C. Normal TSH, low T3, low T4
   D. Elevated TSH, low T3, low T4

6. Obese patients may experience rapid oxygen desaturation during induction of general anesthesia because of

   A. A decrease in lung compliance
   B. A reduction in functional residual capacity (FRC)
   C. A history of obstructive sleep apnea
   D. Restrictive lung disease

7. A 39-year-old woman with a history of headaches, hypertension, palpitations, and nephrolithiasis is undergoing a parathyroidectomy for parathyroid adenoma. During induction, she develops severe hypertension and tachycardia. The most likely diagnosis for these signs is

   A. Adrenal insufficiency
   B. Carcinoid syndrome
   C. Thyroid storm
   D. Pheochromocytoma

8. Phenoxybenzamine is a

   A. Selective α_1-receptor antagonist and a nonselective β-adrenergic receptor antagonist
   B. Reversible α_1-receptor antagonist
   C. Irreversible, nonselective α-adrenergic receptor antagonist
   D. Selective α_2-receptor agonist

9. A 40-year-old woman with a history of Graves disease is in the recovery room after undergoing a CT scan under general anesthesia. While in the recovery room, her blood pressure drops to 80/55 mm Hg, her heart rate increases to 140 bpm, and she becomes agitated and complains of difficulty breathing and feeling hot. The most likely diagnosis for these signs is

   A. Thyroid storm
   B. Carcinoid syndrome
   C. Malignant hyperthermia
   D. Pheochromocytoma

10. Treatment of thyroid storm includes

    A. Dantrolene
    B. Phenoxybenzamine
    C. Octreotide
    D. Propylthiouracil

11. During a postoperative check on a 53-year-old patient who underwent a total thyroidectomy earlier in the day, you notice that he is stridorous and is complaining of muscle cramps. The best treatment for these symptoms is

    A. Administration of calcium gluconate
    B. Opening the neck wound
    C. Reintubation for airway protection
    D. Administration of sodium bicarbonate

12. Patients with obstructive sleep apnea (OSA)

    A. Are at increased risk of left-heart failure
    B. Have the same perioperative complication rate as patients without OSA
    C. May have an increased likelihood of difficult intubation
    D. Rarely require continuous positive airway pressure (CPAP) after bariatric surgery

13. A 39-year-old patient with a BMI of 45 kg/m^2 is scheduled for a Roux-en-Y gastric bypass. She has a history of hypertension. Your perioperative concerns include

    A. Preparation for a rapid sequence induction, since she is at increased risk for aspiration of gastric contents
    B. Placing her in the reverse Trendelenburg position to reduce atelectasis in dependent areas of the lung and move the chest and breast tissue caudally to allow easier access to the mouth for endotracheal intubation
    C. Need to dose water-soluble drugs (e.g., neuromuscular-blocking agents) to actual body weight
    D. More frequent administration of lipid-soluble drugs will be needed

14. During the preoperative evaluation of a critically ill patient with ischemic bowel scheduled for a second look laparotomy and possible abdominal closure, you notice multiple electrolyte abnormalities including hypophosphatemia, hypokalemia, and hypomagnesemia. A possible cause for these electrolyte abnormalities is

   A. Renal failure
   B. Hypoventilation
   C. Hypoparathyroidism
   D. Refeeding syndrome

15. Complications of cricoid pressure include

   A. Esophageal obstruction
   B. Displacement of thoracic spine
   C. Worsening of view of airway in patients with difficult airway
   D. Need for less pressure in parturients

16. You are evaluating a 55-year-old patient with type 2 diabetes mellitus for a total knee replacement. His diabetes is controlled on a regimen of Glucophage (metformin), NPH insulin twice a day, and insulin sliding scale. Perioperative instructions for glucose management should include

   A. Give half of the NPH dose if morning blood glucose level is at least 150 mg/dL
   B. Give regular insulin dose according to morning blood glucose level
   C. Holding metformin for 48 hours preoperatively to avoid risk of fatal lactic acidosis
   D. Starting insulin infusion with target glucose range of 81 to 108 mg/dL

17. Carcinoid tumors

   A. Grow rapidly, and patients are often symptomatic with carcinoid syndrome
   B. Synthesize epinephrine and norepinephrine
   C. Can cause left-sided heart failure due to mitral and aortic valve damage
   D. Can cause right-sided heart failure due to tricuspid and pulmonary valve damage

18. You are taking care of a 67-year-old patient undergoing a parathyroidectomy. The patient is hypercalcemic with a serum calcium of 20 mg/dL. Anesthetic considerations should include all of the following, except

   A. Hypoventilation to decrease ionized calcium level
   B. Careful titration of neuromuscular-blocking agents
   C. Hydration with normal saline and diuresis with furosemide
   D. Care with laryngoscopy because of risk of vertebral compression

19. Clinical manifestations of mineralocorticoid excess include

   A. Hypotension
   B. Metabolic acidosis
   C. Hypokalemia
   D. Tetany

20. Normal daily cortisol production (mg/day) in adults is

   A. 10 to 15
   B. 20 to 30
   C. 50 to 60
   D. 75 to 100

21. A 75-year-old patient with coronary artery disease, hypertension, and chronic obstructive pulmonary disease (COPD) is undergoing a left colectomy for cancer. He had a COPD exacerbation 4 months ago and was on steroids for a week at the time. Steroid replacement

    A. Should be given at a dose greater than 10 times the normal daily cortisol production rate
    B. Should not exceed 100 to 150 mg of cortisol equivalent per day
    C. Is not necessary in this patient
    D. Should include 100 mg of cortisol, tapered over 5 to 7 days

22. Physiologic effects of chronically elevated corticosteroid levels (Cushing syndrome) include all of the following, except

    A. Hypotension
    B. Muscle wasting
    C. Hypokalemia
    D. Glucose intolerance

23. You are taking care of a 45-year-old patient undergoing a left adrenalectomy for a pheochromocytoma. Intraoperative management includes

    A. Use of ketamine as an induction agent to counteract the effects preoperative of α-adrenergic blockade
    B. Long-acting antihypertensive agents should be available to treat hypertension
    C. Judicious fluid replacement as these patients are usually volume-overloaded
    D. Magnesium sulfate infusion to treat hypertension

24. A 75-year-old, 110-kg patient is scheduled for a radical prostatectomy. He has a history of hypertension and type 2 diabetes mellitus. His preoperative ECG is significant for Q waves in leads II, III, and aVF, though the patient denies having a previous myocardial infarction. His medications include insulin, Glucophage (metformin), a β-blocker, and an angiotensin-receptor blocker. Upon induction, his blood pressure drops from 150/80 to 65/40. The most likely cause of hypotension is

    A. Use of angiotensin-receptor blocker
    B. Diabetic autonomic neuropathy
    C. Volume depletion
    D. Myocardial ischemia

25. Patients with type 1 diabetes mellitus may be difficult to intubate because of

    A. Increased supraglottic soft tissue due to chronic hyperglycemia
    B. An association between type 1 diabetes and an anterior larynx
    C. Limited joint mobility
    D. An increased incidence of obesity in patients with type 1 diabetes

CHAPTER 15 ANSWERS

1. **B.**   Type 1 diabetes mellitus results from the autoimmune destruction of insulin-producing β cells of the pancreas and thus these patients always need insulin to prevent hyperglycemic ketoacidosis and other complications. Most patients carrying the diagnoses of diabetes (95%) have type 2 diabetes, which is characterized by a relative lack of insulin plus resistance to endogenous insulin. Type 2 diabetes can be controlled with diet and weight loss, and oral agents, though these patients may also require insulin.

2. **A.**   Complications of diabetes result largely from microangiopathy and macroangiopathy. Diabetes is a well-recognized risk factor for coronary artery disease (CAD). Cardiac autonomic neuropathy may mask angina pectoris and obscure the presence of CAD. Hence, a careful assessment of functional status and any symptoms such as increasing dyspnea on exertion and fatigue may be indicative of significant CAD. While diabetes is a leading cause of renal failure, there is no evidence that a preoperative evaluation with a 24-hour creatinine clearance is helpful. While the risk of complications of diabetes increases with increasing HbA_{1c} levels, and there is evidence that higher HbA_{1c} levels are associated with adverse outcomes following a variety of surgical procedures, there is insufficient evidence to recommend an upper limit of HbA_{1c} prior to elective surgery. The risks associated with poor glycemic control should be balanced against the necessity for surgery.

3. **C.**   In patients with hyperthyroidism, the goal of anesthesia is to avoid an increase in heart rate or sympathetic activation. Ketamine, desflurane, and meperidine cause sympathetic stimulation and tachycardia. Conversely, anesthetics and techniques that reduce or blunt sympathetic activity are preferred. Sevoflurane for anesthesia, and fentanyl and its congeners for analgesia would be favored. Regional anesthesia, when practical, might also be efficacious in avoiding sympathetic activation.

4. **D.**   MEN I syndrome includes the triad of tumors of the pancreas, pituitary, and parathyroid glands and is inherited as an autosomal-dominant trait. Medullary thyroid carcinomas are a component of the MEN II endocrine syndromes, of which there are several subtypes.

5. **D.**

Table 15-1

Thyroid disorder	TSH	T3	T4
Primary hypothyroidism	↑	↓	↓
Secondary* hypothyroidism	↓	↓	↓
Primary hyperthyroidism	↓	↑	↓
Secondary* hyperthyroidism	↑	↑	↑
Subclinical hypothyroidism	↑	Normal	Normal
Subclinical hyperthyroidism	↓	Normal	Normal
Sick euthyroid	Normal	↓	↓

*Secondary hypo/hyperthyroidism may occur as a consequence of hypothalamic or pituitary disease or after surgery on these structures.

6. **B.**   Obesity is associated with obstructive sleep apnea, decreased pulmonary compliance, and lung volumes suggestive of restrictive lung disease. Total pulmonary compliance decreases due to a decrease in both chest-wall compliance and lung compliance. Chest-wall compliance decreases because of excessive adipose tissue over the thorax, while lung compliance decreases because of the increased abdominal mass, which pushes the diaphragm cephalad causing an increase in pulmonary blood volume. The FRC of the lung is the volume of air

present in the lungs at the end of passive expiration and reflects a balance between the elastic recoil of the lungs and the pleural pressure. With obesity, there is a shift in this balance due to adipose tissue in the chest wall and abdomen, resulting in a decreased FRC. The FRC is the reservoir of oxygen during the apneic state associated with the induction of general anesthesia. Thus, the reduction of FRC associated with obesity results in greater oxygen desaturation during the induction of general anesthesia.

7. **D.** While inadequate anesthesia and thyroid storm may result in intraoperative hypertension and tachycardia, the most likely diagnosis is pheochromocytoma. Pheochromocytoma is a catecholamine-secreting tumor and is part of the multiple endocrine neoplasia (MEN) type II syndrome, which consists of pheochromocytoma, medullary thyroid carcinoma, and parathyroid adenoma. Symptoms associated with pheochromocytoma include paroxysmal headache, hypertension, diaphoresis, and palpitations.

8. **C.** Phenoxybenzamine is an irreversible, nonselective α-adrenergic receptor antagonist used preoperatively for adrenergic blockade in patients with pheochromocytomas. It blocks both the postsynaptic α_1 and presynaptic α_2 receptors in the nervous system, thereby reducing sympathetic activity. Clinical signs of the optimal dose of phenoxybenzamine are a stuffy nose and slight dizziness due to postural hypotension. Doxazosin is a reversible, selective α_1-receptor antagonist that is an alternative to phenoxybenzamine for treatment of pheochromocytoma. In patients with pheochromocytoma, α-blockade is always started prior to β-blockade. Starting β-blockade first will lead to unopposed α stimulation causing further increase in the blood pressure.

9. **A.** Thyroid storm is characterized by fever, tachycardia, altered mental status, and hypertension, presenting most often in the postanesthesia care unit or in the immediate postoperative period (24 hours). Hypertension may be followed by congestive heart failure that is associated with hypotension and shock. Thyroid storm is a state of severe hypermetabolism induced by excessive release of thyroid hormones. It can be precipitated by surgery, stress, infection, and drugs including chemotherapeutic agents, anticholinergic, and adrenergic drugs such as pseudoephedrine, amiodarone, and iodinated contrast media. Unlike malignant hyperthermia, it is not associated with muscle rigidity, an elevated creatinine kinase, or acidosis.

10. **D.** Thyroid storm is a medical emergency and if untreated, often fatal. Supportive treatment includes cooling, hydration, and β-blockers to control heart rate. Propranolol has the additional benefit of inhibiting the peripheral conversion of T4–T3. Propylthiouracil and methimazole inhibit the synthesis of T4 by blocking the organification of tyrosine residues. Iodide blocks the release of preformed thyroid hormones, but it should be given only after the loading dose of antithyroid medication to prevent the utilization of iodine in the synthesis of new thyroid hormones. Administration of cortisol is also recommended to prevent complications from potential coexisting adrenal insufficiency.

11. **A.** Hypoparathyroidism resulting from the unintentional removal of the parathyroid glands is a potential complication of thyroidectomy. Low blood calcium levels interfere with normal muscle contraction and nerve conduction, and can result in muscle cramps, weakness, tetany, laryngospasm, and stridor. Treatment consists of normalizing the serum calcium level with intravenous calcium. While a neck hematoma can cause airway compromise due to compression, it is unlikely to cause muscle cramps. Stridor due to bilateral vocal cord paralysis is evident immediately on extubation and would require reintubation to establish a patent airway. Sodium bicarbonate would cause a metabolic alkalosis and potentially worsen symptoms of hypocalcemia by decreasing ionized calcium levels.

12. **C.** Patients with OSA may have an increased likelihood of difficult intubation, since the upper airway abnormalities associated with OSA (increased neck circumference, large tongue, decreased cross-sectional area of the upper airway) may also predispose to difficult intubation. Hypercapnia associated with severe OSA can lead to right-heart failure. OSA is

associated with increased perioperative complications including cardiac arrhythmias, hypertension, myocardial ischemia, respiratory failure, and stroke. Supine positioning and sedative agents make the upper airway even more prone to obstruction. Thus, patients with OSA may require CPAP in the immediate postoperative period.

13. **B.**   Preoperative preparation is essential for caring for the obese patient. Perioperative concerns include difficult intravenous access, possible need for arterial blood pressure monitoring, positioning, difficult endotracheal intubation, and appropriate dosing of medications. Nondiabetic obese patients are not at increased risk of aspiration of gastric contents, as they may have smaller gastric fluid volumes at higher pH than do lean nondiabetic patients. However, obesity may increase the risk of a difficult laryngeal intubation, especially in males and patients with a higher Mallampati score. Placement of the patient in the reverse Trendelenburg position during intubation is advantageous because it reduces atelectasis, increases time to oxygen desaturation after preoxygenation, and moves the chest and abdominal tissue caudally to allow easier access to the mouth for endotracheal intubation. Obese patients have a smaller volume of distribution for water-soluble drugs. Thus, dosing of these drugs should be based on ideal body weight to avoid overdosing. Larger fat stores provide an increased volume of distribution for lipid-soluble drugs. For lipid-soluble drugs, while a loading dose should be based on actual body weight, clearance will be slower because of the larger volume of distribution, and thus, maintenance doses should be administered less frequently.

14. **D.**   Refeeding syndrome can occur in malnourished patients who are acutely fed (either enterally or parenterally). It is caused by increased adenosine triphosphate production and metabolic rate. Hypophosphatemia is the hallmark biochemical feature of refeeding syndrome. Other metabolic and electrolyte disturbances may include abnormal sodium and fluid balance; hypokalemia; hypomagnesemia; thiamine deficiency; and changes in glucose, protein, and fat metabolism. Refeeding syndrome can be avoided by slowly increasing the nutritional intake toward caloric goals.

15. **C.**   Cricoid pressure can be associated with several complications. These complications are more likely in the elderly, children, pregnant women, patients with cervical injury, patients with difficult airways, and when there is difficulty palpating the cricoid cartilage. The technique involves the application of backward pressure on the cricoid cartilage to occlude the esophagus and thus prevents the aspiration of gastric contents during induction of anesthesia. However, strong downward pressure can also displace an unstable cervical spine and worsen visualization of the airway by occluding the glottis. In contrast, parturients may need more pressure to effectively occlude the esophagus.

16. **A.**   The primary goal of intraoperative blood sugar management is to avoid hypoglycemia. The most common perioperative management regimen consists of giving the patient a fraction (usually half) of the morning intermediate-acting insulin dose. If hypoglycemia is a concern, an infusion of dextrose may be started. Short-acting insulin preparations are held because of an increased risk of hypoglycemia and their short duration of action. Metformin has a duration of action of 6 to 24 hours (up to 48 hours with the extended release formulation). While it was previously recommended that metformin be discontinued 48 hours preoperatively to avoid risk of fatal lactic acidosis, more recent data suggest that this risk is low. The optimal level of glucose control in the perioperative setting remains controversial. The American Association of Clinical Endocrinologists (AACE) and the American Diabetes Association (ADA) recommend keeping blood glucose between 140 and 180 mg/dL in critically ill patients. For noncritically ill patients treated with insulin, premeal glucose targets should generally be <140 mg/dL and random blood glucose values should be <180 mg/dL. The NICE-SUGAR trial in critically ill patients showed an increased mortality and increased incidence of severe hypoglycemia in patients randomized to intensive glucose control (target glucose range 81–108 mg/dL).

17. **D.**   Carcinoid tumors are slow-growing tumors that secrete serotonin, kallikrein, and histamine. Excess serotonin secretion can result in carcinoid syndrome, which is characterized by

diarrhea, flushing, palpitations, and bronchoconstriction. However, most patients with carcinoid tumors are not symptomatic because the liver detoxifies the excess serotonin. Patients are symptomatic if they have tumors arising outside of the hepatic portal venous system or when liver metastatic disease has compromised hepatic synthetic function. The sclerosing effect of serotonin on the tricuspid and pulmonary valves can result in right-heart failure. The left heart is generally not affected because of lung metabolism of serotonin. Preoperative echocardiography should be considered in patients with carcinoid syndrome.

18. **A.**   Patients with a serum calcium >14 mg/dL should be managed with saline and diuresis to decrease their calcium level. Neuromuscular-blocking agents should be titrated carefully as severe hypercalcemia can result in muscle weakness. Prolonged hypercalcemia can result in osteoporosis and risk of vertebral compression fractures with laryngoscopy and bone fractures during transport. Hypoventilation should be avoided as acidosis increases ionized calcium levels.

19. **C.**   Hypersecretion of aldosterone results in increased sodium reabsorption in the distal renal tubule in exchange for potassium and hydrogen ions. This results in fluid retention, hypertension, metabolic alkalosis, hypokalemia, and muscle weakness.

20. **B.**   Adults normally secrete 20 to 30 mg of cortisol daily. This may increase to over 300 mg under conditions of stress.

21. **C.**   Patients who have received the equivalent of 5 mg of prednisone or more for a period of more than 2 weeks within the previous 3 months may not be able to respond appropriately to surgical stress due to adrenal suppression. These patients should receive perioperative steroid replacement therapy. The dose of steroids needed is controversial though. One recommended approach is to give a dose between 1 and 5 times the daily cortisol production (no more than 100 to 150 mg of cortisol equivalent) per day, beginning at the time of surgery and taper the replacement over 48 to 72 hours.

22. **A.**   Cushing syndrome is characterized by muscle weakness/wasting, glucose intolerance, hypertension, hypokalemia, weight gain, hypercoagulability, and osteoporosis.

23. **D.**   Intraoperative management of pheochromocytoma resection includes avoidance of drugs (e.g., ketamine, ephedrine) or techniques that may stimulate the sympathetic nervous system. Intubation should be performed after a deep level of anesthesia is achieved and hypoventilation should be avoided. Despite adequate preoperative α- and β-blockade, hypertension may still occur. These should be treated with short-acting, easily titrated agents such as nitroprusside or nicardipine. Phentolamine may also be useful because it blocks α-adrenergic receptors. Magnesium infusions have been shown useful in managing hypertension by inhibiting catecholamine release and by altering adrenergic receptor response. Patients with pheochromocytomas are often hypovolemic and become hypotensive, and hypoglycemic (lack of catecholamine-induced glucose synthesis) after tumor ligation and resection.

24. **B.**   While all of the above may cause hypotension on induction of anesthesia, the most likely cause in this patient is diabetic autonomic neuropathy. Diabetic patients with hypertension, longstanding diabetes, coronary artery disease, and old age are more likely to have autonomic dysfunction. Patients with autonomic neuropathy are unable to compensate for intravascular volume changes with an increased heart rate, and thus are more likely to have hemodynamic instability and even sudden cardiac death. This risk is increased by concomitant use of β-blockers, angiotensin-converting enzyme inhibitors, and angiotensin-receptor blockers.

25. **C.**   Limited joint mobility syndrome is due to glycosylation of tissue proteins due to chronic hyperglycemia. It is characterized by hand stiffness, though other joints (wrists, elbows, feet, spine) may be involved. Involvement of the temporomandibular joint and the cervical spine can result in difficult endotracheal intubation.

16

Ophthalmic, Ear, Nose, and Throat Surgery

Thoha Pham

1. The most accurate statement regarding absorption of topically administered ophthalmic drugs is that they are absorbed

    A. Slower than subcutaneous absorption
    B. Faster that intravenous absorption
    C. Similar to oral absorption
    D. Slower than intravenous absorption

2. Drainage of aqueous humor occurs at all of these sites, except

    A. Canal of Schlemm
    B. Trabecular network
    C. Episcleral venous system
    D. Tear ducts

3. The normal intraocular pressure (IOP) is _____ (mm Hg):

    A. 5
    B. 10
    C. 25
    D. 30

4. Correct consequence of respiratory variables on intraocular pressure (IOP) is

    A. Decrease in Pao_2 will decrease IOP
    B. Increase in Pao_2 will decrease IOP
    C. Decrease in $Paco_2$ will increase IOP
    D. Increase in $Paco_2$ will increase IOP

5. All of the following will serve to decrease intraocular pressure (IOP), except

    A. Nitrous oxide
    B. Acidosis
    C. Morphine
    D. Vecuronium

6. Increases in intraocular pressure (IOP) following succinylcholine administration for tracheal intubation can be minimized by all of the following, except

    A. β-Adrenergic blocker
    B. Nondepolarizing relaxant
    C. Detachment of extraocular muscles from the globe
    D. Lidocaine

7. The ocular effects of ketamine includes

   A. Pupillary constriction
   B. Blepharospasm
   C. Decrease in intraocular pressure
   D. Myoclonus

8. An 82-year-old female patient who resides in a nursing home facility presents for breast biopsy. She states that she uses eye drops to treat glaucoma, but does not know exact names. Patient denies other medical issues, however states that she frequently has acid reflux. Potential anesthetic considerations as a result of eye drops include all of the following, except

   A. Hyperchloremic metabolic acidosis
   B. Hypokalemic metabolic acidosis
   C. Prolonged neuromuscular block with succinylcholine
   D. Atropine-resistant bradycardia

9. An air bubble is injected into the posterior chamber at the conclusion of retinal surgery (pneumatic retinopexy) to facilitate anatomically correct healing. The most appropriate anesthetic management, before the air bubble is injected, is

   A. Increase depth of anesthesia
   B. Discontinue nitrous oxide (N_2O)
   C. Ensure adequate muscle relaxation
   D. Hyperventilate the patient

10. Compared with air, sulfur hexafluoride (SF_6) bubble injected following vitreous surgery

   A. Has a longer duration of action
   B. Is more soluble in blood than nitrogen
   C. Is inert and will not expand
   D. Is contraindicated in outpatient surgery

Questions 11 to 14

A 22-month-old 14.5-kg "preemie" is undergoing strabismus repair under general endotracheal anesthetic (GETA). Following an uneventful inhaled induction with sevoflurane, peripheral IV was obtained, and by oversight, patient was given 20 mg of succinylcholine prior to intubation. Masseter spasm was noted moments later.

11. What parameter is considered the earliest sign and symptom of an ensuing hypermetabolic state following succinylcholine administration?

   A. Hyperthermia
   B. Hypotension
   C. $EtCO_2$ increase
   D. Low oxygen saturation

12. Midway through the surgery, when surgical traction in the operative field is applied, patient's heart rate plummets from 110 bpm down to 55 bpm. The pairing that accurately reflects the afferent and efferent limbs, respectively, of this reflex is

   A. Trigeminal nerve   vagus nerve
   B. Optic nerve   vagus nerve
   C. Vagus nerve   trigeminal nerve
   D. Trochlear Nerve   optic nerve

13. The most appropriate first step in the management of this hemodynamic instability is

    A. Epinephrine
    B. Atropine
    C. Remove traction
    D. Phenylephrine

14. At the conclusion of the surgery, postoperative nausea and vomiting should be anticipated and can be minimized by all of the following, except

    A. Serotonin (5-HT$_3$) antagonist
    B. Propofol infusion
    C. Limiting opioids
    D. Deep extubation

15. The true statement regarding an oculocardiac reflex is

    A. It does not occur in enucleated patients
    B. Incidence is increased in the setting of hypercarbia
    C. Intensity increases with repeated stimulation
    D. Suppressed by general anesthesia

16. All of the following anatomic structures may participate in triggering an acute and abrupt bradycardia during ophthalmic surgery, except

    A. Trigeminal nerve
    B. Vagus nerve
    C. Globe
    D. Optic nerve

17. Appropriate anesthetic management for ophthalmic surgery requires tight control of intra-ocular pressure (IOP) before, during, and after the procedure. The accurate effect of an anesthetic drug or maneuver on IOP is

    A. Decreased by glycopyrrolate
    B. Increased by hyperventilation
    C. Decreased by nitrous oxide
    D. Increased by nondepolarizing muscle relaxants

18. All these nerves can be disrupted by injection of local anesthetics into the retrobulbar space, except

    A. Optic nerve
    B. Oculomotor nerve
    C. Trochlear nerve
    D. Abducens nerve

19. The eye movement that is preserved, or unaffected, following a retrobulbar block with 0.5% bupivacaine is

    A. Abduction
    B. Rotation
    C. Adduction
    D. Elevation

20. Possible complications of a retrobulbar block include all the following, except

    A. Central retinal artery occlusion
    B. Oculocardiac reflex
    C. Puncture of the globe
    D. Horner syndrome

Questions 21 to 22

A patient is given propofol 20 mg intravenously just before placement of a retrobulbar block (0.5% bupivacaine—3 mL) to provide ocular akinesia for ocular surgery.

21. As the surgeon attempts to place a lid speculum, the patient squints, preventing adequate placement. Additional blockade of which muscle can provide additional akinesia?

    A. Orbicularis oculi
    B. Temporalis
    C. Zygomaticus minor
    D. Levator anguli oris

22. Moments later, apnea occurs followed by complete loss of consciousness. The most likely etiology to explain this event is

    A. Subarachnoid injection of local anesthetic
    B. Effects of propofol
    C. Oculocardiac reflex
    D. Intravenous injection of local anesthetic

Questions 23 to 27

A 57-year-old otherwise-healthy male was leaving a dinner party when he was involved in a roll-over car accident during which a foreign object became lodged into his right eye. He is taken to the OR for emergent surgical repair of a penetrating wound to his right globe.

23. The most appropriate anesthetic plan to consider is

    A. Retrobulbar block followed by monitored anesthesia care (MAC)
    B. IV induction of general anesthesia avoiding muscle relaxants
    C. Rapid-sequence induction of anesthesia using large dose rocuronium
    D. Secure the airway with an awake fiberoptic intubation

24. Anesthetic strategies that can minimize intraocular pressure (IOP) increase and lessen his risk of ocular extrusion include all of the following, except

    A. Ketamine
    B. Hyperventilation
    C. Inhaled volatile agent, 2.0 MAC
    D. Controlled hypotension

25. Fifteen minutes after the start of surgery, while the surgeon is retracting the medial rectus muscle, the patient becomes hypotensive and bradycardic. The first-line therapy to address this cardiovascular derangement is

    A. Atropine 1 mg IV
    B. Phenylephrine 100 µg IV
    C. Ask the surgeon to stop
    D. Glycopyrrolate 1 mg IV

26. The patient's vital signs normalize and anesthesia is maintained with desflurane and nitrous oxide. Later in the case, conjunctival instillation of a phenylephrine (10%) solution results in immediate escalation of blood pressure from 105/70 to 220/115 mm Hg, while his pulse falls from 86 to 35 bpm. The ECG reveals new onset of ectopic ventricular complexes. The most appropriate treatment option at this time is

    A. Ask the surgeon to stop
    B. Administer nitroprusside
    C. Administer atropine
    D. Discontinue nitrous oxide

27. At the conclusion of the surgery, patient is extubated and brought to the recovery room (PACU) in a stable condition. Thirty minutes later, when he is more awake, he notes unilateral eye discomfort in the nonsurgical eye. He has associated tearing, conjunctivitis, photophobia, and pain, which is worsened with blinking. These eye symptoms are most likely caused by

    A. Retinal hemorrhage
    B. Oculogyric crisis
    C. Angle-closure glaucoma
    D. Corneal abrasion

28. True statement regarding laryngospasm is

    A. Associated risk of pulmonary edema
    B. The false vocal cords do not spasm
    C. Mediated through the recurrent laryngeal nerve
    D. Increased risk of aspiration

29. A patient in the intensive care unit (ICU) with pulmonary failure requires tracheal intubation. Compared with nasotracheal intubation, oral tracheal intubation carries a higher incidence of

    A. Patient discomfort
    B. Maxillary sinusitis
    C. Transient bacteremia
    D. Otitis media

30. When compared to an adult, the airway anatomy of a 6-week-old infant reveals

    A. Tongue is smaller and floppy
    B. Airway is narrowest at the glottic opening
    C. Position of the larynx is more anterior in the neck
    D. Epiglottis is flat and firm

Questions 31 to 32

A 3-year-old patient arrives for rescheduled tonsillectomy and adenoidectomy with another acute upper respiratory tract infection (URI). Her initial surgery was postponed 3 weeks ago as she had a URI at that time as well. Exam reveals a runny nose with greenish-yellow discharge with an intermittant wet cough. She is afebrile with normal vital signs.

31. Postponement of surgery will reduce the risk of

    A. Laryngospasm
    B. Hemorrhage
    C. Difficult intubation
    D. Gastroesophageal reflux

32. Surgery proceeded without incident; however, 2 hours later in the recovery room (PACU), she vomits a large blood clot followed by ongoing bleeding. She appears pale and anxious. Vitals reveal heart rate = 130 bpm, respiratory rate = 25 bpm, and blood pressure = 77/35 mm Hg. Her capillary refill time is 4 seconds. The most appropriate next step in management at this time is

    A. Insertion of orogastric tube to empty the stomach of blood
    B. Emergent return to the operating room
    C. Administer anxiolysis medication
    D. Provide liberal fluid resuscitation

Questions 33 to 35

A 65-year-old male requires transoral laser microsurgery to address his laryngeal webs. His medical history reveals remote tobacco smoking and recreational drug use in college.

33. Minimizing airway fire hazards associated with laser surgery can be accomplished by use of all of the following, except

    A. Intermittent mode laser emissions
    B. An air/oxygen anesthetic technique
    C. A polyvinylchloride (PVC) endotracheal tube
    D. Saline-soaked sponges over exposed tissues

34. Ten minutes later, the surgeon yells "FIRE!" The most appropriate next step is to

    A. Ventilate with air
    B. Increase F_{IO_2} to 1.0
    C. Instill saline down the endotracheal tube lumen
    D. Remove the endotracheal tube

35. One hour later while recovering in the PACU, the patient is noted to have stridor and difficulty breathing. At this time, the most appropriate next step in his airway management includes

    A. Administration of aerosolized epinephrine
    B. Endotracheal intubation
    C. Administration of helium and oxygen
    D. Intravenous injection of dexamethasone

36. A 10-year-old girl with hoarseness presents for laser microsurgery to address laryngeal papillomas. She is otherwise healthy. The surgeon is requesting a general endotracheal anesthetic (GETA). The gas mixture least likely to support combustion is

    A. Oxygen 35%, air 65%
    B. Oxygen 30%, helium 70%
    C. Oxygen 20%, nitrous oxide (N_2O) 80%
    D. Oxygen 30%, nitrogen (N_2) 70%

37. A 55-year-old woman with a 35 pack-year history of tobacco smoking is undergoing laryngobronchoscopy utilizing the Sanders jet ventilation technique. The principle behind apneic oxygenation is

    A. Contrasting density of inhaled gases
    B. Maintenance of spontaneous ventilation
    C. Air entrainment
    D. Use of helium–oxygen mixtures

38. During apneic oxygenation via a rigid bronchoscope, anesthetic considerations include all of the following, except

    A. Duration of the procedure is limited by the increase in carbon dioxide
    B. Denitrogenation should be performed prior to apnea
    C. $Paco_2$ remains unchanged for the first 15 minutes
    D. Functional residual capacity and body weight influence the rate of desaturation

Questions 39 to 43

A 35 year old male with a toxic multinodular goiter presents for thyroidectomy with radical neck dissection. He denies any other significant medical history. Review of systems reveals orthopnea and dysphagia with a recent change in the caliber of his voice.

39. True statements about this patient include all of the following, except

    A. A flow–volume loop on spirometry can evaluate tracheal compression
    B. The airway may obstruct with sedation
    C. The trachea may collapse postoperatively
    D. An abnormally low forced expiratory volume in 1 second (FEV_1) would be diagnostic of an upper airway obstruction

40. To attenuate risk of a "cannot ventilate, cannot intubate" scenario, an awake airway intubation is discussed. The neural structure that does not need to be blocked in order to provide adequate airway analgesia for a nasal intubation is

    A. Hypoglossal nerve
    B. Sphenopalatine ganglion
    C. Superior laryngeal nerve
    D. Recurrent laryngeal nerve

41. At the conclusion of a complicated 4-hour resection, the patient is extubated and brought to the recovery room. One hour after extubation, the patient complains of dyspnea with stridorous respiration. Initial steps include all of the following, except

    A. Intravenous administration of calcium
    B. Nebulized racemic epinephrine
    C. Inspection of the surgical site
    D. Direct laryngoscopy

42. If bilateral recurrent laryngeal nerves were unintentionally severed, the likely finding on direct laryngoscopy would be

    A. Paralysis of the cricothyroid muscles
    B. Intermediate position of the cords
    C. Midline, closed position of the cords
    D. Pure adductor vocal cord paralysis

43. Instead, postoperative direct laryngoscopy reveals normal position of the cords at rest, widely open glottic opening at maximal inspiration, and symmetrically moving cords during quiet breathing but with weak phonation and inability to speak loudly or shout. The most likely etiology is

    A. Recurrent laryngeal nerve paralysis
    B. Superior laryngeal nerve (SLN) paralysis
    C. External airway compression
    D. Vagus nerve paralysis

Questions 44 to 45

A 27-year-old male arrives to the operating room with laryngotracheal injuries stemming from a motorcycle collision. He presents with hoarseness and dyspnea while sitting, but is unable to lie flat due to worsening dyspnea. He is unable to swallow, and is drooling/spitting moderately blood-stained sputum. His anterior neck is diffusely swollen and exquisitely tender with notable subcutaneous emphysema. Oxygen saturation is 100% with supplemental oxygen via face mask. Review of imaging reveals a thyroid cartilage fracture horizontally and crossing the midline.

44. The most appropriate approach to his airway management is

    A. Tracheostomy
    B. Laryngeal mask airway
    C. Nasotracheal intubation
    D. Cricothyroidotomy

45. His injury would be consistent with trauma to this zone of his neck:

  A. Zone I
  B. Zone II
  C. Zone III
  D. Zone IV

Questions 46 to 47

During thyroidectomy for carcinoma, a 22-year-old patient develops tachycardia to 115 bpm while blood pressure intensifies to 145/100 mm Hg. The inhaled anesthetic is deepened and minute ventilation is increased. Thirty minutes later, tachycardia and hypertension persists despite all efforts (Table 16-1).

Table 16-1

	Pre-op	15 Minutes	30 Minutes
Heart Rate (bpm)	72	115	134
Blood pressure (mm Hg)	118/56	145/100	174/108
O_2 Saturation (%)	99 (room air)	97 ($FIO_2 = 0.60$)	94 ($FIO_2 = 1.0$)
$EtCO_2$ (mm Hg)	-	48	69
Temperature (°C)	36.6	38.5	41.8
Electrocardiogram	Normal sinus rhythm	Sinus tachycardia	Trigeminy

46. The appropriate treatment to consider at this time is

  A. Propranolol
  B. Acetaminophen
  C. Iodine
  D. Dantrolene

47. Diagnosis of malignant hyperthermia is most commonly confirmed by

  A. Caffeine halothane contracture test (CHCT)
  B. Urinalysis
  C. Arterial blood gas
  D. Core temperature >42°C

CHAPTER 16 ANSWERS

1. **D.**   Topically applied drops are quickly absorbed by the mucosal lining of the nasolacrimal duct as well as by blood vessels in the conjunctival sac with a potential to produce systemic effects. Absorption is rapid, faster than oral or subcutaneous administration, but still slower than intravenous.

2. **D.**   Intraocular pressure (IOP) is a reflection of the eye's ability to form and drain aqueous humor. The posterior chamber's ciliary body is the major producer of aqueous humor. Obstruction of the drainage system, whether it is at the canal of Schlemm, the trabecular network, or the episcleral venous system, will elevate IOP. Tear ducts do not contribute to the drainage of aqueous humor.

3. **B.**   Normally, IOP of the eye varies between 10 and 22 mm Hg, and is generally considered abnormal when >25 mm Hg. This pressure is not static, as it can vary by 1 to 2 mm Hg with each cardiac contraction. Diurnal variations of up to 5 mm Hg also exist, with a higher pressure noted upon awakening.

4. **D.**   Hypoventilation ($\uparrow Paco_2$) along with hypoxemia ($\downarrow Pao_2$) will result in increased IOP, whereas hyperventilation ($\downarrow Paco_2$) will serve to minimize choroidal blood flow to decrease IOP. Hyperoxemia ($\uparrow Pao_2$) does not affect IOP significantly.

5. **B.**   Inhaled and injected anesthetics (with the exception of ketamine) along with opioids tend to lower IOP. Nondepolarizing muscle relaxants will decrease IOP, presumably via their relaxant effects on extraocular muscles. Hypoventilation ($\uparrow Paco_2$) results in respiratory acidosis, which will increase IOP (Table 16-2).

Table 16-2 Factors Affecting Intraocular Pressure (IOP)

Increased IOP	• Hypertension (sympathetic stimulation) as occurs during laryngoscopy and intubation • Acidosis • Hypoxia • Increased central venous pressure (coughing, valsalva maneuver)
Decreased IOP	• Hypotension • Inhalational anesthetics (volatile and nitrous oxide) • Opioids • Nondepolarizing muscle relaxants

Table 16-3 Signs of Malignant Hyperthermia

Early	Late
Increased $EtCO_2$	Hyperthermia
Tachycardia	Elevated creatine phosphokinase
Skeletal muscle spasm/rigidity	Myoglobinuria
Tachypnea	Cyanosis
Sweating	Disseminated intravascular coagulation
Acidosis—respiratory and metabolic	Cardiac arrest

6. **C.**   The use of succinylcholine for eye surgery is controversial. Succinylcholine can increase IOP by about 5 to 10 mm Hg for about 5 to 10 minutes after intravenous administration (longer duration of $\uparrow$IOP following intramuscular administration). Pretreatment with nondepolarizing muscle relaxants, lidocaine, or β-blockers may reduce the ocular hypertensive

response to minimize increases in IOP. The increase in IOP after succinylcholine persists whether or not the extraocular muscles are intact, suggesting that cycloplegic effects, rather than physical contraction, are responsible for IOP elevation.

7. **B.** Ketamine may cause nystagmus and blepharospasm and may not be suitable for ophthalmic surgery. Studies with respect to the effect of ketamine on intraocular pressure (IOP) have shown conflicting results, but it appears more likely to increase, as opposed to decrease, ocular pressures. This may depend on whether ketamine is administered through the IM or IV route. Ketamine is not known to affect pupil size. Myoclonus is commonly associated with etomidate and likely should also be avoided when IOP control is essential.

8. **A.** Topical ophthalmic medications undergo sufficient and prompt absorption to produce systemic effects and may cause adverse cross-reactions to medications used in routine anesthesia care. Acetazolamide drops, due to its action as a carbonic anhydrase inhibitor, can induce a hypokalemic metabolic acidosis. Topical echothiophate iodine, an irreversible cholinesterase inhibitor, can reduce plasma cholinesterase activity, prolonging the duration of action of succinylcholine and mivacurium. Absorption of timolol, a nonselective β-adrenergic blocker has been associated with atropine-resistant bradycardia, hypotension, and bronchospasm during general anesthesia. Hyperchloremic acidosis is largely related to large volume resuscitation with normal saline.

9. **B.** In the presence of N_2O, air bubbles will increase in size as N_2O is 35 times more soluble compared to molecular nitrogen (the major component of air), allowing it to diffuse into an air bubble more rapidly than nitrogen is absorbed out of the bubble. If the bubble expands after the incision is closed, intraocular pressure will rise. This complication can be avoided by discontinuing N_2O at least 15 minutes prior to the bubble injection, as the washout of N_2O from the lungs is 90% complete within 10 minutes. Additionally, repeat general anesthesia with N_2O should be avoided until the bubble is fully absorbed, which for air can take up to 5 days.

10. **A.** SF_6 is an inert gas that is much less soluble than nitrogen (the major component of air) in blood and, therefore, will have a longer duration of action (10 days) compared to an air bubble. Bubble size doubles within 24 hours after injection of SF_6 because nitrogen from inhaled air will enter more rapidly into the bubble than sulfur can diffuse out of it. This slow bubble expansion usually does not pathologically affect IOP. However, inspired N_2O, which is 117 times more diffusible than hexafluoride (compared to 35 times more than nitrogen), will rapidly enter the SF_6 bubble such that IOP will rise significantly within 30 minutes after the eye is closed. As with air, repeat general anesthesia with N_2O should be avoided until the SF_6 bubble is fully resorbed.

11. **C.** Although still quite rare, an increased incidence of malignant hyperthermia (MH) has been reported in patients with strabismus (underlying myopathy) such that a high index of suspicion should be maintained. $EtCO_2$ is considered the earliest indicator of a hypermetabolic state with unexpected increases in CO_2 despite constant minute ventilation. Avoiding known triggers can negate the risk of inducing MH, such that succinylcholine is not recommended during strabismus surgery involving infants and children.

12. **A.** Trigeminovagal reflex: the afferent limb of the oculocardiac reflex is via the trigeminal nerve (CN V), primarily through the ophthalmic division (V1). The impulse travels along the long and short ciliary nerves (LCN and SCN) to synapse on the ciliary ganglion. The impulse then continues through the trigeminal ganglion arriving at the sensory nucleus of the trigeminal nerve. The convergence between the afferent and efferent limbs is at the motor nucleus of

the vagus nerve (CN X) of the brain stem. From here, the efferent limb is via the vagus nerve, which eventually synapses on the sinoatrial node of the heart, resulting in an abrupt bradycardia (Fig 16-1).

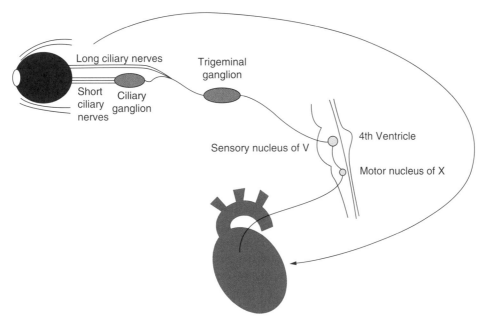

Figure 16-1.

13. **C.**   The oculocardiac reflex (OCR) occurs frequently during strabismus surgery. It can occur following traction of the extrinsic eye muscles, or placement of pressure on the globe. The OCR is most commonly manifested as bradycardia, which regresses almost immediately after the stimulus is removed. Bigeminy, ectopy, nodal rhythms, atrioventricular block, and cardiac arrest have also occurred. Traction on any of the extraocular muscles can evoke this reflex, but it appears that manipulation of the medial rectus muscle is the most consistent trigger. Though the prophylactic use of an anticholinergic (atropine or glycopyrrolate) before the potential evoking stimulus may be recommended, the most effective treatment is the removal of the stimulus.

14. **D.**   The incidence of nausea and vomiting following strabismus surgery can be high, ranging anywhere from 48% to 85%. Minimizing the use of opioids, substituting propofol for inhaled anesthetics, along with the prophylactic use of antiemetics can reduce nausea and vomiting after surgery. Deep extubation has no impact on postoperative nausea and vomiting, and may place patient at risk for aspiration.

15. **B.**   The afferent limb of the oculocardiac reflex (OCR) is the trigeminal nerve such that pressures on the globe, conjunctiva, or orbital structures and traction on the extraocular muscles are potential triggers. This reflex occurs even with an empty globe. Hypercarbia and hypoxemia are factors believed to augment the incidence and severity of the reflex. This reflex is noted to fatigue with repeated stimulation and is not suppressed by general anesthesia.

16. **D.**   The afferent limb of the oculocardiac reflex is the trigeminal nerve such that triggers include pressure on the globe, conjunctiva, or orbital structures as well as traction of the extraocular muscles. The vagus nerve is the efferent limb with connections to the sinoatrial node triggering a reflex bradycardia. The optic nerve is not involved in this reflex activity.

17. C.   Anticholinergics (e.g., glycopyrrolate) may include mydriasis of the pupils, leading to an increase in intraocular pressure. Unlike atropine, however, glycopyrrolate is completely ionized at physiologic pH; thus, the occurrence of CNS-related side effects is lower, as it has difficulty crossing the blood–brain barrier. Anesthetic agents, whether inhaled or injected, reduce IOP, with the possible exception of ketamine. Nondepolarizing neuromuscular-blocking agents produce a slight decrease, while depolarizing relaxants increase IOP. Hyperventilation will cause vasoconstriction with decrease in choroidal blood flow and intraocular pressures.

18. C.   Nerves blocked are those within the optic cone (annulus of Zinn), which include optic (CN II), oculomotor (CN III), and the abducens (CN VI). The trochlear nerve (CN IV) is not affected, since it is located outside of this muscle cone.

19. B.   The trochlear nerve (CN IV) remains intact following a retrobulbar block, since it is located outside of the muscle cone. The trochlear nerve innervates the superior oblique muscle; thus, rotational movement of the eye remains intact.

20. D.   Common complications attributed to a retrobulbar block include retrobulbar hemorrhage with possible central artery occlusion, oculocardiac reflex, puncture of the posterior globe, penetration of the optic nerve, and inadvertent intrathecal injection. Horner syndrome is not commonly seen following retrobulbar blocks; instead, it results from an interruption of the sympathetic nerve supply to the head/face, resulting in a triad of miosis, ptosis, and anhidrosis.

21. A.   Blockade of the orbicularis oculi muscle, which is a sphincter muscle around the eye, can further provide adequate surgical conditions for any ocular procedure with consequent inability to squeeze the lids shut. This can be achieved by blockade of the facial nerve (CN VII).

22. A.   There is 1% to 3% risk of complications with retrobulbar block, ranging from mild to severe. Possible complications include accidental subarachnoid injection, which can cause a "total spinal" leading to apnea, unconsciousness, and cardiorespiratory collapse.

23. C.   Eye injuries commonly occur as a result of trauma, which frequently means providing emergent general anesthesia for patients with full stomachs. It is important to avoid any sudden increases in intraocular pressure (IOP) that may cause extrusion of the ocular contents. Although awake tracheal intubation provides the greatest margin of safety to prevent aspiration, it may in fact promote increase in IOP with inadequate orotracheal anesthesia. Placement of a retrobulbar block is not advised as inadvertent globe puncture may lead to extrusion of orbital contents. For most cases, rapid-sequence or modified rapid-sequence induction is utilized. The choice of succinylcholine offers the advantage of rapid onset of muscle relaxation, but may acutely cause elevation in IOP. Alternatively, the use of a large dose of nondepolarizing neuromuscular-blocking agent will reduce IOP and facilitate tracheal intubation as long as adequate blockade is confirmed prior to laryngoscopy.

24. A.   Hyperventilation, hypotension, and hypothermia decrease IOP, whereas arterial hypoxemia and hypoventilation elevate IOP. External pressure can also be generated by venous congestion of orbital veins, which is accentuated during a valsalva, coughing, and vomiting. Additionally, most inhaled and injected anesthetics (with the exception of ketamine) can also serve to reduce IOP.

25. C.   The oculocardiac reflex best explains this cardiovascular presentation during ophthalmologic surgeries. First-line therapy is always to remove the stimulus, which is mediated via trigeminal afferents.

26. B.   Hypertensive episodes during anesthesia should be tackled logically. Common causes are light anesthesia, hypoxia, and hypercarbia. In this case, excessive systemic uptake of the phenylephrine precipitated severe hypertension. Elevated diastolic pressures with ECG pathology necessitate immediate action to prevent further cardiovascular decline. Administration of sodium nitroprusside is beneficial to quickly reduce the blood pressure and decrease cardiac afterload.

27. **D.** Corneal abrasions produce a foreign body sensation with associated tearing, conjunctivitis, and photophobia. This pain is made worse by blinking. Protection against this occurrence includes application of nonionic petroleum-based ophthalmic ointment to the eye, securely taping the eyelids shut during anesthesia, and discouraging patients from rubbing their eye on emergence. Abrasions can be diagnosed by fluorescein staining, and treatment options include saline flushes, antibiotic ointment, and patching the eye.

28. **A.** Laryngospasm can complicate any routine airway management and is especially prevalent around the time of extubation. It often occurs during stage 2—"excitement stage"—of general anesthesia in combination with an airway irritant such as blood, mucus, laryngoscope blade, suction catheter, surgical debris, or other foreign objects. This protective reflex is mediated by the superior laryngeal nerve and manifested as sustained closure of the glottis. Laryngospasm with complete airway obstruction can be associated with negative pressure pulmonary edema, as patients can create a significant amount of negative intrathoracic pressure during attempts to breathe against an obstructed upper airway. The management consists of positive pressure ventilation, increasing the depth of anesthesia, and occasionally a small dose of a muscle relaxant with or without reintubation.

29. **A.** Tracheal intubation to facilitate mechanical ventilation is common in ICU patients to appropriately manage failure of adequate spontaneous ventilation and/or oxygenation. Both nasal and oral tracheal tubes are relatively safe, for at least several weeks, while patients convalesce. When compared with prolonged oral intubation, nasotracheal intubation may be more comfortable for the patient, more secure (fewer occurrences of accidental self-extubations), and less likely to cause laryngeal damage. Nasal intubation, however, has its own significant adverse events, including significant nasal bleeding, transient bacteremia, sinusitis, and otitis media (from obstruction of the auditory tubes).

30. **C.** Recognizing the anatomical differences between an adult and a pediatric airway is important. One of the most obvious differences is the tongue itself. The pediatric tongue is larger, in relation to the amount of free space in the oropharynx, when compared to the adult tongue. With regards to the pediatric epiglottis, it tends to be large and floppy with a more oblong configuration, making epiglottis control with a laryngoscope blade more challenging. Additionally, the position of the adult larynx is at about the level C5–C6; the pediatric larynx is more cephalad, at about the level of the C3–C4. This is an important anatomical airway consideration, since the higher larynx tends to be more anterior as well (Fig 16-2).

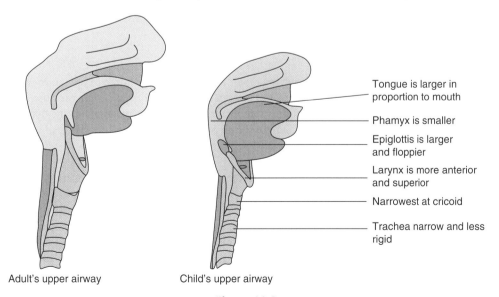

Adult's upper airway Child's upper airway

Tongue is larger in proportion to mouth

Phamyx is smaller

Epiglottis is larger and floppier

Larynx is more anterior and superior

Narrowest at cricoid

Trachea narrow and less rigid

Figure 16-2.

31. A. Laryngospasm associated with airway manipulation is more likely to occur in the presence of a URI such that surgery is typically postponed until resolution of symptoms, typically 1 to 2 weeks. Young children, however, have frequent URIs such that risk:benefit ratio should be considered when determining appropriateness of proceeding versus further postponement.

32. D. Hemorrhage from a bleeding tonsillar bed in the postoperative period is a hazardous complication. Her vitals reveal hypovolemia and as such, initial management should be to resuscitate the patient prior to returning to the operating room to minimize morbidity associated with anemia and hypovolemia in the setting of repeat general anesthesia. Also assume that patient will now have a difficult airway with a "full stomach."

33. C. Anesthesia during laser surgery may be administered with or without an endotracheal tube. If intubation is needed, appropriate laser-resistant endotracheal tubes should be utilized. In this regard, remember that all PVC tubes are flammable and can ignite when contacted by the laser beam. Using the laser intermittently, ventilating the patient with a low concentration of combustible gases, along with protecting adjacent tissues with saline-soaked sponges are all appropriate approaches to minimize the fire hazards.

34. D. Airway fires are an inherent risk with laser surgery, such that a plan of action should be considered before the case begins. The cuff of the endotracheal tube may be filled with saline, as opposed to air, to minimize flammability should the laser beam rupture the cuff. Inspired oxygen concentration is minimized as tolerated (usually Fio_2 of <0.50), as oxygen readily supports combustion. In the event of an airway fire, the anesthesia circuit should be immediately disconnected to interrupt further delivery of oxygen, followed by removal of the tube from the patient's airway. If the flame persists, the field should next be flooded with normal saline.

35. B. Post airway fires, it is most appropriate to leave the patient intubated for continued observation as the presence of laryngeal and pharyngeal edema can result in failed extubation. Therefore, this patient should be reintubated with a regular endotracheal tube and monitored for the next 24 hours. Corticosteroids can be considered for severe edema with absent cuff leak, but generally is not given prophylactically.

36. B. The mixture of gases delivered into the endotracheal tube may affect the risk of combustion during general anesthesia and laser surgery of the airway. N_2O is highly combustible and should be strictly avoided. Fio_2 should be reduced to as low as possible with an air–oxygen mixture. Helium, if available, is ideal as it is inert and noncombustible. Though N_2 is also considered safe, the mean time to ignition with nitrogen has been found to be significantly shorter when compared to the same concentration of helium.

37. C. In 1960s, Sanders described ventilation technique using a 16-gauge jet placed down the side arm of a rigid bronchoscope, relying on air entrapment to continue oxygenation with an open bronchoscope. An intermittent jet of oxygen administered from a high-pressure source (50 psi) entrains room air to maintain supranormal oxygen concentrations in the upper airways, which creates a diffusion gradient to the alveolar spaces. This gradient is maintained as alveolar oxygen is constantly consumed.

38. C. Apneic oxygenation relies on mass movement oxygenation. With the onset of apnea, a low pressure develops in the airspace of the lungs, as more oxygen is absorbed (230 mL/min) than CO_2 is released (200 mL/min). If the airways are open, 100% oxygen supplied to the upper airways will follow the pressure gradient and flow into the lungs, replacing the oxygen consumed. The uptake of oxygen into the blood will then remain at relatively normal levels, recognizing that the lack of ventilation will eventually cause marked hypercapnia and acidosis.

39. D. The configuration of the flow–volume curve during spirometry testing can be used to demonstrate abnormalities of the larger central airways (larynx, trachea, and main stem bronchi). The FEV_1/FVC ratio can provide diagnostic value, as disproportionate reduction in the FEV_1 as compared to the FVC is the hallmark of obstructive lung diseases. Concern should be made regarding airway collapse following sedation or induction of anesthesia when extrathoracic lesions are present. If long-standing, tracheomalacia may leave the trachea weak and collapsible postoperatively (Fig 16-3).

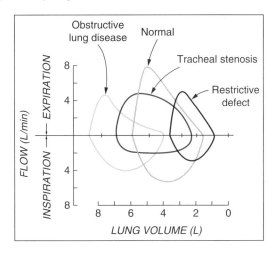

Figure 16-3.

40. A. Anesthesia of the nasal mucosa and nasopharynx is achieved via blockade of trigeminal branches, particularly the sphenopalatine ganglion and ethmoid nerves. Blockade of the glossopharyngeal and superior laryngeal nerves provide anesthesia to the mouth, oropharynx, and base of the tongue. The hypopharynx, larynx, and trachea are innervated via a branch of the vagus nerve (CN X), specifically the recurrent laryngeal nerve, which can be blocked via a transtracheal approach. On the other hand, blockade of the hypoglossal nerve (CN XII) will only serve to paralyze the intrinsic muscles of the tongue without adding to anesthesia of the airway (Fig 16-4).

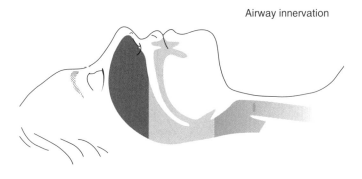

Airway innervation

Trigeminal (V) n.   Glossopharyngeal (IX) n.   Vagus (X) n.

Figure 16-4.

41. A. Inspection of the neck is generally considered the first step, as it may reveal a life-threatening and reversible cause of airway obstruction such as a compressing hematoma. Direct visualization of vocal cords may point toward recurrent laryngeal nerve damage contributing to dyspnea. Though hypocalcemia due to removal of the parathyroid glands can occur, signs and symptoms will usually present much later in the perioperative course (24–96 hours), and unlikely to be contributing to dyspnea in the PACU. Inhaled racemic epinephrine is commonly used when stridor is present after extubation.

42. **B.**   The recurrent laryngeal nerves provide motor innervation to all the intrinsic muscles of the larynx, except the cricothyroid muscle, which is innervated by the superior laryngeal nerve. Damage to bilateral recurrent laryngeal nerves will affect abduction and adduction of the cords, resulting in both vocal cords adopting an intermediate, or paramedian, position. Patient would also have associated aphonia with risk of airway obstruction with inspiration as the cords flap together. Unilateral damage will present with hoarseness.

43. **B.**   In the case of lesions to the SLNs, adduction and abduction of the vocal cords remain intact. SLN lesions instead lead to weak tensor strength (cricothyroid muscle), leaving the voice hoarse, weak, breathy, and with the inability to scream or shout. Other associated findings would be loss of sensation above the cords, leaving patient vulnerable to inhalation of any material present in the pharynx.

44. **A.**   Blunt-neck trauma is most commonly a result of a motor vehicle collision associated with rapid acceleration or deceleration injuries, which may include crushing injuries of the trachea, esophagus, vascular structures, and cervical spine. A laryngeal fracture can lead to life-threatening airway obstruction and as such should be treated in an emergent manner. Signs and symptoms of dyspnea, emphysema, and inability to lie flat reflect a fragile airway. Definitive airway management following airway trauma is a surgical airway, most commonly a tracheostomy. Cricothyroidotomy is not recommended following laryngotracheal injuries, as the landmarks are usually difficult to assess, since the cricoid is often the level of the injury.

45. **B.**   The neck is divided into three zones: zone I, including the thoracic inlet, up to the level of the cricothyroid membrane, is treated as an upper thoracic injury. Zone III, above the angle of the mandible, is treated as a head injury. In this case, fracture of the thyroid cartilage represents an injury of the neck in zone II. For ease of memory, consider that the cricoid cartilage demarcates the border between zones I and II and the angle of the mandible separates zone II from zone III (Fig 16-5).

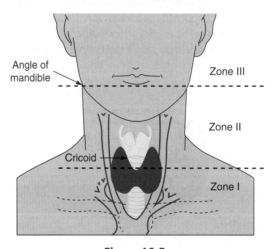

Figure 16-5.

46. **D.**   Increasing $EtCO_2$ and temperature may reveal possible malignant hyperthermia. With onset of cardiac arrhythmias, and the increasing likelihood of the development of malignant hyperthermia with rapidly climbing $EtCO_2$ and hyperthermia, treatment with dantrolene should be considered and pursued. Other signs that can strengthen the diagnosis are muscle rigidity and myoglobinuria.

47. **A.**   More than 30 different mutations are linked to malignant hyperthermia susceptibility. Genetic testing is available to establish a diagnosis, but the CHCT remains the criterion standard.

17

Obstetric Anesthesia

Thoha Pham

1. Beyond midgestation, pregnant women are at increased risk of gastroesophageal reflux and aspiration of gastric contents for all these reasons, except

   A. Decreased competence of the lower esophageal sphincter
   B. Delayed gastric emptying associated with the onset of labor
   C. Delayed gastric emptying due to opioid administration
   D. Increased incidence of constipation

2. Changes in the cardiovascular system associated with pregnancy include

   A. Increase in central venous pressure
   B. Increase in cardiac output
   C. Increase in systemic vascular resistance
   D. Increase in blood pressure

3. During pregnancy, the disproportionate increase in plasma volume versus erythrocyte volume accounts for

   A. Increase in the mean arterial pressure
   B. Increase in stroke volume
   C. Increase in cardiac output
   D. Relative anemia of pregnancy

4. By the third trimester of pregnancy, cardiac output increases to nearly 50% due to which of these alterations?

   A. Increase in stroke volume and increase in heart rate
   B. Decrease in stroke volume and increase in heart rate
   C. Increase in stroke volume and decrease in heart rate
   D. Decrease in stroke volume and decrease in heart rate

5. The largest increase in cardiac output is seen during this peripartum period:

   A. During induction of anesthesia
   B. During the start of labor
   C. Immediately after delivery
   D. At conception

6. A 20-year-old G_1P_0 female at 42^5 weeks of gestation presents to labor and delivery floor with rupture of membranes and onset of early labor. She appears uncomfortable and becomes extremely anxious with peripheral IV placement, and begins to hyperventilate. If allowed to continue hyperventilation, it will cause

   A. Increased placental perfusion
   B. Decreased maternal arterial pH
   C. Increased fetal arterial pH
   D. Decreased maternal uterine artery flow

7. In the above patient, labor is nonprogressive with signs of fetal distress on heart rate monitoring. Spinal anesthesia with 2-chloroprocaine 3% (2 mL) is provided for emergent cesarean section. On postpartum day 2, she complains of leg numbness, which quickly progressed to flaccid paralysis. On examination, inability to move her lower extremities with complete loss of pain and temperature sensation below T4 with normal sensation to light touch was noted. The most likely cause of this complication is

   A. 2-Chloroprocaine neurotoxicity
   B. Inadvertent subdural injection
   C. Anterior spinal artery syndrome
   D. Brown-Séquard syndrome

Questions 8 to 9

A 23-year-old female, in early labor, was transferred from an outside hospital at 37 weeks' gestation with a history of a congenital bicuspid aortic valve. The patient reports dyspnea throughout her pregnancy, and had a recent syncopal event. Subsequently, transthoracic echocardiogram revealed a mean aortic valve gradient of 45 mm Hg and an aortic valve area of 1.2 cm².

8. Two hours later, she endorses abdominal pain (8/10) and is requesting analgesia. The most appropriate option for her pain management during labor and delivery is

   A. Spinal anesthetic with bupivacaine
   B. Epidural anesthesia with adequate volume preloading
   C. Inhaled nitrous oxide
   D. Oral analgesics

9. Despite an appropriate increase in her cardiac output and plasma volume, her systemic blood pressure does not increase during the course of her pregnancy because of

   A. Decrease in systemic vascular resistance
   B. Compression of the vena cava
   C. Decrease in venous capacitance
   D. Decrease in heart rate

10. Iatrogenic contributions to maternal supine hypotension syndrome can be minimized by

   A. Left hip elevation
   B. Left-uterine displacement
   C. Regional anesthesia
   D. General anesthesia

11. The most significant change in maternal lung volume that occurs in the third trimester of pregnancy includes

   A. Decrease in vital capacity
   B. Increase in residual volume
   C. Decrease in functional residual capacity (FRC)
   D. Decrease in closing capacity (CC)

12. Which of the following is *not* associated with oxytocin administration?

    A. Myocardial ischemia
    B. Respiratory depression
    C. Hypotension
    D. Tachycardia

13. During maintenance of a general inhaled anesthetic for an urgent nonobstetric surgery, one would expect this difference in the pregnant patient versus a nonpregnant patient:

    A. Slower emergence from anesthesia
    B. Minimal changes in depth of anesthesia
    C. There is to be no difference
    D. Faster induction of anesthesia

14. When providing general anesthesia during pregnancy, minimum alveolar concentration (MAC) is

    A. Increased
    B. Decreased
    C. Unchanged
    D. Unclear

15. The speed of time to hypoxia following apnea is faster in the late-trimester parturient due to all of the following factors, except

    A. Reduced functional residual capacity
    B. Increased minute ventilation
    C. Preoxygenation
    D. Increased oxygen consumption

16. The correct respiratory physiologic change associated with pregnancy is

    A. Increase in arterial pH
    B. Increase in HCO_3
    C. Increase in $Paco_2$
    D. Increase in tidal volume

17. The P_{50} for maternal hemoglobin

    A. Increases due to elevated levels of 2,3-diphosphoglycerate (DPG)
    B. Remains unchanged
    C. Increases to maintain pH
    D. Decreases to enhance oxygen delivery to tissues

18. At sea level, the most likely arterial blood gas (ABG) sample of a parturient at 35 weeks' gestation when she rests in the supine position breathing room air is

    A. pH = 7.35, Pao_2 = 90, $Paco_2$ = 45, HCO_3 = 20
    B. pH = 7.40, Pao_2 = 100, $Paco_2$ = 40, HCO_3 = 24
    C. pH = 7.44, Pao_2 = 90, $Paco_2$ = 30, HCO_3 = 20
    D. pH = 7.50, Pao_2 = 105, $Paco_2$ = 30, HCO_3 = 20

19. A 27-year-old G_2P_1 at 39^2 weeks' gestation is electing to have spinal anesthesia for a repeat cesarean section. Five minutes after bupivacaine spinal injection, the patient becomes hypotensive and is complaining of tingling in her fingers with subjective difficulty breathing. Her oxygen saturation remains 100% and blood pressure is 95/55. The most likely etiology is

   A. Engorgement of epidural veins contributed to inadvertent intravascular injection of the local anesthetics
   B. Decrease in volume of CSF in the subarachnoid space facilitated higher spread of local anesthetics
   C. Severe patient anxiety
   D. Increased peripheral nerve sensitization to local anesthetics

20. During pregnancy, hepatic changes contribute to

   A. Decreased albumin levels contributing to higher free blood levels of highly protein-bound drugs
   B. Decreased liver function tests due to decreased blood flow
   C. Decreased concentration levels of coagulation factors leading to easy bruisability
   D. Decreased activity of plasma cholinesterase resulting in significantly longer duration of action of succinylcholine

Questions 21 to 23

After 18 hours of laboring and adherence to a strict nonpharmacologic natural birth plan, the patient experiences late decelerations and fetal distress, requiring emergent cesarean section.

21. To minimize the risk of aspiration and resultant pneumonitis,

   A. Place patient in left-uterine displacement
   B. Give H_2-receptor antagonist to decrease the pH of gastric fluid present in the stomach
   C. Give metoclopramide to reverse opioid-induced gastric hypomotility
   D. Give a nonparticulate antacid to decrease the pH of the gastric fluid

22. The most common cause of late decelerations in fetal heart rate (FHR) (down to 90 bpm) is

   A. Fetal vagal reflex
   B. Compression of the fetal head
   C. Umbilical cord compression
   D. Fetal alkalosis

23. After performing a single-shot intrathecal anesthetic consisting of 7.5 mg of preservative-free bupivacaine and 25 µg of fentanyl, the surgical incision is made and systemic hypotension (78/44 mm Hg) ensued. To avoid significant decreases in uterine blood flow, first-line therapy to consider is

   A. Provide additional inhaled nitric oxide (NO) to vasodilate the uterine vasculature
   B. Increase maternal cardiac output with use of epinephrine
   C. Increase intravascular volume with fluids
   D. Use reverse Trendelenburg to decrease aortocaval compression

Questions 24 to 25

With increasing concern of variable decelerations, a male fetus is delivered with vacuum assistance. The amniotic fluid was noted to be meconium stained. Initial evaluation reveals a cyanotic limp infant with a heart rate of 80 bpm, poor respiratory efforts, and grimacing in response to suctioning.

24. Patient's Apgar score would be

    A. 0
    B. 3
    C. 5
    D. 10

25. Appropriate initial steps in the resuscitation efforts would include all of the following, except

    A. Tracheal suctioning
    B. Provide radiant heat source
    C. Positive-pressure ventilation
    D. Supplemental oxygen

26. Regarding forceps-assisted delivery

    A. High-forceps delivery has the highest success rate
    B. Prevents clavicle fracture associated with dystocia
    C. Hastens postpartum maternal recovery
    D. Is associated with increased incidence of fetal facial nerve trauma

27. True statement regarding fetal circulation includes

    A. The ductus venosus shunts blood away from the pulmonary circuit.
    B. Deoxygenated blood is carried in the umbilical vein.
    C. The foramen ovale shunts blood from right to left ventricles.
    D. Intracardiac pressures are equalized across both right and left ventricles.

28. Successful transition from fetal to neonatal circulation is required after birth to support extra-uterine life. This depends primarily on these factors, except

    A. Removal of the placenta
    B. Decreased systemic vascular resistance
    C. Decreased pulmonary vascular resistance
    D. Closure of the intra- and extracardiac shunts

29. In considering placental exchange and fetal uptake, all statements are true, except

    A. Minimizing the maternal blood concentrations of a drug is the most important method of limiting the amount that ultimately reaches the fetus
    B. Drugs that readily cross the blood–brain barrier will also cross the placenta
    C. Placental exchange of substance occurs principally via ion transport from the maternal circulation to the fetus
    D. Ion trapping explains why fetal-to-maternal lidocaine ratios are higher during fetal acidemia than during normal fetal well-being

30. Which of the following best explains why lidocaine has a higher fetal-to-maternal plasma ratio when compared with bupivacaine?

    A. Bupivacaine has a smaller molecular weight
    B. Lidocaine has higher protein-binding
    C. Bupivacaine has a lower dissociation constant (pK_a)
    D. Lidocaine is less lipid soluble

31. In order to provide analgesia for all stages of labor, one must accommodate the evolving and varied course of labor and delivery. The *least* accurate statement regarding the anatomy of labor is

    A. Pain during labor and delivery is often described in two stages
    B. Somatic and visceral innervation of the uterus and cervix enters the spinal cord via T10 to L1
    C. Innervation of the perineum is primarily via the pudendal nerve
    D. Somatic and visceral afferent sensory fibers from the uterus and cervix travel with greater, lesser, and least splanchnic nerves via the celiac plexus

32. The regional or neuraxial technique that would *not* be expected to provide appropriate analgesic benefit during the first stage of labor is

    A. Lumbar epidural
    B. Pudendal nerve block
    C. Lumbar sympathetic block
    D. Paracervical block

Questions 33 to 37

A 37-year-old G_9P_4 patient at 38 weeks of gestation presents for management of labor and delivery. She denies any medical history and admits to minimal prenatal care. The patient is moderately hypertensive (160/95) with associated pitting edema at her ankles.

33. The statement about her disorder that is most likely true is

    A. Eclampsia is imminent
    B. Preeclampsia is a syndrome manifested after the 36th week of gestation
    C. HELLP syndrome is the mildest form of eclampsia
    D. Definitive treatment of preeclampsia is delivery of the fetus and placenta

34. The patient is started on oxytocin to augment her labor, and the patient is now requesting a labor epidural. Anesthetic considerations include

    A. The presence of hypertension and edema requires further workup before proceeding
    B. No workup is required prior to performing epidural anesthesia, as this will treat her hypertension
    C. Neuraxial anesthesia should be avoided, as there is increased risk of bleeding
    D. Avoid systemic opiates, as the risk of respiratory depression is too high

35. After a review of her laboratory results, a lumbar (L3–L4) epidural was placed without incident (including lack of CSF, and negative test dose after administration of 45 mg lidocaine with 1:200,000 epinephrine). Epidural anesthesia is then initiated with a bolus of 15 mg of bupivacaine. Variable decelerations are noted minutes later on fetal heart rate monitoring. If scalp pH reveals fetal acidosis, compared with a normal pH, the anesthetic absorbed by the fetus will be present in

    A. Higher concentration, most in ionized form
    B. Lower concentration, most in ionized form
    C. Higher concentration, most in unionized form
    D. Unchanged concentration, equal fraction of ionized and nonionized

36. The patient has now been receiving a dilute infusion (bupivacaine 0.125% with 2 µg/mL fentanyl) for the past 3 hours and reports good pain relief with a bilateral T5 sensory level. Her blood pressure is now 85/45 mm Hg, and her heart rate is 120 bpm. The fetal heart rate pattern begins to show late decelerations. The most appropriate management in this patient includes

    A. Immediate bedside cesarean delivery
    B. Administration of phenylephrine
    C. Administration of ephedrine
    D. Discontinuation of the epidural infusion

37. As augmentation of labor continues, patient's blood pressure slowly climbs again, with waning epidural analgesic benefit. Highest pressure was noted to be 166/112 mm Hg with heart rate sustained over 100 bpm. The most appropriate pharmacologic option for *acute* treatment of severe hypertension in a preeclamptic patient is

    A. Magnesium
    B. Dopamine
    C. Labetalol
    D. Hydralazine

38. Four hours postdelivery, and after the epidural is removed, the patient now requires emergent anesthesia for surgical removal of retained placental products. The appropriate anesthetic management includes all of the following, except

    A. Antibiotic administration
    B. Total intravenous anesthesia
    C. General endotracheal inhaled anesthetic
    D. Sodium citrate

39. Forty-eight hours postdelivery, the patient is febrile, complaining of chills with severe occipital and neck pain worsened with sitting and standing, but not improved when lying in bed. The finding you would *not* expect to find on examination is

    A. Urinary retention
    B. Low back pain
    C. Nausea and vomiting
    D. Normal white blood cell (WBC) count

40. Postdural puncture headache (PDPH) occurs more frequently

    A. In elderly (>50 year old) vs. young patients
    B. In underweight vs. overweight patients
    C. With a cutting-point vs. pencil-point spinal needles
    D. With larger- vs. smaller-gauge spinal needles

41. Decrease in fasciculations can be seen following induction doses of succinylcholine for emergent cesarean section. The factor that can blunt this response is

    A. Increased cardiac output
    B. Prior magnesium administration
    C. Prior nitrous oxide inhalation
    D. Metabolic alkalosis

42. Administration of all the following will provide uterine relaxation, except

    A. Sevoflurane
    B. Nitrous oxide
    C. Nitroglycerine
    D. Terbutaline

43. Adverse effects of inhaled β-tocolytic therapy for preterm labor to the mother include all of the following, except

    A. Hypoglycemia
    B. Pulmonary edema
    C. Tachycardia
    D. Ventricular arrhythmias

44. During a general anesthetic for emergent cesarean section, administering of all of the following could contribute to increased operative blood loss, except

    A. Nitroglycerine
    B. Ritodrine intravenously
    C. 1 MAC Desflurane
    D. Hyperventilation

45. With regard to sodium thiopental, the following statements are accurate, except

    A. Peak concentration in the brain occurs at 1 minute postinjection
    B. Rapid redistribution allows for return of consciousness in $<$10 minutes
    C. Infusions maintain appropriate surgical conditions with fast recovery due to ultra-short action
    D. Repeating the induction dose results in fetal depression

46. The following statements are true regarding umbilical cord blood, except

    A. Provides a picture of the acid–base balance in the infant at the moment of birth
    B. Double clamping of the umbilical cord at birth will preserve a segment of cord blood in isolation, which can remain stable for up to 24 hours
    C. Cord blood that is still in continuity with the placenta will have shifting acid–base balance due to ongoing placental metabolism and gas exchange
    D. Normal paired arterial and venous specimens can provide evidence against an intrapartum hypoxic–ischemic event to the newborn

47. Maternally administered drugs that decrease beat-to-beat variability of fetal heart rate include all of the following, except

    A. Ritodrine
    B. Atropine
    C. Prochlorperazine
    D. Bupivacaine

48. A 24-year-old G_4P_2 parturient is undergoing a general anesthetic for emergency cesarean section due to uterine rupture. All these findings would suggest an amniotic fluid embolism (AFE), except

    A. Decreased $EtCO_2$
    B. Increased maternal pH
    C. Bleeding diathesis
    D. Upsloping $EtCO_2$ tracing

49. A 42-year-old G_1P_0 at 29^4 weeks' gestation is undergoing intracranial clipping of a large arteriovenous malformation, following sudden onset of a severe headache with associated nausea/vomiting. Patient is intubated in the interventional radiology suite and ventilated with settings of TV = 500 mL, respiratory rate = 14 bpm, PEEP = 5 cm H_2O, and F_{IO_2} = 1.0. Arterial blood gas (ABG) 30 minutes later reveals pH = 7.55, Pao_2 = 502, $Paco_2$ = 19, and HCO_3 = 21. These findings are associated with all of the following, except

    A. Decreased fetal cerebral oxygen delivery
    B. Decreased placental transfer of oxygen
    C. Rightward shift of the oxygen dissociation curve
    D. Decreased umbilical blood flow

50. True statement concerning hyperglycemia during pregnancy is

    A. Increases risk of fetal microsomia
    B. Fetal oxygen requirements remain decreased
    C. May contribute to neonatal hypoglycemia
    D. Increases risk of sepsis during cesarean delivery

51. True statement regarding neuraxial opioids for labor and delivery is

    A. Opioids should never be used as a sole agent
    B. Most common side effect is fetal bradycardia
    C. Intrathecal morphine is associated with quick peak in concentration and early onset maternal respiratory depression
    D. Systemic absorption is similar to intramuscular (IM) administration

52. All of the following drugs readily cross the placenta, except

    A. β-Agonist antagonists
    B. Local anesthetics
    C. Insulin
    D. Morphine

53. Following a 0.6 mg/kg intravenous dose of rocuronium to facilitate rapid-sequence induction in a parturient requiring surgical delivery, one would expect

    A. Minimal placental transfer of rocuronium to the newborn
    B. Shorter duration of relaxation with concurrent magnesium administration
    C. Unsuitable intubating conditions as recommended doses are 1.5 mg/kg
    D. Use of rocuronium has been shown to affect Apgar scores and fetal muscle tone at birth and should be strictly avoided

54. During cesarean section under general endotracheal anesthesia, venous air embolism (VAE)

    A. Is associated with high end-tidal CO_2
    B. Should be treated with nitrous oxide
    C. Is associated with expired nitrogen
    D. Induces severe hypertension

Questions 55 to 58

A 30-year-old otherwise-healthy G_2P_0 (167 cm, 68 kg) presents at 34^1 weeks' gestation with the rupture of membranes, single footling in breech presentation with fetal bradycardia. The decision for emergent cesarean delivery under general anesthesia is made, and the patient is quickly prepared for a rapid sequence induction. However, patient's larynx is noted to be very anterior, and is unable to be intubated after multiple direct laryngoscopy attempts.

55. The appropriate next step considering persistent fetal bradycardia (<80 bpm) is

    A. Administer 1 mg/kg of rocuronium intravenously
    B. Use bag-mask ventilation and allow surgical delivery to proceed
    C. Wake the patient up for awake fiberoptic intubation
    D. Reposition the patient in Trendelenburg with left-uterine displacement

56. The fetus is quickly delivered (skin-to-skin time of 18 minutes). However, 10 minutes after delivery, her uterus is noted to be boggy and bleeding persists. The appropriate treatment option is

    A. Bolus oxytocin (Pitocin) 20 U intravenously
    B. Bolus methylergonovine (Methergine) 0.2 mg intravenously
    C. Misoprostol (Cytotec) 800 mg intramuscularly
    D. 15-Methyl $PGF_{2\alpha}$ (Hemabate) 0.25 mg intramuscularly

57. Two hours later, the patient remains apneic and intubated in the intensive care unit. She is sedated and mechanically ventilated (TV = 450, RR = 12, F_{IO_2} = 0.4) with the arterial blood gas revealing a pH of 7.45, Pa_{O_2} of 100 mm Hg, and Pa_{CO_2} of 37 mm Hg with a base excess of zero. Her examination reveals absent deep-tendon reflexes throughout. ECG reveals intermittent ventricular bigeminy. This situation could be explained by

   A. Hypermagnesemia
   B. Severe hypovolemic shock
   C. Hypocalcemia
   D. Pituitary necrosis

58. At 3 weeks' postpartum, the patient has absence of lactation and denies return of her menstrual cycle. Review of systems is positive for intolerance to cold, constipation, hair loss, and 2-pound weight gain. The best explanation for this constellation of symptoms is

   A. Amenorrhea–galactorrhea syndrome
   B. Sheehan syndrome
   C. Fibromyalgia
   D. Meigs syndrome

CHAPTER 17 ANSWERS

1. **D.**   Increasing levels of progesterone along with an enlarging uterus contributes to incompetence of the lower esophageal sphincter placing parturients at increased risk of aspiration. This risk increases further as delayed gastric emptying is associated with both the onset of labor (sympathetic effects) and μ-opioid administration for analgesia. Aspiration precautions must be utilized when providing anesthesia for women beyond midgestation.

2. **B.**   During pregnancy, cardiovascular changes include increase in blood volume, plasma volume, cardiac output, stroke volume, and heart rate. Despite these increases, the systemic blood pressure, during a normal uncomplicated pregnancy, does not increase due to decrease in systemic vascular resistance. Similarly, there is no change in central venous pressures despite the increase in plasma volume due to increase in venous capacitance (Table 17-1).

Table 17-1 Normal Hemodynamic Changes during Pregnancy

Parameter	Pregnancy	Labor
Blood volume	Increase of 50%	Increase
Heart rate	Increase of 10–15 bpm	Increase
Blood pressure	Decrease of 10 mm Hg	Increase
Stroke volume	Increase—1st and 2nd trimester Decrease—3rd trimester	Increase of 300 mL/contraction
Cardiac output	Increase of 30%–50%	Additional increase of 50%
Systemic vascular resistance	Decrease	Increase

3. **D.**   Maternal intravascular fluid volume increases in the first trimester, and at term, the plasma volume is increased by about 45%, while the erythrocyte volume increases only 20%, accounting for the relative anemia of pregnancy despite the higher hematocrit. This serves to decrease blood viscosity and improve flow. This increase in maternal blood volume also allows women to better tolerate the blood loss associated with delivery.

4. **A.**   Cardiac output in the third trimester is increased by nearly 50% due to an increase in both the stroke volume and heart rate to meet augmented maternal and fetal metabolic demands.

5. **C.**   The largest increase in cardiac output is seen immediately after delivery as the increase in blood volume persists with an additional increase in intravascular volume (300–500 mL) from the contracting uterus. This autotransfusion further increases cardiac output. Patients with fixed stenotic valvular lesions therefore should continue to be monitored closely after delivery.

6. **D.**   Hyperventilation with oxygen consumption creates significant changes in acid–base status that can be hazardous to the fetus. Extremely low $Paco_2$ levels result in vasoconstriction and global reduction in placental perfusion and blood flow. The alkalemia also shifts

the oxygen–hemoglobin dissociation curve to the *left*, impairing the release of oxygen from maternal blood to fetal blood. Both factors will decrease the availability of oxygen delivery to the fetus (Fig 17-1).

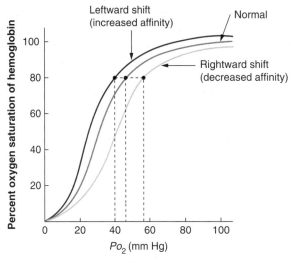

Figure 17-1.

7. **C.**   The anterior spinal cord achieves its blood supply from the anterior spinal artery, which is single and unpaired. Due to this, injury or thrombosis can lead to a unique constellation of symptoms consisting of loss of motor function, pain, and temperature below the level of the injury, bilaterally. The posterior columns, carrying fine touch and proprioception, are preserved as paired posterior spinal arteries supply.

8. **B.**   The presence of moderate–severe aortic stenosis makes it especially crucial to minimize sympathetic output and hemodynamic deterioration. Though a regional anesthetic is capable of attenuating the release of catecholamines during painful labor, one must be vigilant to prevent hypotension. The abrupt hypotension following spinal anesthesia with local anesthetics may result in cardiac hypoperfusion and ischemia. Epidural anesthesia, with its slow onset to effect, is usually well tolerated, especially with adequate volume loading. Inhaled nitrous oxide and oral analgesics are unlikely able to provide adequate analgesia to maintain hemodynamic stability in this patient with a fixed valve lesion.

9. **A.**   Although there is an increase in cardiac output and plasma volume, the systemic blood pressure in normal maternal physiology does not actually increase due to decreases in systemic vascular resistance. In fact, the mean arterial pressures generally decrease by approximately 10 to 15 mm Hg. Certainly, her fixed stenotic lesion also contributes.

10. **B.**   The mechanism of supine hypotension syndrome is decreased venous return as a result of aortocaval compression by the gravid uterus when the pregnant woman assumes the supine position. Removal of the compression with left-uterine displacement can minimize this incidence, which is particularly important for patients undergoing regional or general anesthesia because usual compensatory increases in systemic vascular resistance will be blocked.

11. **C.**   With increasing enlargement of the uterus, the diaphragm is forced cephalad, which is responsible for decreasing the FRC. While supine, FRC can become less than CC for many small airways resulting in atelectasis. Expiratory reserve volume and residual volume are also decreased while both vital capacity and CC remain unchanged.

12. **B.**   Oxytocin remains a first-line agent in the prevention and management of uterine atony. Oxytocin has important cardiovascular side effects, including hypotension and tachycardia, setting the stage for myocardial ischemia. Slow continuous intravenous administration of oxytocin minimizes maternal hemodynamic instability and also encourages maintenance of uterine tone.

13. **D.** Decreased functional residual capacity (FRC) with increased minute ventilation results in an escalation in rate at which changes of alveolar concentration of inhaled anesthetics can be achieved, increasing speed of induction, emergence, and changes in depth of anesthesia.

14. **B.** MAC progressively decreases during pregnancy—at term by as much as 40%—for all volatile anesthetic agents.

15. **C.** Increased oxygen consumption and decreased reserve due to reduced functional residual capacity can result in a rapid fall in arterial oxygen tension during apnea. This occurs despite careful preoxygenation, which importantly provides a time buffer.

16. **D.** Minute ventilation is increased above prepregnant levels primarily by a significant increase in tidal volume with smaller increases in respiratory rate. Resting maternal $Paco_2$ decreases from 40 to about 32 mm Hg, though arterial pH approaches normal levels with increased renal excretion of bicarbonate ions. At term, Pao_2 generally does not change significantly, though may be slightly decreased, reflecting airway closure and atelectasis.

17. **A.** Elevated levels of 2,3-DPG decreases maternal hemoglobin affinity for oxygen, shifting the P_{50} curve to the *right* (increasing it from 27 to 30 mm Hg) to enhance oxygen delivery to tissues.

18. **C.** An increased metabolic rate in addition to the pregnancy-induced increase in minute ventilation results in a markedly decrease in $Paco_2$ from 40 to 30 mm Hg. Such that a $Paco_2$ of 40 to 45 on ABG would indicate CO_2 retention. However, respiratory alkalosis is minimized due to metabolic compensation with increased renal excretion of bicarbonate and thus a lower HCO_3 as compared to the nonparturient. At 35 weeks' gestation, a normal maternal pH is approximately 7.44. Lastly, maternal position can affect Pao_2, even in healthy parturients. In the upright position and breathing room air, Pao_2 will be slightly greater than 100 mm Hg, as the increase in cardiac output is greater than the increase in oxygen consumption. However, as functional residual capacity decreases during pregnancy and is often less than closing capacity in the supine position, Pao_2 will frequently fall below 100 mm Hg, while supine likely reflecting atelectasis.

19. **B.** Engorgement of epidural veins occurs with progressive enlargement of the uterus contribute to decrease in size of the epidural space and can predispose to intravascular injection with attempted epidural anesthesia. Additionally, CSF volume is decreased in the subarachnoid space, facilitating the spread of local anesthetics. Therefore, in pregnancy, there is a decrease in dose requirements of local anesthetics for neuraxial procedures.

20. **A.** Similar to physiologic anemia of pregnancy, dilution of serum albumin will result in higher free blood levels of highly protein-bound drugs (e.g., fentanyl and midazolam), resulting in a more robust clinical effect as compared to the nonpregnant state. Though plasma cholinesterase activity is also decreased, this is unlikely to be of clinical significance with regard to the duration of action of succinylcholine.

21. **D.** Cephalad displacement of the pylorus, decreased gastrointestinal motility, and decreased pH of gastric contents all contribute to significant risk of aspiration and resultant pneumonitis during labor and delivery. H_2-receptor antagonists, unlike antacids, do not alter the pH of gastric contents already present in the stomach. Avoidance or particulate antacids can minimize pulmonary damage should aspiration occurs. Though metoclopramide can increase gastric motility to decrease the gastric volume, opioid-induced hypomotility is resistant to this treatment.

22. **C.** Late decelerations are shallow, uniformly shaped decelerations that are characterized by a gradual decrease from and return to baseline of the fetal heart rate. The nadir of late decelerations usually is between 5 and 30 bpm below the baseline. Late decelerations typically begin near the end of a contraction; with return to baseline, FHR always occurring after the

contractions have ended. Uteroplacental insufficiency (e.g., umbilical cord compression, maternal supine hypotension syndrome) contributes to late decelerations. Cephalopelvic disproportion and fetal head compression are associated with early decelerations (Fig 17-2).

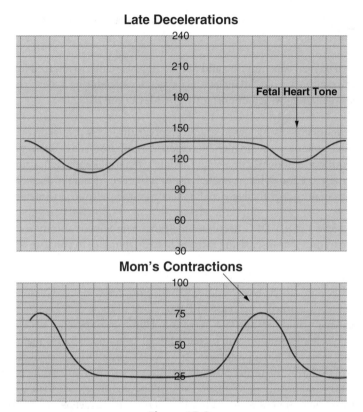

Late Decelerations

Mom's Contractions

Figure 17-2.

23. **C.**   The uterine vasculature is not autoregulated and remains essentially maximally dilated under normal conditions during pregnancy. Epidural or spinal anesthesia does not pathologically alter uterine blood flow as long as maternal hypotension is avoided. Acceptable options include left-uterine displacement to minimize aortocaval compression, increase IV fluids to improve volume status, Trendelenburg position to encourage venous return, and α-adrenergic agents to increase maternal arterial blood pressure. Prompt correction of maternal hypotension will lead to best neonatal outcome.

24. **B.**   The Apgar is a scoring system for evaluating an infant's physical condition at birth. The infant's heart rate (1 pt), respiration (1 pt), muscle tone (0 pt), response to stimuli (1 pt), and color (0 pt) are rated at 1 minute and again at 5 minutes after birth. Each factor is scored 0, 1, or 2; the maximum total score is 10 (Fig 17-3).

APGAR SCORE		0	1	2
	Heart rate	Absent	Slow < 100/min	> 100/min
	Respiratory rate	Absent	Slow, weak cry	Good cry
	Muscle tone	Flaccid	Some flexion of extremities	Well flexed
	Reflex, irritability	No response	Grimace	Cry
	Color	Blue, pale	Body pink, extremities blue	Completely pink

Score _____

Figure 17-3.

25. **C.**   A team that is skilled at reviving newborn infants should be at the delivery if meconium staining is found in the amniotic fluid. Newborns should be placed under radiant heat sources to support body temperature, as heat loss can be rapid. If the baby is active and crying, no treatment is needed. If the baby is not active and crying right after delivery, the trachea should be suctioned. Avoiding positive-pressure ventilation before suctioning can minimize further aspiration into the lungs.

26. **D.**   The invention of the forceps has had a profound influence on obstetrics, providing an alternative modality to surgical delivery during cases of difficult, nonprogressing, or obstructed labor. High-forceps delivery refers to attempted delivery prior to head engagement, which carries high risk and is no longer an accepted practice. Certainly, there is risk to both mother and child. Maternal risks include increased postpartum recovery time and pain, while in the fetus, forceps assistance can cause minor injuries such as cuts and bruises, or more serious damages such as facial nerve injury, clavicle fracture, and intracranial hemorrhage.

27. **D.**   The fetal circulation is markedly different from the adult circulation as gas exchange does not occur in the lungs but instead occurs in the placenta. The placenta provides oxygen-rich blood via the umbilical vein to the fetal circulation and removes deoxygenated blood via umbilical arteries. In addition, the fetal cardiovascular system is designed in such a way that the most highly oxygenated blood is delivered preferentially to vital organs (brain and heart) while minimizing flow to nonvital fetal organs (liver and lungs). The presence of intra- and extracardiac shunts achieves these circulatory adaptations in the fetus; the ductus venosus shunts oxygenated blood away from the liver, while the ductus arteriosus shunts blood away from the fetal pulmonary bed. The foramen ovale effectively shunts blood from the right to the left atrium, resulting in equalization of right and left sides of the heart (Fig 17-4).

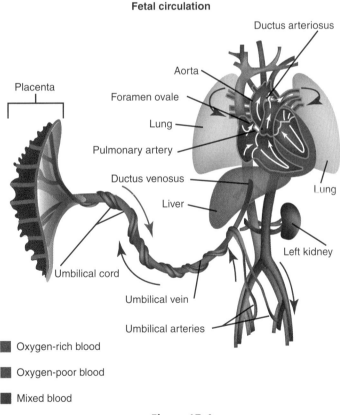

Fetal circulation

Figure 17-4.

28. **B.**   Successful transition from fetal to neonatal circulation starts when the umbilical cord is clamped and cut such that the placenta no longer acts as the "lungs" to provide oxygen. The ductus venosus closes physiologically as soon as the umbilical vein is obstructed with the clamping of the cord. With the loss of the placenta, a large low-resistance bed, systemic vascular resistance rapidly increases. With the first breath, the lungs inflate with a fall in pulmonary vascular resistance and increase pulmonary blood flow. The rise in pulmonary venous return results in left-atrial pressure being slightly higher than right-atrial pressure to close the foramen ovale. Decrease in circulating prostaglandins and the higher blood oxygen content of blood result in vasoconstriction of the ductus arteriosus.

29. **C.**   Placental exchange of substances occurs principally by diffusion from the maternal circulation to the fetus and vice versa, which depends on maternal–fetal concentration gradients, maternal protein-binding, molecular weight, lipid solubility, and the degree of ionization of that substance.

30. **D.**   Local anesthetics easily cross the placenta, which is affected by several independent factors, including maternal–fetal hemodynamics, permeability of the placenta, concentration of free drug in the maternal plasma, and physiochemical properties of the drug itself. Lidocaine is less lipid soluble than bupivacaine, which is reflected in their lipid–water partition coefficients. Protein-binding also plays a role in the diffusion of drugs across the placenta. The unbound form of the drug is freely transferred, whereas protein-binding limits diffusion. High protein-binding, as in the case of bupivacaine, leads to much lower fetal-to-maternal plasma ratio. Local anesthetics are weak bases and therefore have minimal ionization at physiologic pH. The closer the pK_a is to the physiologic pH, the more it will be affected by the acid–base status of the fetus.

31. **D.**   Somatic and visceral afferents from the uterus and cervix travel with sympathetic nerve fibers en route to the spinal cord. These fibers pass through the inferior, middle, and superior hypogastric plexuses to arrive at the sympathetic chain. The first stage of labor is largely visceral (T10–L1) due to uterine contractions. As labor progresses, the parturient encounters the second stage of labor with additional somatic pain complaints as the fetus descends into the pelvis causing distension of the vagina, perineum, and pelvic floor muscles. This somatic pain is transmitted via the pudendal nerve (S2–S4).

32. **B.**   Lumbar sympathetic blocks and paracervical blocks, though rarely performed for labor analgesia, are appropriate targets during the first stage of labor. However, paracervical blocks are rarely used in current practice because of an association with fetal bradycardia. Epidural and combined spinal–epidural techniques are ideal, in that they are able to block the visceral afferent fibers responsible for the first stage of labor and the somatic nerve fibers through which the second stage is transmitted. The obstetrician can also provide pudendal blocks during delivery to mitigate somatic pain during the second stage, though cannot mitigate visceral first stage pain.

33. **D.**   Preeclampsia is a syndrome manifested after the 20th week of gestation, which is characterized by systemic hypertension ($>$140/90 mm Hg), proteinuria ($>$0.5 g/day), generalized edema, and complaints of a headache. HELLP syndrome (*h*emolysis, *e*levated *l*iver enzymes, *l*ow *p*latelets) is a severe form of preeclampsia. Eclampsia is present when seizures are superimposed on preeclampsia, and it is potentially life-threatening. Causes for maternal mortality in women with preeclampsia include congestive heart failure, myocardial infarction, coagulopathy, and cerebral hemorrhage. Definitive treatment is the delivery of the fetus and placenta, after which preeclampsia usually abates within 48 hours.

34. **A.**   The presence of hypertension with associated edema requires further workup including complete blood count with platelets and prothrombin time/international normalized ratio to ensure adequate hemostasis can be achieved. Usually, platelets $>$100 K/µL carry little

increased risk, and one may safely proceed with epidural placement. Platelet count <50 K/µL is generally considered a contraindication to neuraxial interventions due to high risk of epidural hematoma. Epidural anesthesia is often viewed as the technique of choice for labor pain as the parturient remains awake and alert without sedative side effects. However, systemic opiates are reasonable if epidural is contraindicated for whatever reason, including patient refusal. A general or regional anesthetic should not be used in attempts to lower maternal blood pressure.

35. **A.**   Transfer of drugs from mother to fetus takes place at the level of the placenta mainly by diffusion. Thus, keeping maternal blood levels of drugs as low as possible is a major strategy for decreasing the amount of drug that reaches the fetus. In addition, since most of the blood in the umbilical vein travels directly to the liver, a large portion of the drug will be metabolized before reaching vital fetal organs. Furthermore, drug in the umbilical vein that bypasses the liver via the ductus venosus to access the inferior vena cava will be diluted with blood from the lower extremities, and this further reduces concentration of drugs in the fetal blood. Two things work against these "safety features": (1) fetal acidosis during times of distress causes increased perfusion of the heart and brain and thus increases delivery of drug to these important organs. (2) Fetal pH is lower than maternal pH and results in basic drugs (such as local anesthetics) becoming more ionized when they reach fetal circulation. This effectively traps them on the fetal side of the circulation, since ionized molecules cannot easily cross the placenta. This also maintains a gradient for diffusion. This is known as "ion trapping" and can be quite a significant effect especially during times of fetal distress (when pH gets even lower).

36. **B.**   Late decelerations are worrisome as it is a sign of fetal hypoxemia, which requires prompt treatment. Uteroplacental resuscitation measures should be implemented immediately in an attempt to improve uteroplacental perfusion and oxygen delivery to the fetus. Supplemental oxygen should be provided to the mother, and she should be placed in a lateral position to avoid aortocaval compression. Maternal hypotension should be treated promptly with an IV fluid bolus and/or administration of a vasopressor. In this case, phenylephrine may also improve her tachycardia. Emergent cesarean delivery is indicated only if these utero resuscitative measures are not successful. Discontinuation of the epidural infusion is recommended only if the patient has an excessively high sensory level.

37. **C.**   Definitive treatment is delivery of the fetus and placenta. In the interim, magnesium and antihypertensive drugs may be required. Magnesium is effective by decreasing the irritability of the CNS to decrease the risk of seizures. Though it mildly reduces blood pressure due to its vasodilatory effect, it is not an effective agent for severe hypertension. Antihypertensives are usually required when the diastolic pressure is >110 mm Hg. Hydralazine and labetalol are the most commonly administered. Hydralazine has the advantage of being a vasodilator; thus, it can improve uteroplacental and renal blood flow. Labetalol, with its adrenergic blockade may improve tachycardia. Keep in mind that labetalol has a much faster onset of action (5 minutes) vs. hydralazine (30 minutes) as such may be more appropriate for acute management of severe hypertension.

38. **B.**   All women in the peripartum period should be given a nonparticulate antacid such as sodium citrate 30 mL to neutralize gastric contents. A rapid-sequence induction should be performed following adequate preoxygenation. If a woman is in shock, etomidate is preferable to thiopental or propofol as an induction agent. Equipotent doses of all the volatile agents depress uterine contractility to an equivalent, dose-dependent extent. Following retained placenta, there is an increased incidence of endometritis; however, there is no consensus opinion on whether antibiotic prophylaxis is routinely indicated.

39. **D.**   Epidural abscesses are associated with headache, fevers/chills, nausea/vomiting, low back pain, and bowel or bladder dysfunction that can range from retention to incontinence. Hematologic evaluation would likely reveal an immune response with elevated WBC.

40. C.   Since the first reported case in 1898, PDPH has been a problem for patients following dural puncture. Research over the last 30 years has shown that use of larger-gauge needles, particularly of the pencil-point design, is associated with a lower risk of PDPH than larger traditional cutting-point (Quincke) needle tips. Keep in mind that gauge and bore diameter of a needle are inversely related such that a 22G is smaller compared to a 16G. A careful history should rule out other causes of headache. A postdural component of headache is the sine qua non of PDPH. High-risk patients include those <50 years, postpartum, and puncture with small gauge (large bore diameter) needles.

41. B.   Magnesium acts as a physiologic calcium blocker to provide uterine relaxation in addition to electrical conduction disruption such that levels can be predicted strength of deep-tendon reflexes. Similarly, postsuccinylcholine fasciculations are blunted.

42. B.   Nitroglycerin may be used as an alternative to terbutaline sulfate (β_2 agonist) or general endotracheal anesthesia with halogenated agents for uterine relaxation. Inhaled anesthetics produce dose-dependent uterine vasodilatation with a decrease in uterine contractility. Uterine relaxation produced by inhalation agents may be helpful for removal of retained placenta. However, uterine vasodilatation might lead to increased blood loss during obstetric surgery or delivery. Nitrous oxide does not change uterine contractility in doses provided during delivery. Initiating treatment with incremental doses of nitroglycerin may relax the uterus sufficiently while minimizing potential complications (e.g., hypotension).

43. A.   Maternal side effects due to β_2-agonist therapy (e.g., terbutaline, ritodrine) for tocolysis include cardiopulmonary complications (e.g., arrhythmias, tachycardia, hypotension, and pulmonary edema) and metabolic hyperglycemia.

44. D.   Alkalization of the blood causes vasoconstriction, to provide a semblance of hemostasis. Inhaled anesthetics, ritodrine, and nitroglycerine are all potent vasodilators that can contribute to her ongoing blood loss.

45. C.   Sodium thiopental is an ultra-short-acting barbiturate commonly used to induce general anesthesia prior to intubation. Following a low dose, the drug rapidly reaches the brain and causes unconsciousness within 30 to 45 seconds. At 1 minute, the drug attains a peak concentration of about 60% of the total dose in the brain. Thereafter, the drug distributes to the rest of the body, and in about 5 to 10 minutes, the concentration is low enough in the brain such that consciousness returns. Thus, a one-time bolus displays first-order kinetics. Larger doses, or infusions, undergo slow zero-order elimination kinetics such that thiopental is not used to maintain anesthesia in surgical procedures ($T_{1/2}$ 11.5–26 hours) due to slow recovery. As such, larger or repeated doses can depress the baby.

46. B.   Umbilical cord blood gas analysis is recommended in all high⊠risk deliveries. For most accurate interpretation, paired umbilical arterial and venous samples should be taken soon after birth from a segment of cord that has been doubly clamped to isolate it from the placenta. This cord blood will remain stable for up to 1 hour. Infants with pH <7.0 at birth who are not vigorous are at high risk of adverse outcome. Analysis of paired arterial and venous specimens can give insights into the etiology of the acidosis. In combination with other clinical information, normal paired arterial and venous cord blood gas results can usually provide a robust defense against a suggestion that an infant had an intrapartum hypoxic–ischemic event.

47. A.   The fetal heart rate varies beat to beat, with a normal heart rate ranging between 110 and 160 bpm. This normal variability is thought to reflect the integrity of the vagal neural pathway from the fetal cerebral cortex to the cardiac conduction system. Fetal well-being is safeguarded when this beat-to-beat variability is present. Conversely, fetal distress is associated with minimal (or absent) variability of the fetal heart rate. Opioids, benzodiazepines, sedative-hypnotics, local anesthetics, phenothiazines, and anticholinergics administered to the mother have been shown to eliminate or reduce this variability, even in the absence of distress. This drug-related effect does not appear to be deleterious, but may cause difficulty in interpreting fetal heart rate monitors.

48. B. Normally, amniotic fluid does not enter the maternal circulation because it is contained safely within the uterus, sealed off by the amniotic sac. An AFE occurs when the barrier between amniotic fluid and maternal circulation is broken, allowing it to abnormally enter the maternal venous system. The devastating consequence of circulating fetal debris (carried by amniotic fluid) occurs only rarely. Newer theories contend that AFE more closely resembles an anaphylactic reaction to fetal debris rather than a true embolic event. Cardinal signs include bronchospasm/wheezing, hypoxemia, shock/maternal acidosis, coagulopathy/disseminated intravascular coagulation, and altered mental status.

49. C. Hyperventilation and hypocapnia have profound effects on cerebral blood flow (CBF), resulting in a 2% decline in CBF for each 1 torr decline in $Paco_2$. In the same manner, low CO_2 concentrations will cause vasoconstriction of the uterine vessels impairing uterine blood flow. In addition, maternal hypocapnia will shift the oxyhemoglobin dissociation curve to the *left*, further impairing oxygen release and transfer to the fetus. Carbon dioxide tensions in arterial blood plays an important role in determining blood flow and delivery to the pregnant uterus; hypocarbia can lead to poor oxygen and nutrient delivery with a resulting fetal hypoxic distress (Fig 17-5).

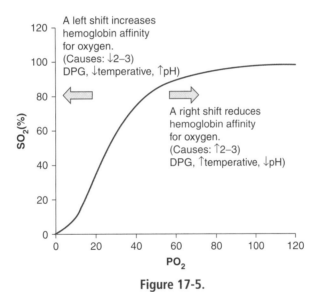

Figure 17-5.

50. D. Hyperglycemia during pregnancy contriXbutes to higher birth weights (macrosomia) with cephalopelvic insufficiency and shoulder dystocia requiring surgical delivery via cesarean section. Fetal hyperglycemia induces fetal hyperinsulinemia, resulting in elevated metabolic rates that lead to increased oxygen demand, risking ischemia. This hypoxemia in turn contributes to the development of a metabolic acidosis and may trigger polycythemia with increased production of red blood cells. At birth, however, with separation from the maternal hyperglycemic circulation, neonatal hypoglycemia develops secondary to high levels of neonatal insulin.

51. D. Opioids can be added to local anesthetics or alternatively can be used as a sole agent (epidural or intrathecal) to provide peripartum analgesia. Side effects of neuraxial opioids include pruritus, nausea/vomiting, hypotension, urinary retention, fetal bradycardia, and maternal respiratory depression. Among these, pruritus occurs most commonly. The epidural space contains an extensive vascular plexus with extensive systemic absorption such that absorption of epidural morphine, fentanyl, or sufentanil produces opioid serum concentrations that are similar to an equivalent dose of IM injection.

52. **C.**   Glycopyrrolate, insulin, heparin, and neuromuscular blockers are unable to cross the placenta, whereas opioids, local anesthetics, atropine, ephedrine, and β-blockers readily cross the placenta to enter the neonatal circulation.

53. **A.**   Reversal of neuromuscular blockade may be unsatisfactory in patients receiving magnesium for preeclampsia as magnesium can enhance the neuromuscular blockade. Though doses of 1 mg/kg have been used safely for rapid sequence induction of anesthesia, this dose has not been tested for safety in pregnancy. Therefore, only a dose of 0.6 mg/kg is recommended in this patient population despite the knowledge that rocuronium (similar to all paralytics) does not readily cross the placental barrier, as evidenced by low umbilical-to-venous plasma concentrations.

54. **C.**   VAE has a very high incidence during cesarean sections secondary to entrainment of room air from ruptured or severed veins. The sudden development of hypotension, hypoxia, and a drop in end-tidal CO_2 suggests the presence of a VAE. Supportive therapy includes flooding the surgical field with normal saline and placing the patient in Trendelenburg position with a left-lateral tilt. Medical gases such as carbon dioxide, nitrous oxide, and helium will aggravate this condition by expanding the pulmonary vascular bubbles that can create an air lock with mechanical flow obstruction. If central venous catheter or pulmonary artery catheter is in place, the trapped air may be aspirated. Expired nitrogen is the most sensitive VAE-detection method, as the largest component of air is nitrogen.

55. **B.**   General anesthesia is used most commonly in emergency surgical deliveries for fetal distress. Endotracheal intubation following rapid-sequence induction remains the principal approach. Pregnancy-related features (obesity, enlarging breasts, short neck) make intubation challenging such that inability to intubate the trachea is a major cause of morbidity and mortality. Current opinion is that after two failed attempts at direct laryngoscopy, one should proceed with surgery as repeated trauma and edema may prevent ability to ventilate as well. Severe fetal distress requires emergent delivery as opposed to preparing for an awake fiberoptic intubation.

56. **D.**   15-Methyl $PGF_{2\alpha}$ is a smooth-muscle constrictor with additional sites of action on bronchial smooth muscles, which may promote bronchospasm. Direct intravenous bolus injection of oxytocin (>5 units) has been associated with maternal hypotension and death, thus should only be infused over time in a dilute solution (e.g., 40 units/L). Methylergonovine is a potent vasoconstrictor that can cause vasospasm and severe hypertension if given intravenously, such as usual administration intramuscularly. Misoprostol is a prostaglandin analog that can be given up to 1 mg rectally or sublingually, but is to be used with caution in patients under general anesthesia due to aspiration risk.

57. **A.**   Overdose of magnesium during the peripartum period can lead to arreflexia and cardiac conduction abnormalities, resulting in bradycardia and ectopy. Metabolic acidosis would be seen in cases of severe hypovolemic shock. Examination findings expected with hypocalcemia would include hyperreflexia, as opposed to arreflexia.

58. **B.**   During pregnancy, hypertrophy and hyperplasia of lactotrophs result in enlargement of the anterior pituitary, but without a corresponding increase in blood supply. As such, major hemorrhage or hypotension during labor and delivery can result in anterior pituitary ischemia and necrosis. Sheehan syndrome specifically is hypopituitarism caused by ischemic necrosis during the peripartum period.

Pediatric Anesthesia

Dipty Mangla and Ashish Sinha

1. Correct statement regarding neonatal physiology is

    A. Neonates have a greater volume of distribution for water-soluble drugs
    B. Total body water is higher in adults
    C. Dose of propofol (mg/kg) is lower in neonates than in adults
    D. Neonates have a higher body fat content than adults

2. A 4-year-old child weighing 16 kg is scheduled for hernia repair under general anesthesia. Assuming he was NPO for 8 hours, his total fluid deficit will be about _____ (mL):

    A. 380
    B. 420
    C. 460
    D. 500

3. The total dose of midazolam that may be given orally as premedication is

    A. 0.2 mg/kg, maximum 10 mg
    B. 0.2 mg/kg, maximum 20 mg
    C. 0.5 mg/kg, maximum 15 mg
    D. 0.5 mg/kg, maximum 20 mg

4. A newborn baby of 37 weeks of gestation has a heart rate of 90 bpm, is crying, is pink with blue extremities, and shows some flexion. Her Apgar score would be

    A. 6
    B. 7
    C. 8
    D. 9

5. After initial evaluation of the baby described above, the next step in managing her would be

    A. Provide positive-pressure ventilation
    B. Chest compressions
    C. Warming blanket
    D. Cardiology consult

6. All of the following drugs can be given through endotracheal tube, except

    A. Epinephrine
    B. Lidocaine
    C. Surfactant
    D. Calcium

7. The disease or syndrome with known association with malignant hyperthermia is

    A. Huntington chorea
    B. Fabry disease
    C. King Denborough syndrome (KDS)
    D. Burns

8. An 8-year-old child is brought to the emergency room with testicular torsion. The parents tell you he ate a sandwich 6 hours ago. Surgeon wants to operate immediately. Your response should be

    A. Take him to the OR, deem it emergent, rapid-sequence intubation
    B. Wait for 2 more hours, deem it urgent, rapid-sequence intubation
    C. He is adequately fasting, elective, intubation
    D. Wait for 2 hours, elective, intubation

9. Which of the following statements about pediatric airway is true?

    A. More caudal position of larynx as compared to adult
    B. More acute angulation of epiglottis
    C. Glottic opening is the narrowest part of airway
    D. Longer trachea as compared to adults

10. A 10-week-old baby, who was born prematurely at 30 weeks of gestation, undergoes circumcision uneventfully under general anesthesia. After the baby recovers from anesthetics in post-anesthesia care unit, he can/should be

    A. Admitted and monitored for 24 hours
    B. Discharged home with parents
    C. Discharged home if parents live within a 30-minute radius
    D. Admitted to the ICU

11. Hypertrophic pyloric stenosis is associated with

    A. Metabolic acidosis
    B. Metabolic alkalosis
    C. Hyperkalemia
    D. Hyperchloremia

12. A child with which of the following diseases/syndromes should be evaluated for heart disease?

    A. Omphalocele
    B. Gastroschisis
    C. Hypertrophic pyloric stenosis
    D. Tracheobronchitis

13. The earliest and the most pathognomic feature of malignant hyperthermia (MH) is

    A. Increased temperature
    B. Increased end-tidal CO_2
    C. Increased heart rate
    D. Increased respiratory rate

14. The most common type of tracheoesophageal fistula (TEF) is

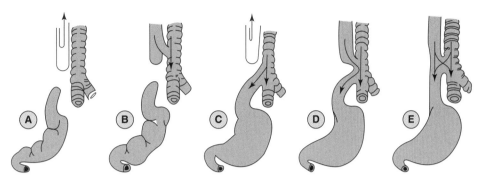

Figure 18-1.

15. Down syndrome is associated with all of the following, except

   A. Large tongue
   B. Atlantooccipital instability
   C. Hyperthyroidism
   D. Increased incidence of seizures

16. The first sign of intrathecal injection following the placement of caudal epidural with 0.25% bupivacaine in a 1-year-old child would be

   A. Hypotension
   B. Bradycardia
   C. Falling oxygen saturation
   D. Tachycardia

17. A 2-year-old child weighing 13 kg is scheduled for inguinal hernia repair. The calculated dose of 0.25% bupivacaine for a caudal epidural would be approximately _____ (mL):

   A. 13
   B. 7
   C. 10
   D. 20

18. All the following are physiologic changes that occur at birth, except

   A. Closure of foramen ovale
   B. Closure of ductus arteriosus
   C. Decreased right-ventricular afterload
   D. Decreased left-ventricular afterload

19. Neonates lose heat by all the following mechanisms in the operating room, except

   A. Conduction to cold surfaces
   B. Exposure to cold operating room
   C. Dry airway gases
   D. Metabolism of brown fat

20. A 4-year-old child with tetralogy of Fallot is scheduled for incision and drainage of a foot abscess. All the following measures can be used to improve his oxygenation, except

   A. Phenylephrine
   B. Nitroglycerine
   C. Nitric oxide
   D. Epinephrine

21. Which of the following heart rates is inappropriate for the age?

    A. 50 bpm at 12 years of age
    B. 120 bpm for a neonate
    C. 100 bpm for a 1-year-old
    D. 80 bpm for a 3-year-old

22. The age at which the glomerular filtration rate in a child is same as in adults is

    A. 6 months
    B. 1 year
    C. 1.5 years
    D. 2 years

23. Normal blood glucose level in a neonate is _____ (mg/dL):

    A. 20 to 40
    B. 40 to 60
    C. 60 to 70
    D. 50 to 80

24. The recommended size of an endotracheal tube for a 1-year-old child is

    A. 2.5
    B. 3.0
    C. 4.0
    D. 5.0

25. As compared to a 10-year-old child, a 1-year-old child will have higher

    A. Oxygen consumption
    B. Functional residual capacity
    C. Tidal volume
    D. Vital capacity

26. The total blood volume in a preterm is _____ (mL/kg):

    A. 90 to 100
    B. 70 to 80
    C. 50 to 60
    D. 80 to 90

27. A 2-year-old is scheduled for elective tonsillectomy and adenoidectomy. His mother tells you he has runny nose. Your decision whether to proceed will be based on all the following, except

    A. If he is afebrile
    B. If he is not actively wheezing
    C. Cancel the surgery since it is elective
    D. Reluctance of parent for admitting the child, if needed

28. Urine output in a 6-year-old child undergoing surgery under general anesthesia should be _____ (mL/kg/h):

    A. 0.5
    B. 1
    C. 1.5
    D. 2

29. Perioperative management of a child with a femur fracture and sickle cell disease includes all of the following, except

    A. Hydration
    B. Treat infections
    C. Transfuse to hemoglobin of 14 mg/dL
    D. Avoid metabolic acidosis

30. Anesthetic management of a 12-year-old with Down syndrome includes all of the following, except

    A. Continue antiseizure medications
    B. Heavy sedation since all such patients are combative
    C. Prepare for manual in line neck stabilization
    D. Radiographs of the neck should be reviewed to rule out atlantooccipital instability

31. An 8-year-old boy, weighing 30 kg, is undergoing resection of a Wilms tumor in the operating room. His starting hemoglobin is 12 g/dL. If the threshold for transfusion is 8 g/dL, the allowable blood loss is _____ (mL):

    A. 820
    B. 840
    C. 860
    D. 880

32. A 5-year-old otherwise-healthy child is undergoing strabismus surgery with a laryngeal mask airway (LMA) in place. Thirty minutes into the procedure, his heart rate is 60 bpm, blood pressure is 90/60 mm Hg, and the pulse oximeter reads 98%. The next step in management should be

    A. Replace the LMA with an endotracheal tube
    B. Inform surgeon, administer atropine
    C. Nothing, this is normal for this child
    D. Increase the F_{IO_2} to 1.0

33. The afferent limb for oculocardiac reflex is

    A. Vagus nerve
    B. Trigeminal nerve
    C. Glossopharyngeal nerve
    D. Facial nerve

34. Positive-pressure ventilation with a face mask is contraindicated in which of the following condition?

    A. Laryngospasm
    B. Congenital diaphragmatic hernia
    C. Trauma
    D. Asthma

35. Treatment of postintubation croup in a child who underwent adenoidectomy is

    A. Inhalation of mist
    B. Steroids
    C. Racemic epinephrine
    D. All of the above

36. The most important measure to avoid subglottic edema in children is

    A. Use of an appropriate-size endotracheal tube
    B. Lubricating the endotracheal tube prior to intubation
    C. Administering intravenous lidocaine for all intubations
    D. Administering intravenous steroids for all intubations

37. Important difference between epiglottitis and laryngotracheobronchitis (croup) is

    A. Croup responds to racemic epinephrine and steroids
    B. Croup occurs in older children
    C. Higher temperatures are seen in croup patients
    D. Etiology of croup is bacterial

38. Anesthesia in a patient with Pierre Robin syndrome can be complicated by

    A. Renal failure
    B. Tendency to develop malignant hyperthermia
    C. Cardiac failure
    D. Difficult airway

39. Basic metabolic rate in children is

    A. Least at 1 year of age
    B. Same as adults
    C. Highest till 2 years of age
    D. Decreases after puberty

40. The percentage of patients developing malignant hyperthermia (MH) after masseter spasm is

    A. 0% to 24%
    B. 25% to 49%
    C. 50% to 74%
    D. 75% to 100%

41. All of the following are true for children with congenital diaphragmatic hernia (CDH), except

    A. Pulmonary hypoplasia may be present
    B. Dextrocardia is common
    C. Bag and mask ventilation is contraindicated
    D. Surgical management takes precedence over medical management

42. To protect lungs in a child with tracheoesophageal fistula, all the following should be done, except

    A. Avoid feeding
    B. Upright position
    C. Intermittent suction of upper blind esophageal pouch
    D. Prophylactic intravenous steroids

43. The main factor responsible for physiologic closure of a patent ductus arteriosus is

    A. Increased $Paco_2$
    B. Increased Pao_2
    C. Increased pulmonary artery pressure
    D. Administration of nonsteroidal anti-inflammatory agents

44. The most effective method for maintaining normothermia in an operating room is

    A. Warm humidified gases
    B. Warm intravenous fluids
    C. Warming blankets
    D. Increasing the room temperature

45. A 2-year-old child undergoing myringotomy develops laryngospasm in the operating room. The patient is breathing spontaneously with face mask at an F_{IO_2} of 0.6. Next step in the management would be

    A. Increasing F_{IO_2} to 1.0
    B. Jaw thrust
    C. Endotracheal intubation
    D. Intramuscular succinylcholine

46. Normal pulmonary dead space in a neonate is _____ (mL/kg):

    A. 1
    B. 2
    C. 3
    D. 4

47. Which of the following statements regarding fetal hemoglobin is true?

    A. It is composed of two α and two β chains
    B. It has more affinity for oxygen than adult hemoglobin
    C. Patients with sickle cell disease and high fetal hemoglobin have poor prognosis
    D. None of the above

48. Compared to adults, oxygen desaturation is more frequent in pediatric population because of

    A. Lower functional residual capacity (FRC) in children
    B. Higher oxygen consumption in adult
    C. Lower heart rate in adults
    D. Lower functional residual capacity in adults

49. The most consistent sign of intravascular injection following caudal epidural with 0.25% bupivacaine with 1:200,000 epinephrine is

    A. Tachycardia
    B. ST segment changes
    C. Bradycardia
    D. Hypertension

50. The dose of nondepolarizing muscle relaxants in a neonate is

    A. Decreased as compared to adults
    B. Increased as compared to adults
    C. Same as adults
    D. Cannot be predicted

CHAPTER 18 ANSWERS

1. **A.** Total body water in a term neonate is 75% of the total body weight, as compared to 60% in adult males and 55% in adult females. Water-soluble drugs will have an increased volume of distribution because of increased body water. Propofol dose (mg/kg) will be higher in neonates and infants than adults.

2. **B.** Maintenance fluid requirements to replace fluid deficits accounting for a period of fasting can be calculated by the following formula.

Table 18-1 Calculation of maintenance fluid requirements

Weight	Hourly Fluid Requirement
<10 kg	4 mL/kg
10–20 kg	40 mL + 2 mL/kg > 10 kg
>20 kg	60 mL/kg + 1 mL/kg > 20 kg

Thus using above formula, total fluid deficit would be $40 + (6 \times 2) = 52$ mL/h.
Accounting for 8 hours of fasting, total fluid deficit will be $52 \times 8 = 416$ mL.

3. **D.** Preoperatively, midazolam is the most common medication given for sedation and anxiety. Midazolam can be given orally in a dose of 0.25 to 0.5 mg/kg (maximum dose of 20 mg) in children. Sedative premedication is generally omitted for neonates, infants, and sick children. Oral ketamine (4–6 mg/kg) can also be used as premedication. For uncooperative children, intramuscular midazolam (0.1–0.15 mg/kg, maximum of 10 mg) and ketamine (0.02 mg/kg) can be used.

4. **B.** Apgar scores recorded at 1 minute and 5 minutes after birth remains a valuable method for assessment of the well-being of a neonate.

Table 18-2 Apgar Score

Sign	Points		
	0	1	2
Heart rate (bpm)	Absent	<100	>100
Respiratory effort	Absent	Slow, irregular	Good crying
Muscle tone	Flaccid	Some flexion	Active motion
Reflex irritability	No response	Grimace	Crying
Color	Blue or pale	Body pink, blue extremities	All pink

Apgar score in this case would be $1 + 2 + 1 + 2 + 1 = 7$.

5. A. Indications of positive-pressure ventilation in a newborn include apnea, gasping respirations, persistent central cyanosis with 100% oxygen, and heart rate less than 100 bpm. Assisted ventilation by bag and mask should be at a rate of 30 to 60 bpm with 100% oxygen. If after 30 seconds the heart rate is less than 80 bpm, chest compressions should be started and the neonate should be intubated (Fig 18-2).

Newborn Resuscitation

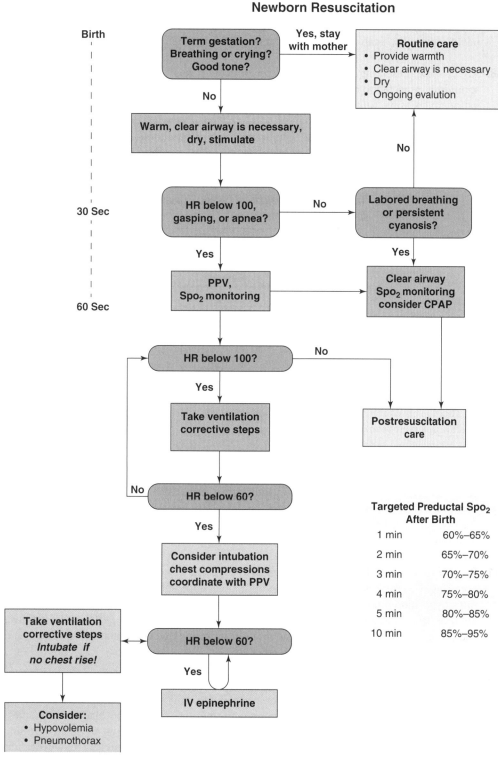

Figure 18-2. Reused with permission from Kattwinkel J, Perlman JM, Aziz K, et al. 2010 American Heart Association Guidelines for Cardiopulmonary Resuscitation and Emergency Cardiovascular Care Science. Part 15: Neonatal Resuscitation. *Circulation*. 2010;122:S909–S919.

6. **D.** Lidocaine, epinephrine, atropine, and vasopressin can be delivered down a catheter whose tip extends beyond the endotracheal tube. The dose of drugs through endotracheal tube is 2 to 2.5 times the intravenous dose. Surfactant can be given through endotracheal tube in children with severe bronchopulmonary dysplasia.

7. **C.** Musculoskeletal diseases associated with a relatively high incidence of malignant hyperthermia include Duchenne muscular dystrophy, myotonia, and KDS. KDS is seen primarily in young boys who exhibit short stature, mental retardation, cryptorchidism, kyphoscoliosis, pectus deformity, slanted eyes, low-set ears, webbed neck, and winged scapulae.

8. **A.** A male presenting with sudden onset of acute scrotal pain in the absence of trauma should be suspected to have testicular torsion. Testicular torsion requires immediate investigation and possible surgery to preserve potentially viable testis. Surgery should be performed within 6 hours of onset of pain to save the testicle. The salvage rate decreases to 50% if surgery is delayed between 6 and 12 hours. Children with suspected torsion of testis are assumed to have a full stomach and should have a rapid-sequence endotracheal intubation. The surgery is emergent and the patient needs to be taken to the OR.

Table 18-3 Preanesthesia Fasting Guidelines for Pediatric Patients

Product	Minimal Fasting Time
Clear liquids	2 hours
Breast milk	4 hours
Infant formula, Jell-O	6 hours
Solid food	8 hours

9. **B.** Neonates and infants have a larger head and tongue, an anterior and cephalad epiglottis and larynx, and a short trachea and neck. The larynx is at a vertebral level of C4 versus C6 in adults. The narrowest portion of larynx in children is at the level of cricoid cartilage as compared to glottic opening in adults. An adult's epiglottis is flat and broad, and its axis is parallel to that of trachea, whereas an infant's epiglottis is typically narrower, omega-shaped, and angled away from the axis of trachea.

10. **A.** Premature infants who are less-than-50-weeks postconceptional age at the time of surgery are prone to postoperative apneic episodes for up to 24 hours. Besides prematurity, other risk factors for postanesthetic apnea include hematocrit <30% (anemia), hypothermia, and neurological abnormalities. Thus, elective or outpatient procedures should be deferred until the preterm infant reaches the age of at least 50 weeks' postconception. These patients should be monitored for 12 to 24 hours postoperatively with pulse oximetry.

11. **B.** Hypertrophic pyloric stenosis causes stasis of gastric contents and thus leads to persistent vomiting. This can lead to depletion of sodium, potassium, chloride, and hydrogen ions, causing a hypochloremic metabolic alkalosis. Patients are first medically stabilized (correction of volume-deficit and metabolic alkalosis), and then a pyloromyotomy is performed. Hydration should be done with a sodium chloride solution supplemented with potassium (avoidance of ringer lactate as it is metabolized to bicarbonate).

12. **A.** Both gastroschisis and omphalocele are congenital disorders characterized by defects in the abdominal wall. Omphaloceles have a hernia sac, and are often associated with other congenital anomalies (trisomy 21, diaphragmatic hernia, cardiac and bladder anomalies). Gastroschisis, on the other hand, does not have a hernia sac, and is often an isolated finding. The latter is a more serious condition, as the absence of a hernial sac can lead to dehydration, hypothermia, and infection.

13. **B.** MH is a rare but potentially fatal hypermetabolic disorder triggered by exposure to volatile inhalational anesthetics or succinylcholine. The incidence of MH is 1:15,000 in pediatric population and 1:50,000 in adults. Signs of MH include masseter muscle rigidity, tachycardia, tachypnea, hypercarbia (increased CO_2 production—earliest sign), and hyperthermia (late sign). Hypertension and arrhythmias may be seen (sympathetic overactivity). Generalized muscle rigidity is not consistently present, and presence of dark-colored urine indicates myoglobinuria.

14. **C.** Among the different types of TEF, the most common is the type IIIB. This is where the upper esophagus ends in a blind pouch and a lower esophagus that connects to the trachea. At birth, TEF is suspected by failure to pass a catheter into the stomach and visualization of the catheter coiled in the blind upper esophageal pouch. Typically, breathing leads to gastric distension and feeding leads to choking and cyanosis. TEF patients are, therefore, prone to pulmonary aspiration. Coexistence of cardiac congenital anomalies is common. TEF patients may have associated *v*ertebral defects, *a*nal atresia, and *r*adial dysplasia, known as the VATER syndrome. Addition of *c*ardiac and *l*imb anomalies is called the VACTERL variant.

15. **C.** Down syndrome or trisomy 21 is one of the most common congenital syndromes in pediatric population. Anesthetic considerations in these patients include presence of short neck and large tongue (possible difficult airway), irregular dentition, mental retardation, hypotonia, congenital heart disease in 30% to 40% of patients (particularly endocardial cushion defects and ventricular septal defect), subglottic stenosis, tracheoesophageal fistula, chronic pulmonary infections, seizures, duodenal stenosis, and delayed gastric emptying.

16. **C.** Unlike older children and adults, subarachnoid and epidural blockade in infants and small children is characterized by hemodynamic stability, even when the level of block reaches upper dermatomes. Young children rely more on the diaphragm for maintaining tidal volumes; thus, apnea may be the first sign of total spinal in infants and small children.

17. **B.** Armitage formula can be used for calculation of caudal bupivacaine in a child with appropriate weight for his age.

    0.5 mL/kg for a lumbosacral block
    1 mL/kg for a thoracolumbar block
    1.25 mL/kg for a midthoracic block
    0.25% Bupivacaine up to a maximum of 20 mL

18. **D.** Fetal circulation is associated with increased pulmonary vascular resistance, decreased pulmonary blood flow, decreased systemic vascular resistance, and right to left blood flow through patent ductus arteriosus and foramen ovale. At birth, the onset of spontaneous ventilation and elimination of placental circulation decreases pulmonary vascular resistance and increases pulmonary blood flow. Simultaneously, systemic vascular resistance increases, left-atrial pressure increases, foramen ovale closes functionally, and right-to-left shunting ceases. When anatomic closure is achieved and the cardiac anatomy is normal, shunting through ductus arteriosus ceases.

19. **D.** Neonates are susceptible to increased heat losses due to thin skin, low fat content, and a higher relative body surface area. Cold operating room, wound exposure, unwarned intravenous fluid administration, dry anesthetic gases, and the direct effect of anesthetic agents on temperature regulation can further accelerate heat loss. Hypothermia is associated with delayed awakening from anesthesia, cardiac irritability, respiratory depression, increased pulmonary vascular resistance, altered drug responses, delayed wound healing, and coagulation and platelet dysfunction. Metabolism of brown fat is responsible for heat production in infants.

20. **D.** Tetralogy of Fallot consists of right-ventricular obstruction, right-ventricular hypertrophy, and a ventricular septal defect with an overriding aorta. About 20% of patients also have pulmonic stenosis. Anesthetic management of a child with tetralogy of Fallot includes adequate preoperative hydration, avoiding factors that can increase pulmonary vascular resistance, maintaining systemic vascular resistance (SVR), and avoid increases in heart rate that may worsen infundibular stenosis. Hypercyanotic spells are treated by volume administration, sedation, and administration of drugs that increase SVR such as phenylephrine. Propranolol may be given to relieve infundibular spasm. Epinephrine in this situation may worsen cyanosis by increasing HR and decreasing SVR.

21. **A.** Normal cardiovascular variables in children:

Table 18-4

Parameter	Neonate	Infant	5 Years	Adult
Oxygen consumption (mL/kg/min)	6	5	4	3
Systolic blood pressure (mm Hg)	65	90–95	95	120
Heart rate (bpm)	130	120	90	80

22. **D.** Premature neonates have decreased creatinine clearance, impaired sodium retention, glucose excretion, and bicarbonate reabsorption, and poor diluting and concentrating ability. Normal kidney function may develop anywhere from 6 months to 2 years of age. Therefore, it is extremely important to pay meticulous attention to fluid management in children less than 2 years of age.

23. **B.** Laboratory value of blood glucose in children:

Table 18-5

	Newborn	1 Week	1 Month	1 Year
Glucose (mg/dL)	40–60	50–80	60–100	60–100

24. **C.** The approximate diameter inside the endotracheal tube can be estimated by a formula based on age:

$$\text{Tube diameter in mm} = (\text{Age in years}/4) + 4$$

Exceptions include premature neonates (2.5- to 3.0-mm tube) and full-term neonates (3.0- to 3.5-mm tube).
Formula for the length of endotracheal tube at the lip:

$$\text{Length} = 12 + \text{Age}/2$$

25. **A.** Metabolic rate and oxygen consumption are higher in infants than in older children. Rest of the parameters in the question remain the same per weight basis in younger and older children. Respiratory rate is increased in neonates and gradually falls to adult levels by adolescence. Airway resistance is increased in neonates due to a relative paucity of small airways. The high metabolic rate and oxygen consumption limit oxygen reserves during periods of apnea (e.g., intubation) and predispose neonates and infants to atelectasis and hypoxemia.

26. **A.** Developmental changes in blood volume:

Table 18-6

Age	Blood Volume (mL/kg)
Preterm	90–105
Term neonate	78–86
1–12 Months	73–78
1–3 Years	74–82
4–6 Years	80–86
7–18 Years	83–90
Adults	68–88

27. **C.** Presence of an acute purulent upper respiratory infection, fever, change in mental status, or signs of lower respiratory tract infection (wheezing, rales), especially in a child, is sufficient to postpone the surgery.

Factors affecting decision for elective surgery in a child with upper respiratory tract infection are as follows:

Pros

- Presence of runny nose alone
- Active, happy child
- Older child
- Clear lungs

Cons

- Recent development of symptoms within 1 to 2 days
- Lethargic child
- Purulent nasal discharge
- Wheezing, rales
- Child <1 year, ex-premature
- Major surgery

28. **A.** Urine output should be monitored in all children undergoing surgeries involving major fluid shifts. The fluid therapy should be aimed at maintaining a urine output of 1 mL/kg/h.

29. **C.** Optimal preoperative preparation in patients with sickle cell anemia includes adequate hydration, treatment of infections, and an acceptable hemoglobin concentration. Preoperative transfusion therapy in sickle cell patients is individualized to the patient and to the surgical procedure. The goal of transfusion therapy is to achieve a hematocrit of 35% to 40%, with 40% to 50% normal hemoglobin. Hemoglobin desaturation or low-flow states (stasis) should be avoided in sickle cell patients. Therefore, tourniquet use should be avoided during surgical procedures. Conditions that could cause hemoglobin desaturation or stasis include hypothermia or hyperthermia, acidosis, hypoxemia, hypotension, or hypovolemia.

30. **B.** Patients with Down syndrome exhibit a short neck, irregular dentition, mental retardation, hypotonia, large tongue, congenital heart disease (in 40% of patients, endocardial cushion defects, ventricular septal defect), subglottic stenosis, tracheoesophageal fistula, chronic pulmonary infections, and seizures. Down syndrome patients often have a difficult airway (use of smaller size of the endotracheal tube). Excessive neck flexion during laryngoscopy or intubation may result in atlantooccipital dislocation because of the laxity of the ligaments. Postoperative stridor and apnea are common in these patients. Antiseizure medications should be continued perioperatively.

31. B.   Maximum allowable blood loss during surgery can be calculated by the following formula:

$$\text{Maximum allowable blood loss} = \text{Patient's hemoglobin} - \text{Allowed hemoglobin}/\text{Average of the two} \times \text{EBV}$$

$$\text{EBV or expected blood volume} = 70 \text{ mL/kg} \times \text{weight of the child}$$

32. B.   Traction on extraocular muscles or pressure on the eyeball can result in cardiac dysrhythmias (bradycardia, ventricular ectopy, ventricular fibrillation). This reflex, called the oculocardiac reflex, consists of a trigeminal afferent and a vagal efferent pathway. The reflex can occur in patients undergoing ocular procedures such as cataract extraction, enucleation, and retinal detachment repair. In awake patients, the oculocardiac reflex may be associated with somnolence and nausea. Management of the oculocardiac reflex consists of (1) immediate notification to the surgeon and temporary cessation of surgical stimulation, (2) confirmation of adequate ventilation, oxygenation, and depth of anesthesia, (3) administration of intravenous atropine (10 µg/kg) if the conduction disturbance persists, and (4) infiltration of the rectus muscles with local anesthetic. Also, retrobulbar block performance can elicit the oculocardiac reflex.

33. B.   Traction on extraocular muscles or pressure on the eyeball can result in cardiac dysrhythmias (bradycardia, ventricular ectopy, ventricular fibrillation). This reflex, called the oculocardiac reflex, consists of a trigeminal afferent and a vagal efferent pathway. The reflex can occur in patients undergoing ocular procedures such as cataract extraction, enucleation, and retinal detachment repair. In awake patients, the oculocardiac reflex may be associated with somnolence and nausea. Management of the oculocardiac reflex consists of (1) immediate notification to the surgeon and temporary cessation of surgical stimulation; (2) confirmation of adequate ventilation, oxygenation, and depth of anesthesia; (3) administration of intravenous atropine (10 µg/kg) if the conduction disturbance persists; and (4) infiltration of the rectus muscles with local anesthetic. Also, retrobulbar block performance can elicit the oculocardiac reflex.

34. B.   Positive pressure with a face mask can be a lifesaving temporizing measure in situations such as laryngospasm, hypoxia, and even difficult intubation. However, it is contraindicated in situations where there is an increased risk of aspiration. In patients with congenital diaphragmatic hernia and tracheoesophageal fistula, positive-pressure ventilation with a face mask is relatively contraindicated.

35. D.   Perioperative postintubation croup occurs in 0.1% to 1% of children. Factors associated with increased risk of croup include a larger outer diameter of endotracheal tube relative to airway, frequent patient position changes, multiple intubation attempts, traumatic intubation, and children aged 1 to 4 years. Treatment includes humidified mist, nebulized racemic epinephrine, and dexamethasone.

36. A.   Perioperative postintubation croup occurs in 0.1% to 1% of children. Factors associated with increased risk of croup include a larger outer diameter of endotracheal tube relative to airway, frequent patient position changes, multiple intubation attempts, traumatic intubation, and children aged 1 to 4 years. Treatment includes humidified mist, nebulized racemic epinephrine, and dexamethasone.

37. A.   Croup is upper airway obstruction characterized by a barking cough. It could be postintubation croup or a result of viral infection. Incidence of infectious croup is increased in children aged 3 months to 3 years. Infectious croup progresses slowly, and patients rarely require intubation. It is treated with nebulized racemic epinephrine and dexamethasone. Acute epiglottitis is a bacterial infection commonly due to *Haemophilus influenzae* type B. It affects children of 2 to 6 years old. Acute epiglottitis can rapidly progress from a sore throat to complete airway obstruction. Endotracheal intubation (spontaneous breathing inhalational induction in sitting position) and antibiotic therapy can be lifesaving.

38. **D.** Pierre Robin syndrome is a genetic disorder characterized by hypoplastic mandible, pseudo macroglossia, and high arched and cleft palate. Large tongue and small mouth can lead to both difficult ventilation and intubation.

39. **C.** Children have a higher metabolic rate than adults until 2 years of age. Pediatric patients have a larger surface area per kilogram than adults (increased surface area/weight ratio). Besides the higher surface area accounting for the higher metabolic rate, children (especially neonates) also loose heat to a greater extent.

40. **B.** Masseter muscle spasm (MMS) may be seen in pediatric patients after the administration of succinylcholine. About 50% of patients in whom MMS develops prove to be susceptible to MH by muscle testing.

41. **D.** During fetal development, the gut can herniate into the thorax through diaphragmatic defects, with left-sided herniation is the most common type (90%). The reported incidence of diaphragmatic hernia is about 1:5000 live births. Clinical features of diaphragmatic herniation include hypoxia, a scaphoid abdomen, and evidence of bowel in the thorax (confirmed with auscultation or radiography). Pulmonary hypoplasia and malrotation of the intestines are commonly associated. While the ipsilateral lung is particularly affected, the herniated gut can compress and retard the maturation of both the lungs. Pulmonary hypertension is common. CDH is often associated with dextrocardia. The goal of initial management of CDH is to avoid a surgical intervention when the infant is hypoxic and acidotic. Instead, medical management is directed to stabilizing the infant's cardiorespiratory status by improving oxygenation, correcting metabolic acidosis, reducing the right-to-left shunting, and increasing pulmonary perfusion.

42. **D.** Interventions to protect the lungs from aspiration in the presence of tracheoesophageal fistula include
    - Avoidance of feedings
    - Upright positioning of the infant to decrease the likelihood of gastroesophageal reflux (30-degree elevation)
    - Antibiotic therapy and physiotherapy if pneumonia is diagnosed
    - Intermittent suctioning of the upper blind esophageal pouch

43. **B.** At birth, initiation of spontaneous ventilation and elimination of the placental circulation decrease pulmonary vascular resistance and increase pulmonary blood flow. At the same time, systemic vascular resistance increases, left-atrial pressure increases, foramen ovale closes functionally, and the right-to-left shunting ceases. When anatomic closure is achieved and cardiac anatomy is normal, shunting through ductus arteriosus also ceases.

44. **C.** Hypothermia is defined as a body temperature less than 36°C. Prewarming for half an hour with convective forced-air warming blankets effectively prevents phase I (initial rapid decline in body temperature) hypothermia by eliminating the central–peripheral temperature gradient. Methods to minimize phase II hypothermia (slower decrease in body temperature) from heat loss include use of forced-air warming blankets and warm-water blankets, heated humidification of inspired gases, warming of intravenous fluids, and raising ambient operating room temperature. Passive insulators such as heated cotton blankets or the so-called space blankets have little utility in preventing hypothermia.

45. **A.** Laryngospasm is a forceful and involuntary spasm of the laryngeal musculature caused by stimulation of the superior laryngeal nerve. Initial treatment of laryngospasm includes gentle positive-pressure ventilation with 100% oxygen and forward jaw thrust. Intramuscular

or intravenous succinylcholine and controlled ventilation may be required in recalcitrant laryngospasm.

46. **B.**   Normal dead space in a neonate is 2 mL/kg.

47. **B.**   Approximately 70% to 80% of the hemoglobin at birth is fetal hemoglobin (HbF). The concentration of HbF decreases significantly by 3 to 6 months of age. HbF has a high affinity for oxygen, which shifts the oxyhemoglobin saturation curve to left. Sickle cell patients with more HbF have a better prognosis.

48. **A.**   Alveolar maturation is not complete until about 8 years of age. Increased airway resistance and decreased compliance lead to increased work of breathing and thus respiratory muscles easily fatigue. The chest wall collapses during inspiration, and residual lung volumes are low at expiration. The resulting decrease in FRC and increased oxygen consumption lead to rapid desaturation in the event of hypoxia. In addition, the hypoxic and hypercapnic ventilatory drives are not well developed in neonates and infants.

49. **B.**   Bupivacaine is cardiotoxic, and an inadvertent intravascular injection can lead to ST segment changes, cardiac arrhythmias, and cardiac arrest. When epinephrine is added to bupivacaine, tachycardia is usually seen, but at times this sign can be unreliable (higher heart rate in infants).

50. **A.**   Because of shorter circulation times than adults, all pediatric patients have a shorter onset time (up to 50% less) of muscle relaxants. Nonetheless, intravenous *succinylcholine* (1–1.5 mg/kg) has the fastest onset among muscle relaxants. Significantly larger volume of distribution is attributed to larger dose requirements in infants. With the notable exclusion of succinylcholine, mivacurium, and possibly *cisatracurium*, infants require significantly less muscle relaxant than older children. Moreover, based on weight, older children require higher doses than adults for some neuromuscular blocking agents (e.g., mivacurium and *atracurium*). As with adults, a more rapid intubation can be achieved with a muscle relaxant dose that is 1.5 to 2 times the ED_{95} dose at the expense of prolonging the duration of action.

19

Critical Care

David Stahl, Daniel Johnson, and Edward Bittner

1. A 78-year-old otherwise-healthy woman arrives in the postanesthesia care unit after an urgent cystoscopy and ureteral stent placement for an impacted ureteral stone. In the operating room, there were no complications and only minimal blood loss. One hour later, she is febrile to 102.3°F, tachycardic with a heart rate of 117 bpm, and hypotensive with a noninvasive blood pressure of 73/42 mm Hg. Blood cultures are drawn and broad-spectrum antibiotics are initiated. A central venous catheter is placed, and the central venous pressure is measured at 2 mm Hg. The best next step in the management of her shock is

   A. Start dobutamine for increased inotropy
   B. Fluid resuscitation to restore adequate preload
   C. Blood transfusion to a goal hemoglobin concentration of 12 g/dL
   D. Initiate nitroglycerin infusion to off-load the right ventricle

2. Shock is most accurately defined as

   A. Inadequate tissue perfusion to meet the oxygen demand of end organs
   B. Hypotension not responsive to intravenous fluid administration
   C. An irreversible process of multisystem organ failure
   D. Decreased blood flow resulting from inadequate cardiac output

3. A 73-year-old man with a history of chronic obstructive pulmonary disease (COPD) on home oxygen was initially admitted to the medical floor for a COPD exacerbation. Over the past few hours, he has developed altered mental status and hypotension. He is transferred to the ICU, intubated, and vasopressors are started to support his blood pressure. A pulmonary artery catheter is placed via the right internal jugular vein. Initial readings reveal central venous pressure = 23 mm Hg, positive airway pressure = 34/15 mm Hg, pulmonary capillary wedge pressure = 4 mm Hg, and CO = 1.9 L/min. The most likely diagnosis is

   A. Hypovolemic shock from inadequate fluid resuscitation
   B. Septic shock from pneumonia
   C. Anaphylactic shock from medications given during intubation
   D. Cardiogenic shock from right-ventricular failure

4. A 54-year-old man is postoperative day 1 after a pancreaticoduodenectomy for pancreatic cancer, complicated by a small intraoperative bile leak. He is febrile to 39.5°C, rigorous, and hypotensive with a blood pressure of 71/32 mm Hg. He is admitted to the ICU. Laboratory work reveals a leukocytosis with bandemia. Despite 4 L of intravenous crystalloid, he remains hypotensive. The most accurate diagnosis for his condition is

   A. Postoperative infection
   B. Sepsis
   C. Severe sepsis
   D. Septic shock

5. Dopamine acts on all of the following receptors, except

    A. α_1

    B. β_1

    C. β_2

    D. DA_1

6. All of the following may be caused by β-agonist effects of vasopressors, except

    A. Increased inotropy

    B. Bronchodilation

    C. Inhibition of renin secretion

    D. Uterine relaxation

7. You are called to the ER to assist in the intubation and management of a 26-year-old man who sustained significant closed head injury during a motorcycle collision. Following uneventful intubation, you accompany the patient and neurosurgery team to the CT scanner where you see a large subarachnoid hemorrhage with effacement of the sulci and 9-mm midline shift. While preparations are made to proceed directly to the operating room, the neurosurgeon asks if you can increase the patient's mean arterial blood pressure (MAP) from 70 to 90 mm Hg to improve cerebral perfusion. The best vasopressor to accomplish this increase in MAP is

    A. Dopamine

    B. Phenylephrine

    C. Norepinephrine

    D. Epinephrine

8. Acute renal failure is defined as

    A. Urine output of less than 0.5 mL/kg/hr or increase in serum creatinine by 50% in 24 hours

    B. Urine output of less than 1 mL/kg/hr or increase in serum creatinine by 100% in 24 hours

    C. Urine output of less than 1 mL/kg/hr or increase in serum creatinine by 200% in 24 hours

    D. Urine output of less than 0.25 mL/kg/hr or increase in serum creatinine by 50% in 24 hours

9. A 28-year-old man is admitted to the intensive care unit after a motorcycle collision from which he suffers multiple injuries including traumatic aortic injury requiring open repair, multiple long-bone fractures, and a closed head injury. On arrival, his blood pressure is maintained on a norepinephrine infusion. His urine output has been <5 mL/hr for the past 8 hours despite adequate fluid resuscitation and a renal ultrasound study that was normal. His pH on arterial blood gas analysis is 6.9 with a base deficit of 16 and a potassium of 5.4 mEq/L. The decision is made to institute renal replacement therapy for recalcitrant acidosis. The best course of action is

    A. Institution of continuous renal replacement therapy (CRRT) as it has been shown to improve mortality at 30 days when compared to intermittent hemodialysis (IHD)

    B. Institution of IHD as it has been shown to improve in-hospital mortality when compared to CRRT

    C. Institution of IHD as it has been shown to more effectively clear acidosis

    D. Institution of CRRT as it has been shown to be more hemodynamically stable than IHD

10. Delirium as defined by the *DSM-IV* includes which of the following major tenants?

    A. Decreased attention and altered cognition

    B. Agitation and pulling at lines

    C. Altered mental status and dementia

    D. Chronic perceptual disturbances and depressed mood

11. Delirium in the ICU setting is

    A. A relatively benign condition
    B. Associated with increased mortality
    C. Associated with a decreased risk of eventual development of dementia
    D. Often successfully treated with benzodiazepines

12. An 88-year-old man is admitted to the intensive care unit after a right-hip hemiarthroplasty to repair an intertrochanteric femur fracture sustained during a fall from standing. On post-operative day 1, he is confused and intermittently agitated with a disorganized thought process. His nurse completed the CAM-ICU screen and reports that the result was positive. The next steps in the management should include all of the following, except

    A. Continually reorienting the patient to his surroundings
    B. Minimizing sedatives if possible
    C. Removing all opioids from his pain regimen
    D. Optimizing sleep health by minimizing nighttime wakeups and encouraging daily wakefulness

13. All of the following conditions are associated with delirium in the ICU, except

    A. Advanced age
    B. Orthopedic surgery
    C. Sepsis
    D. Sleep deprivation

14. Which of the following is a benefit of enteral nutrition when compared to parenteral nutrition?

    A. Decreased cost
    B. Decreased length of mechanical ventilation
    C. Decreased rates of infection
    D. All of the above are benefits of enteral nutrition

15. Enteral nutrition should be initially avoided in a

    A. 54-year-old man who presents with acute alcoholic pancreatitis
    B. 23-year-old G1P0 with hyperemesis gravidarum
    C. 76-year-old woman with a full-thickness esophageal perforation
    D. 34-year-old woman hospitalized with an acute exacerbation of ulcerative colitis

16. A 36-year-old G3, now P3, after a normal spontaneous vaginal delivery is complicated by postpartum hemorrhage. Her vitals are checked, and she is noted to be tachycardic with a HR of 132 bpm and hypotensive with a BP of 76/35 mm Hg. The rapid response team is called. As a result of calling the rapid response team, which of the following outcomes can most reasonably be expected?

    A. She is less likely to have a cardiopulmonary arrest on the postpartum floor
    B. She is less likely to have a cardiopulmonary arrest in the hospital
    C. She is less likely to be transferred to an ICU
    D. She is more likely to survive to hospital discharge

17. The most significant risk of intensive insulin therapy (goal blood glucose 80–100 mg/dL) when compared to moderate glucose control (goal blood glucose <180 mg/dL) is

    A. Myocardial infarction
    B. Seizure
    C. Patient dissatisfaction
    D. Hypoglycemia

18. A 54-year-old man is admitted to the intensive care unit for monitoring after a complicated left colectomy for diverticulitis. He has a history of type 2 diabetes mellitus on metformin. On arrival to the ICU, his blood glucose on an arterial blood gas is 254 mg/dL. One hour later, it is 435 mg/dL. The next appropriate step in his management is

    A. Recheck blood glucose in 1 hour
    B. Restart home metformin
    C. Start IV insulin therapy with a goal glucose <180 mg/dL
    D. Start IV insulin therapy with a goal glucose <120 mg/dL

19. A 93-year-old woman is admitted to the ICU with a leaking 7.8-cm abdominal aortic aneurysm. A multidisciplinary discussion is initiated between the patient, family, bedside nurse, ICU team, and surgery team to decide on the next course of action. Select the answer which best identifies the ethical principle at hand in each quote:

    A. Autonomy—patient: "I accept that refusing an operation means I will likely die soon, but I want to die at home with my family around me if at all possible"
    B. Beneficence—ICU attending: "I worry that if you have this operation it will be unlikely that you will ever return to living at home without significant assistance"
    C. Nonmaleficence—surgeon: "The best chance of you surviving is to have the aneurysm repaired"
    D. Justice—patient's daughter: "Is there another way to do the operation that is less risky?"

20. An 86-year-old man with end-stage congestive heart failure and chronic obstructive pulmonary disease is admitted to the intensive care unit after a fall down one flight of stairs from which he sustains a large subarachnoid hemorrhage. After lengthy discussion with the family, including the patient's wife who has been previously designated his health-care proxy, a decision is made to change goals of care to comfort measures alone. The patient is started on a morphine infusion for pain and to control dyspnea; he is extubated and the family is present at the bedside. About an hour later, the patient's daughter emerges from the room, and tearfully asks, "How much longer can this go on? Can't you do something to speed up the process?" You correctly reply

    A. "We can add additional sedation which will make him pass more quickly"
    B. "I can give him a bolus of morphine to stop him from breathing"
    C. "We can increase the rate of the morphine infusion if he appears to be in pain"
    D. "We can give him a strong muscle relaxant called rocuronium, which will stop him from breathing"

21. An 89-year-old woman is postoperative day 23 from an open repair of a thoracoabdominal aortic aneurysm. She is bacteremic for a second time, and continues to require vasopressor support, mechanical ventilation, and continuous renal replacement therapy. After the most recent of many multidisciplinary family meetings, the decision is made to withdraw life-sustaining treatment and focus on comfort measures alone. As you are discussing with the bedside nurse the logistics of removing vasopressor support, a nursing student asks, "Isn't that going to kill her?" The most correct response is

    A. "Since our goal is not to end her life, it is not technically killing her"
    B. "As long as her heart beats after we turn off the medications, it is not euthanasia"
    C. "As long as the family has given us permission it is OK"
    D. "Stopping these treatments simply discontinues our prolongation of her natural death"

22. A 45-year-old construction worker falls from a three-story building suffers multiple traumatic injuries including a partial amputation of his left leg, resulting in substantial hemorrhage. He is admitted to the intensive care unit directly from the emergency room having received 4 U of packed red blood cells and 2 U of fresh-frozen plasma. Following further resuscitation and operative repair of his left leg, his serum creatinine is noted to be 2.13 mg/dL, and urine output is 0.3 mL/kg/h. The most likely etiology of his renal failure is

   A. Prerenal failure from hypotension
   B. Prerenal failure from thromboembolic disease
   C. Intrinsic renal failure from rhabdomyolysis
   D. Postrenal failure from ureteral obstruction

23. A 28-year-old woman with a history of Hodgkin lymphoma and external beam radiation is admitted to the intensive care unit after repair of an esophageal perforation. She is maintained strictly NPO. Addition of dextrose to her maintenance intravenous fluids will most likely

   A. Fail to suppress protein catabolism
   B. Improve her blood glucose control
   C. Increase her insulin requirement
   D. Improve her cardiac metabolic balance

24. Which of the following tissues does *not* rely on glucose metabolism in the setting of starvation?

   A. Neural tissue
   B. Cardiac tissue
   C. Renal medullary tissue
   D. Erythrocytes

25. Which of the following parenteral nutrition orders would be least likely to precipitate hypercarbic respiratory failure in a patient with severe chronic obstructive pulmonary disease?

   A. Protein = 40 g/L, dextrose = 125 g/L, fat = 0 g/L
   B. Protein = 30 g/L, dextrose = 150 g/L, fat = 0 g/L
   C. Protein = 50 g/L, dextrose = 60 g/L, fat = 50 g/L
   D. Protein = 50 g/L, dextrose = 100 g/L, fat = 25 g/L

26. A 25-year-old man is admitted to the intensive care unit after exploratory laparotomy and repair of multiple bowel injuries from several gunshot wounds. Several hours after admission, the respiratory therapist calls to alert you that his peak airway pressures have increased significantly. The bedside nurse also reports an increase in his vasopressor requirement, and a decrease in urine output. On examination, his abdomen is tense, with a midline dressing intact, and clear breath sounds bilaterally. The most likely diagnosis is

   A. Acute myocardial infarction leading to pulmonary edema
   B. Hypovolemia from inadequate fluid resuscitation
   C. Hemorrhage from an unrecognized injury
   D. Abdominal compartment syndrome from bowel edema or hemorrhage

27. One of the feared adverse effects of reinstituting nutrition in a malnourished patient is refeeding syndrome. The most common electrolyte abnormality seen in refeeding syndrome is

   A. Hypophosphatemia from an increase in intracellular movement of phosphate
   B. Hypokalemia from extracellular buffering of alkalosis
   C. Hypomagnesemia from renal losses
   D. Hyponatremia from excess free water retention by the kidney

28. A 59-year-old man with acute chronic pancreatitis complicated by pseudocyst and necrotizing pancreatitis has been receiving total parenteral nutrition (TPN) for 3 weeks. An error in the ordering system prevents the pharmacy from receiving his order in time to make that day's supply. If his TPN is abruptly discontinued, he is at highest risk for

   A. Hyponatremia
   B. Hypokalemia
   C. Hypoglycemia
   D. Hyperkalemia

29. Acute respiratory distress syndrome (ARDS) patients' plateau pressures should be maintained at or below

   A. 50 cm H_2O
   B. 60 cm H_2O
   C. 40 cm H_2O
   D. 30 cm H_2O

30. Helium–oxygen mixtures can be useful therapies for patients with upper airway obstruction. Compared with air, helium–oxygen mixtures have lower

   A. Density
   B. Viscosity
   C. Oxygen content
   D. Nitrous oxide content

31. In assist-control ventilation (ACV)

   A. Breaths triggered by the ventilator result in the full preset tidal volume being delivered, while breaths triggered by the patient are unsupported by the ventilator
   B. All breaths result in the full preset tidal volume being delivered, regardless of whether they are initiated by the ventilator or by the patient
   C. All breaths must be initiated by the patient
   D. The patient is incapable of triggering breaths

32. A 78-year-old man is admitted from the surgical floor to the intensive care unit for respiratory distress. He is postoperative day 1 from open reduction and internal fixation of a right femoral shaft fracture sustained during a motor vehicle collision. His heart rate is 118 bpm, blood pressure is 104/62 mm Hg, Spo$_2$ is 68% on a non-rebreathing mask at 15 L/min of oxygen, and respirations are 42/min. On examination, he is unresponsive to commands and to sternal rub. The ICU team is deciding whether to initiate noninvasive positive-pressure ventilation (NIPPV) or to perform endotracheal intubation. NIPPV is contraindicated because

   A. The patient's neurologic examination suggests that he is incapable of protecting his airway
   B. NIPPV is incapable of improving significantly low oxygen saturations
   C. The patient is claustrophobic
   D. The patient has certainly suffered a pulmonary embolism (PE), and NIPPV is not helpful in this situation

33. In the first several days following traumatic brain injury requiring mechanical ventilation, an optimal regimen for anxiolysis includes

   A. Diazepam bolus every hour
   B. Lorazepam infusion
   C. Hydromorphone infusion
   D. Propofol infusion

34. In pressure-support ventilation (PSV), inspiration ends (and expiration begins) when

    A. A preset tidal volume has been achieved
    B. A preset airway pressure has been achieved
    C. Flow decreases to a preset level
    D. A preset amount of time has passed

35. A patient can be diagnosed with acute respiratory distress syndrome (ARDS) if he or she has an acute onset of illness, bilateral infiltrates on chest X-ray, lack of evidence of left heart failure, and a Pao_2/Fio_2 (P/F) ratio of less than or equal to

    A. 500 mm Hg
    B. 400 mm Hg
    C. 350 mm Hg
    D. 200 mm Hg

36. A 25-year-old woman has been in the ICU for 6 days after sustaining multiple life-threatening traumatic injuries. She is suffering from septic shock and acute respiratory distress syndrome (ARDS). On examination, she is dyssynchronous with the ventilator, coughing, grimacing in pain, and tearful. Spo_2 is 88% on a Fio_2 of 100%, and the BP is 108/58 mm Hg on a low-dose infusion of norepinephrine. The most appropriate plan for management of the patient's pain, anxiety, and ventilator dyssynchrony is

    A. Hydromorphone PRN and a continuous infusion of cisatracurium
    B. Fentanyl infusion and a continuous infusion of cisatracurium
    C. Midazolam and fentanyl infusions
    D. Lorazepam PRN

37. A patient is at greatest risk for requiring endotracheal intubation and mechanical ventilation if the Spo_2 is 91% while breathing

    A. Room air
    B. 4 L/min of oxygen via nasal cannula
    C. 15 L/min of oxygen via a non-rebreathing mask with reservoir bag
    D. Noninvasive positive-pressure ventilation with an Fio_2 of 35%

38. Weaning from mechanical ventilation is expedited by

    A. Daily spontaneous breathing trials
    B. Synchronized intermittent mandatory ventilation (SIMV)
    C. Administration of bronchodilating medications around the clock
    D. Daily bronchoscopy

39. Synchronized intermittent mandatory ventilation (SIMV) was an improvement on intermittent mandatory ventilation (IMV) because it

    A. Can provide full ventilation support to an apneic patient
    B. Can utilize volume-preset or pressure-preset ventilation
    C. Allows the patient to breathe spontaneously
    D. Reduces the likelihood of breath stacking and volutrauma

40. Tracheostomy should be considered to reduce the risk of subglottic stenosis after an endotracheal tube has been in place for

    A. 5 days
    B. 10 days
    C. 2 to 3 weeks
    D. 8 to 10 weeks

41. A 45-year-old alcoholic male was admitted to the medical floor with severe pancreatitis. On hospital day 5, his respiratory status significantly deteriorates and he is transferred to the ICU. The SpO_2 is 89% on a non-rebreather mask at 15 L/min oxygen. Upon arrival in the ICU, he is sedated and intubated. Initial ventilator settings should include a set tidal volume of

A. 2 mL/kg
B. 6 mL/kg
C. 10 mL/kg
D. 14 mL/kg

42. A 20-year-old trauma patient requires a large dose infusion of propofol while intubated in the ICU. When the propofol is reduced to attempt a spontaneous breathing trial, the patient thrashes wildly and tries to pull out his arterial and central venous lines. A titratable agent that could prove useful for management of this patient's agitation while not depressing his respiratory drive is

A. Methadone
B. Dexmedetomidine
C. Nitrous oxide
D. Fentanyl transdermal patch

43. For pressure-preset ventilation (also known as "pressure-control ventilation"), the independent variable and dependent variable, respectively, are

A. Tidal volume and FIO_2
B. Tidal volume and frequency
C. SpO_2 and airway pressure
D. Airway pressure and tidal volume

44. A mechanically ventilated, 70-kg patient has an arterial blood gas of pH = 7.06, PCO_2 = 83 mm Hg, and PO_2 = 140 mm Hg on volume control ventilation (tidal volume = 450 mL, respiratory rate = 8, FIO_2 = 50%, and positive end–expiratory pressure [PEEP] = 8 cm H_2O). The most appropriate next step in the management is

A. Increase PEEP
B. Increase FIO_2
C. Increase the respiratory rate
D. Administer sodium bicarbonate

45. The primary benefit of positive end–expiratory pressure (PEEP) during mechanical ventilation is

A. Improved elimination of CO_2
B. Improved venous return and cardiac output
C. Prevention and reversal of alveolar collapse (atelectasis)
D. Reduction in peak inspiratory pressure

46. A patient with a chronic obstructive pulmonary disease exacerbation has an initial arterial blood gas (ABG) with pH = 7.05, PCO_2 = 95 mm Hg, and PO_2 = 54 mm Hg on 6 L of oxygen via nasal cannula. The patient is awake, alert, and in moderate respiratory distress with significant wheezing. Bronchodilators and continuous positive airway pressure (CPAP) 10 cm H_2O via face mask with FIO_2 of 50% are initiated. One hour later, the ABG is pH = 7.10, PCO_2 = 90 mm Hg, and PO_2 = 92 mm Hg. The patient remains awake and alert and is now in less distress. The most appropriate next step in the management is

A. Increasing the FIO_2
B. Increasing CPAP to 15 cm H_2O
C. Changing the mode to bi-level positive airway pressure (BiPAP)
D. Stopping CPAP and delivering oxygen via high-flow nasal cannula

47. An ICU patient with severe acute respiratory distress syndrome (ARDS) remains dyssynchronous with the ventilator despite administration of high-dose propofol and fentanyl infusions and changes in the mode of ventilation. The patient's gas exchange has deteriorated over the course of the day, and hypotension requiring vasopressor support has developed in the setting of increasing the propofol dose. The next best step is to

   A. Increase propofol
   B. Change to pressure-support ventilation
   C. Aggressively diurese the patient
   D. Administer a nondepolarizing neuromuscular-blocking agent

48. A 35-year-old man is receiving care in the ICU after sustaining an 80% total body surface area burn from a house fire 5 weeks ago. The surgical team wishes to transition from large dressing changes in the operating room to smaller dressing changes in the ICU. The patient's analgesic regimen consists of extended-release morphine 60 mg by mouth every 12 hours and hydromorphone 2 to 4 mg IV every 2 hours PRN for breakthrough pain. The most appropriate agent for providing sedation and analgesia during the dressing changes in the ICU is

   A. Oral gabapentin
   B. Oral clonidine
   C. Intravenous morphine
   D. Intravenous ketamine

49. A 30-year-old man is admitted to the ICU intubated after a 14-hour spine surgery in the prone position. When he emerges from anesthesia, he bites down on his endotracheal tube, tries frantically to breathe, and panics when he is unable to draw a breath. The nurse boluses propofol and achieves adequate sedation. Five minutes later, the SpO$_2$ rapidly falls from 99% to 65% and the patient appears cyanotic. Pink froth is seen in the endotracheal tube. This complication could have been avoided by

   A. Placing a bite block between the patient's teeth
   B. Administration of less IV fluid during the spine surgery
   C. Omitting the propofol bolus
   D. Positioning the patient in reverse Trendelenburg

50. Effective treatment for carboxyhemoglobinemia includes

   A. Sodium nitrite
   B. Ventilation with 100% oxygen
   C. Ventilation with air
   D. Sodium thiosulfate

1. **B.**   The patient has clinical evidence of shock for which the most common cause is sepsis (likely urosepsis in this case). Primary treatment of vasodilatory shock consists of repleting intravascular volume until adequate preload can be restored, followed by, vasopressor support to maintain adequate end-organ perfusion. The patient's history as otherwise healthy does not rule out cardiogenic shock but makes it less likely, particularly in the setting of fever. Institution of dobutamine for increased inotropy may be useful in cardiogenic shock but is unlikely to improve vasodilatory shock where cardiac output is typically already elevated. Nitroglycerin infusion can be useful in cases of cardiogenic shock secondary to right-ventricular failure, but in such a case, an elevated central venous pressure would be expected. Finally, while blood transfusion may be indicated to increase oxygen-carrying capacity and oxygen delivery in certain shock states, there is no evidence for a goal hemoglobin concentration of 12 g/dL. Fluid resuscitation should begin with crystalloid until more data can be gathered on the patient's condition.

2. **A.**   Shock is a common state in the intensive care unit which has many causes. The common result is inadequate tissue perfusion to end organs, resulting in an imbalance between oxygen supply and demand. If treated early, shock is reversible. However, if untreated, shock can progress to irreversible multisystem organ failure and death. While hypotension is a common component of shock, lack of fluid responsiveness is not a part of the definition, nor is inadequate cardiac output.

3. **D.**   In medically complex patients, the etiology of shock can be difficult to diagnose. While by history, one could presume this patient has hypovolemic, septic, or anaphylactic shock, the pulmonary artery catheter indicates elevated right-sided filling pressures with relatively low left-sided pressures, and hypotension, which are consistent with right-ventricular failure and cardiogenic shock.

4. **D.**   The American College of Chest Physicians/Society of Critical Care Medicine (ACCP/SCCM) Consensus Conference Definitions for sepsis would classify this patient as having septic shock. The consensus definition for sepsis is a confirmed or suspected infection plus two of the SIRS criteria (temperature $<36°C$ or $>38°C$, heart rate >90 bpm, respiratory rate >20 breaths/min or $Paco_2 < 32$ mm Hg, leukocyte count $<4,000$ cells/L or $>12,000$ cells/L). Severe sepsis is defined as sepsis together with dysfunction of at least one organ system. Septic shock is defined as sepsis plus hypotension (systolic blood pressure <90 mm Hg) despite fluid resuscitation. This patient has a suspected infection, meets at least two of the SIRS criteria, and remains hypotensive despite fluid resuscitation, making the most correct answer septic shock.

5. **C.**   Dopamine has direct agonist action on α_1, β_1, and DA_1 receptors, as well as indirect agonism of α_1 and β_1 receptors via release of endogenous norepinephrine. DA_1 effects are predominately seen in low doses of dopamine and cause renal arteriole dilation. β_1 effects are seen at moderate doses of dopamine and increase myocardial contractility and heart rate. Increased myocardial work and oxygen demand resulting from the agonist actions of dopamine can lead to myocardial ischemia. α_1 Effects are seen at high doses of dopamine and lead to increased systemic vascular resistance.

6. **C.**   Agents that act on β receptors have effects on a wide variety of organs. β_1 activation causes an increase in inotropy and chronotropy as well as stimulation of renin secretion. β_2 agonism results in bronchodilation as well as dilation of other smooth muscles, including the uterus.

7. **B.**   Phenylephrine acts directly on α_1 receptors to increase systemic vascular resistance, arterial blood pressure, and cerebral blood flow. Phenylephrine does not cross the blood–brain

barrier and therefore does not affect the cerebral vasculature, making it the vasopressor of choice in brain-injured patients.

8. **A.** There are many definitions of acute renal failure (or acute kidney injury). The most consistent definition is a urine output of less than 0.5 mL/kg/hr or a 50% increase in serum creatinine over 24 hours. Both the Acute Dialysis Quality Initiative (ADQI) criteria (also known as the RIFLE criteria) and the Acute Kidney Injury Network (AKIN) criteria include these in the first stage of acute kidney injury.

9. **D.** CRRT has not been shown to be more efficacious or improve mortality in ICU patients when compared to IHD; however, CRRT is associated with less hypotension presumably because of smaller intravascular fluid shifts when compared to IHD. In this patient who has a persistent vasopressor requirement, CRRT will likely provide more hemodynamic stability, while enabling clearance of both his acidosis and hyperkalemia.

10. **A.** Delirium is defined by the *DSM-IV* as an alteration of consciousness with (1) decreased ability to focus or sustain attention associated, (2) a disturbance in cognition or perception not accounted for by baseline dementia. Agitation and pulling at lines may be signs of hyperactive delirium but are not diagnostic of delirium. Dementia is a chronic condition that is diagnostically separate from delirium, which is an acute condition. Depressed mood is not part of the definition of delirium, although flat affect may be seen in hypoactive delirium.

11. **B.** While previously thought of as a relatively benign condition or a mere inconvenience to ICU providers, delirium has been associated with prolonged mechanical ventilation, prolonged ICU and hospital stay, and increased mortality. Delirium is also associated with eventual development of dementia. Risk of delirium is increased when benzodiazepines are used for sedation.

12. **C.** While opioids may indeed contribute to delirium, inadequate pain control is also associated with delirium. It may be beneficial to optimize pain control with other nonopioid adjuncts such as acetaminophen, but removal of all opioids may not be practical or helpful. Encouraging sleep health, reorienting the patient to his surroundings, and minimizing sedatives are all important treatments for delirium.

13. **B.** Advanced age, sepsis, and sleep deprivation have all be associated with delirium. Orthopedic surgery has not been independently associated with delirium. Other conditions associated with delirium include baseline cognitive impairment, increasing severity of illness, multisystem organ failure, immobilization, pain, mechanical ventilation, and use of sedatives (especially benzodiazepines).

14. **D.** Enteral nutrition is less expensive, easier to administer, and maintains normal enteric physiology and flora better than parenteral nutrition. Enteral nutrition is also associated with lower rates of infection, and more recently has been shown to decrease the length of mechanical ventilation and hospital stay (even in a subset of patients who have limited enteral intake).

15. **C.** While previous concerns have been raised about enteral feeding in a number of disease states, more recent evidence demonstrates the benefits outweigh the risks in cases of acute pancreatitis, hyperemesis gravidarum, and inflammatory bowel disease, as well as cases of enteric fistulas, short-bowel syndrome, and bone marrow or other chemotherapy patients. Patients with an esophageal perforation are managed without enteral nutrition in the acute setting.

16. **A.** The institution of multidisciplinary rapid response teams were in reaction to the high number of cardiopulmonary arrests seen in the in-hospital setting. Despite this intervention, there are no data to demonstrate decreased incidence of cardiopulmonary arrest in the hospital, prevention of ICU admission, or decreased mortality. However, patients evaluated by the

rapid response team are more likely to be moved to the ICU sooner, and therefore less likely to have a cardiopulmonary arrest outside of the ICU, such as on the postpartum floor.

17. **D.** Initial studies of intensive insulin therapy (goal blood glucose approximately 80–100 mg/dL) suggested decreased ICU mortality. Unfortunately, subsequent trials have failed to reproduce the benefit of decreased mortality and have demonstrated substantial increases in rates of hypoglycemia. While myocardial infarction and seizure may be presentations of hypoglycemia, the more likely underlying cause in the case of intensive insulin therapy is hypoglycemia.

18. **C.** The patient has a rapidly increasing blood glucose level that warrants control immediately. Restarting home metformin, while reasonable, is unlikely to have an acute effect on his hyperglycemia. IV insulin therapy is indicated in this patient. While earlier studies demonstrated a mortality benefit to intensive insulin therapy, subsequent data have shown an increased risk of hypoglycemia and failed to show a mortality benefit. It would be most reasonable to start IV insulin with a goal blood glucose of <180 mg/dL.

19. **A.** End-of-life discussions should protect a patient's right to die with dignity. Understanding the ethical principals at play can help guide balanced solutions. Autonomy recognizes the right of the individual (in this case, the patient) to self-determination. In this case, accepting refusal of treatment with a rational understanding respects the patient's autonomy. Beneficence is the principle of taking the action that best serves the patient's interest. The ICU attending, while expressing beneficence is also expressing nonmaleficence, is the concept of avoiding harm to patients. The surgeon is more clearly expressing the ideal of beneficence. Justice refers to the distribution of scarce resources. The question from the patient's daughter of doing the procedure in a less-risky manner is more likely reflective of beneficence and nonmaleficence.

20. **C.** The goal of medications at the end of life should be the treatment of specific symptoms, not the direct hastening of death. In this case, treating pain or dyspnea with morphine is quite appropriate. The principle of the "double effect," that is, two consequences caused by a single action, is also appropriate at the end of life. In this instance, morphine may have the desired effect of treating pain (following the ethical principle of beneficence) but may also hasten death (following the ethical principle of nonmaleficence). It is not ethically appropriate to add sedation to hasten death, or to bolus morphine or a paralytic to stop breathing.

21. **D.** It is important to communicate to family members and providers that withdrawal of life-sustaining treatment is no different from having a patient (or family member) refuse life-sustaining treatment in the first place, and respects the principle of autonomy. Furthermore, withdrawal of life-sustaining treatment is not active euthanasia but rather cessation of the prolongation of natural death. This is true regardless of the physiologic consequences. Whereas, medications at the end of life are often given with the understanding of the "double effect" principle, namely that medications given to alleviate pain and suffering may also speed death; withdrawal of life-sustaining treatment does not have a specific goal other than to respect the patient and family member's autonomy, or to cease medically futile care.

22. **A.** In this vignette, the patient's massive hemorrhage likely leads to prerenal failure from both hypotension and hypovolemia. Evaluation of the urine would likely reveal an elevated specific gravity and a fractional excretion of sodium of <1%. Thromboembolic disease is possible, particularly with long-bone fractures, although much more rare. Rhabdomyolysis is also possible due to muscle injury but less likely. Finally, while urine output does not rule out obstruction, there is no mention of an injury that would increase suspicion of renal-outflow obstruction.

23. **A.** Addition of dextrose to intravenous fluids during acute illness does not suppress protein catabolism. Even the addition of adequate calories may not entirely prevent protein catabolism in a critically ill patient. The amount of dextrose in standard maintenance fluids is unlikely to

improve her glucose control or substantially alter her insulin requirements. The heart preferentially relies on fatty acid metabolism, which is likely unchanged in the setting of additional IV dextrose.

24. **B.** Within approximately 24 hours of the onset of fasting, glycogen supplies are depleted and gluconeogenesis becomes increasingly important. Neural tissue, renal medullary tissue, and erythrocytes continue to utilize glucose, sparing tissue proteins, while other cells preferentially utilize fatty acids such as cardiac myocytes.

25. **C.** The respiratory quotient (RQ) is defined as the ratio of the amount of carbon dioxide produced relative to the amount of oxygen consumed (Vco_2/Vo_2). The RQ changes with the type of caloric intake. Carbohydrates have an RQ of 1, whereas proteins have an RQ of 0.8 to 0.9, and lipids have an RQ closer to 0.7. Given that a higher RQ reflects greater CO_2 production, and therefore, increased need for CO_2 elimination, the parenteral nutrition with the least calories from carbohydrates will be least likely to precipitate hypercarbic respiratory failure.

26. **D.** While all of these diagnoses are important to exclude, the most critical in this case is abdominal compartment syndrome. The increase in peak airway pressures, worsening hypotension, and decreased urine output in the setting of recent abdominal surgery with a tense abdomen raise concern for abdominal compartment syndrome. Bladder pressure can be measured as an indicator of intra-abdominal pressure. Myocardial infarction is unlikely in a 25-year-old, and clear lung sounds make pulmonary edema also unlikely. Hypovolemia and hemorrhage are also both possible, but intra-abdominal compartment syndrome should be ruled out first.

27. **A.** Hypophosphatemia is commonly seen in critically ill patients. As a part of the refeeding syndrome, there is increased synthesis of intracellular adenosine triphosphate, resulting in increased intracellular transport of phosphates. Hypokalemia may also be seen in refeeding syndrome but is related to intracellular transport and secondary effects of endogenous and exogenous insulin. Hypomagnesemia may also occur in refeeding syndrome. Hyponatremia is not commonly associated with refeeding syndrome.

28. **C.** Given the patient's long-term TPN use, he is at highest risk for hypoglycemia, as his constant source of glucose has been acutely removed. If TPN is to be discontinued, then it should be slowly tapered over a period of hours. If TPN is to be abruptly discontinued, then it should be replaced with a dextrose-containing fluid. Patients who receive insulin in their TPN are also at risk of hyperglycemia.

29. **D.** Multiple studies have shown a mortality benefit when patients with ARDS are ventilated with tidal volumes of 6 mL/kg ideal body weight and have plateau pressures maintained at or below 30 cm H_2O.

30. **A.** Helium–oxygen mixtures have a lower density than air, which promotes improved laminar gas flow across obstructed airways. The mixtures have a similar viscosity to air. Helium–oxygen mixtures do not have oxygen content lower than 21% (the oxygen content of air). Neither the mixtures nor the air contains nitrous oxide.

31. **B.** The essence of ACV is that *all* breaths receive the full preset tidal volume regardless of whether the breaths are initiated by the ventilator or by the patient. With ACV if the ventilator is set at Vt = 500 mL, the frequency is set at 10 breaths/min, and the patient exhibits no respiratory effort, the ventilator will deliver 500 mL breaths 10 times per minute. If that same patient makes 8 respiratory efforts in addition to the 10 mandatory breaths, the ventilator will deliver 500 mL breaths 18 times per minute. Choice A is not correct because in assist-control mode, all breaths are fully supported. Choice C is not correct because in assist control, if the patient makes no respiratory effort, the ventilator will provide breaths at the preset frequency. Choice D is not correct because assist control does allow patients to trigger breaths.

32. A. Unresponsive patients are poor candidates for NIPPV because of the risk of regurgitation and aspiration of stomach contents. When considering NIPPV, one must consider whether the patient will be able to protect the airway. Choice B is incorrect because NIPPV can, in fact, improve significantly low oxygen saturation, particularly in cases of chronic obstructive pulmonary disease exacerbations or congestive heart failure. Choice C is incorrect because the question does not mention claustrophobia. While it is difficult for patients with claustrophobia to tolerate NIPPV, modern devices that fit over the nose alone have alleviated this problem to some degree. Choice D is incorrect because it is not certain that the patient has suffered a PE. The clinical scenario is suggestive of PE (trauma, long-bone fracture, status postsurgery), but patients with postoperative pulmonary edema and other etiologies of respiratory failure can present in a similar way.

33. D. Propofol infusion is an excellent choice for anxiolysis in mechanically ventilated patients after acute brain injury because of its favorable pharmacokinetics and pharmacodynamics. The ICU team can stop the propofol infusion frequently and reevaluate the patient's neurologic exam. Choice A is incorrect because hourly boluses of diazepam would result in accumulation of the drug and interfere with neurologic examinations. Choice B is incorrect because a lorazepam infusion is also likely to interfere with neurologic examination. Choice C is incorrect because the question is about anxiolysis, not analgesia.

34. C. In PSV, inspiration is triggered by a patient's respiratory effort. A continuous airway pressure is maintained by gas flow that decreases throughout inspiration. When flow decreases to a preset fraction of the peak flow (usually 25% of peak flow), gas flow into the inspiratory limb ends and expiration begins. Choice A describes volume-preset ventilation, often called "volume control." Choice B is incorrect because in PSV, a preset airway pressure is *maintained* throughout inspiration. Choice D is incorrect because in PSV, decrease in flow (not a preset time) determines the length of inspiration.

35. D. The American-European Consensus Conference (AECC) on ARDS defined ARDS as (1) acute onset and (2) P/F ≤200 mm Hg, bilateral infiltrates on chest X-ray, and a pulmonary artery occlusion (wedge) pressure ≤18 mm Hg or clinical absence of left-atrial hypertension. The pulmonary process was defined at Acute Lung Injury if the above criteria were met but the P/F was 201 to 300 mm Hg. In 2012, the ARDS Definition Task Force removed Acute Lung Injury from the definition and replaced it with the categories mild, moderate, and severe ARDS defined by P/F ratios of 201 to 300, 101 to 200, or ≤100, respectively. The new definition is known as the Berlin definition of ARDS. Only choice D has a P/F ratio low enough to be called ARDS by the AECC or the Berlin definition.

36. C. The combination of an opioid with a benzodiazepine addresses both pain and anxiety and is effective in helping many ARDS patients achieve synchrony with the ventilator. While they can have a significant effect on hemodynamics, both fentanyl and midazolam (in modest doses) are relatively well tolerated by the septic patient suffering from hypotension requiring vasopressors. Choices A and B are incorrect because they involve neuromuscular blockade without any amnestic/anxiolytic agent. Choice D is incorrect because the patient appears to be in pain and lorazepam lacks analgesic properties. Additionally, cough suppression is a quality of opioids that are lacking in benzodiazepines.

37. C. The non-rebreathing mask with reservoir bag can deliver an F_{IO_2} of nearly 100% when oxygen flow is 15 L/min or greater. An Spo_2 of 91% on an F_{IO_2} of 100% should alert the clinician to the likely need for endotracheal intubation and mechanical ventilation. Choice A is clearly incorrect as the F_{IO_2} is only 21%. Choice B is incorrect because the F_{IO_2} is only 35% and can be further increased. Choice D is incorrect assuming that other variables are safe and stable ($Paco_2$, mental status, ability to protect airway). Many chronic obstructive pulmonary disease patients in the ICU benefit from short-term support from noninvasive positive-pressure ventilation and do quite well with Spo_2 readings in the low 90s.

38. A. Many studies have sought to determine the factors that result in the fastest time to weaning from mechanical ventilation. The daily spontaneous breathing trial has emerged as a simple maneuver that consistently results in fewer days on mechanical ventilation. Choice B is incorrect because SIMV has not been shown to reduce days on mechanical ventilation. Choice C is not correct because blanket administration of bronchodilating medications has not been shown to expedite weaning from the ventilator. Choice D is not correct because unnecessary bronchoscopy exposes the patient to the risks of the procedure without benefit.

39. D. Choices A, B, and C describe features that are common to both IMV and SIMV. SIMV allows a patient's respiratory effort to initiate mandatory ventilator-supported breaths; while in IMV, the mandatory breaths are delivered on a preset schedule without regard for the patient's spontaneous breaths. Therefore, ventilation with IMV has a higher risk of breath stacking and volutrauma, as a patient can take a large spontaneous breath just prior to the ventilator delivering a mandatory breath.

40. C. The risk of subglottic tracheal stenosis increases after an endotracheal tube has been in place for 2 to 3 weeks. There is a trend toward performing early tracheostomy, which may facilitate weaning from the ventilator. Waiting 8 to 10 weeks to perform tracheostomy on an intubated patient would put the patient at undue risk for tracheal stenosis.

41. B. This severe pancreatitis patient is at high risk for acute respiratory distress syndrome (ARDS). When compared with the tidal volume of 12 mL/kg, 6 mL/kg was shown to reduce mortality in patients with ARDS. Choice A is incorrect because 2 mL/kg is not larger than anatomic dead space, so it would lead to progressive respiratory acidosis and hypoxia. Choices C and D are incorrect because these tidal volumes are too large for a patient at risk for ARDS.

42. B. Dexmedetomidine is a titratable, intravenous α_2-receptor agonist with sedative and anxiolytic effects. Compared with propofol, benzodiazepines, and barbiturates, it causes less respiratory depression. This makes the drug well suited for cases in which the patient oscillates between apnea/unresponsiveness on large doses of propofol or benzodiazepines, and extreme agitation on lower doses. Young trauma patients being weaned from mechanical ventilation often tolerate the endotracheal tube very poorly, and some benefit from dexmedetomidine in the period leading up to extubation. Choice A is incorrect because methadone, with its complex pharmacokinetic profile, is difficult to titrate over a short period of time and would not provide direct anxiolysis. Choice C is incorrect because nitrous oxide is an impractical agent for use in the ICU. Choice D is incorrect because a transdermal fentanyl patch would be difficult to titrate over a short period of time and would not provide direct anxiolysis.

43. D. With mechanical ventilation, the "independent variable" is manipulated or "set" by the operator, while the dependent variable results from the system and cannot be "set" by the operator. In pressure-preset ventilation, the inspiratory airway pressure is set to a desired value, and thus is an independent variable. The tidal volume is not set; rather, it results from a combination of variables within the system, including the set inspiratory airway pressure, lung compliance, chest-wall resistance, and the set inspiratory time. Thus, tidal volume is a dependent variable. In volume-preset ventilation, or "volume control ventilation," the opposite is true; the independent variable is tidal volume, and the dependent variable is airway pressure. Choice A is incorrect because tidal volume is not an independent variable and FIO_2 is not a dependent variable. Choice B is incorrect because tidal volume is not an independent variable and frequency is not a dependent variable. Choice C is incorrect because SpO_2 is never an independent variable and airway pressure is not a dependent variable in pressure-preset ventilation.

44. C. This is a case of nearly pure respiratory acidosis. The pH is very low as a result of a significantly elevated PCO_2. The management of a respiratory acidosis consists of increasing the minute ventilation by increasing either respiratory rate (choice C) or tidal volume (not given as an answer choice). Choices A and B are incorrect because neither would result in an increased minute ventilation. Choice D is incorrect because giving bicarbonate will temporarily increase the pH, but will not address the underlying problem of inadequate elimination of CO_2.

45. **C.**   PEEP helps to expand collapsed alveoli, which improves ventilation/perfusion matching by reducing shunt. Choice A is incorrect because PEEP does not directly impact ventilation, which determines the elimination of CO_2. Choice B is incorrect because PEEP typically reduces venous return, which in turn reduces the cardiac output. Choice D is incorrect because in general, the peak inspiratory pressure will increase when PEEP is added.

46. **C.**   The patient is tolerating CPAP well, and oxygenation has improved, but ventilation remains inadequate. By changing modes to BiPAP, inspiratory pressure will be added, which will likely increase ventilation and improve the hypercarbic respiratory acidosis. Choices A, B, and C are incorrect because the patient's arterial oxygen level is adequate, and increasing the FIO_2 or CPAP would cause an increase in Pao_2.

47. **D.**   In cases of severe ARDS and ventilator dyssynchrony refractory to high-dose sedatives and opioids, neuromuscular blockade is appropriate. The risk of polymyoneuropathy of critical illness is increased by the use of neuromuscular-blocking agents, but the immediate risks of hypoxemia and hypoventilation are more pressing. Choice A is incorrect because the patient is already on high-dose propofol with adverse effect (worsening hypotension). Choice B is incorrect because the patient is already failing on full ventilator support. A change to pressure-support ventilation would almost certainly result in worsened oxygenation. While diuresis has a role in the care of patients with refractory hypoxemia, choice C is incorrect because the patient is hypotensive. Adding hypovolemia to a distributive shock patient could result in hemodynamic collapse.

48. **D.**   Ketamine is an *N*-methyl-D-aspartate antagonist with dissociative and analgesic effects. It also has sympathomimetic effects, so it will often cause an increase in heart rate and blood pressure. It has minimal effect on respiratory drive. This combination of qualities makes it well suited for procedural sedation in ICU patients, especially for those patients who have developed tolerance to opioids and GABAergic agents. Choices A and B are clearly incorrect because oral medications are impractical for procedural sedation in the ICU. Choice C is incorrect because the patient is already on large doses of hydromorphone and morphine, is likely to have developed tolerance to opioids, and therefore, is unlikely to have a significant response to additional morphine administration.

49. **A.**   This patient is suffering from negative-pressure pulmonary edema resulting from the patient's strong respiratory effort, which generates a large negative intrathoracic pressure in the setting of an occluded airway. In this setting, the large negative pressure in the alveoli pulls fluid from pulmonary capillaries into the airspaces. This can result in the immediate onset of severe pulmonary edema, shunt, and hypoxia. A bite block prevents occlusion of the endotracheal tube.

50. **B.**   The half-life of carboxyhemoglobin is reduced significantly by ventilation with 100% oxygen. Choices A and D are treatments for cyanide poisoning. Ventilation with air would greatly prolong the time to resolution of carboxyhemoglobinemia.

CHAPTER 20

Postoperative Anesthesia Care

Sheri Berg and Edward Bittner

1. The most common cause of postanesthesia care unit (PACU)–related malpractice claims is

   A. Undertreated pain
   B. Critical respiratory incidents
   C. Nerve injury from regional blocks
   D. Cardiovascular events

2. Which of the statements regarding the American Society of Anesthesiologists (ASA) Standards for Postanesthesia Care is true?

   A. A physician is responsible for the discharge of a patient from the postanesthesia care unit (PACU)
   B. Medical supervision and coordination of patient care in the PACU should be the responsibility of an anesthesiologist
   C. Use of a PACU scoring system is recommended
   D. All of the above

3. The most common cause of postoperative airway obstruction is

   A. Loss of pharyngeal tone in a sedated patient
   B. Weak diaphragmatic contraction
   C. Redundant pharyngeal tissue
   D. Laryngeal edema

4. A 36-year-old man who underwent a laparoscopic cholecystectomy develops upper airway obstruction in the PACU. You suspect that residual neuromuscular blockade is a major contributing factor. Which of the following would exclude the presence of residual neuromuscular blockade?

   A. Oxygen saturation of 98% on 2-L nasal cannula
   B. Normal tidal volumes while spontaneously breathing
   C. Normal end-tidal carbon dioxide concentration while spontaneously breathing
   D. None of the above

5. After reversal of neuromuscular blockade, pharyngeal function returns to baseline when the adductor pollicis train-of-four (TOF) ratio is greater than

   A. 0.9
   B. 0.7
   C. 0.5
   D. 0.4

6. Which of the following is considered the "gold standard" when using clinical assessment to evaluate for residual neuromuscular blockade?

    A. Tongue protrusion
    B. Ability to lift the head off the bed for 5 seconds
    C. Ability to lift the legs off the bed for 5 seconds
    D. Hand-grip strength

7. Which of the following metabolic states can contribute to residual neuromuscular blockade?

    A. Hypocalcemia
    B. Hypomagnesemia
    C. Hyperthermia
    D. Alkalosis

8. You are called to evaluate a 14-year-old girl in the postanesthesia care unit (PACU) with decreased oxygen saturation. The nurse tells you her anesthesia team "extubated her deep." You determine that she is in laryngospasm. Which of the following would be the most appropriate first step in her management?

    A. Wait for 5 minutes, watch her, and reassess
    B. Administer 2 mg/kg of propofol
    C. Provide a jaw thrust and apply continuous positive airway pressure (CPAP)
    D. Administer 0.5 mg/kg of succinylcholine

9. A 40-year-old woman undergoes an 8-hour spine surgery and is left intubated for concern of airway edema. Which of the following statements regarding the assessment of airway edema is correct?

    A. The absence of facial edema excludes the presence of airway edema
    B. The presence of air movement around the endotracheal tube with the cuff deflated excludes the presence of airway edema
    C. The absence of scleral edema excludes the presence of airway edema
    D. The cuff-leak test cannot exclude the presence of airway edema

10. Strategies to reduce the risk of airway obstruction in patients with obstructive sleep apnea (OSA) include all of the following, except

    A. Administration of benzodiazepines in place of opioids to reduce anxiety
    B. Application of postoperative continuous positive airway pressure (CPAP)
    C. Use of continuous regional anesthetic techniques
    D. Preoperative screening to identify patients at high risk

11. You are called to evaluate a 65-year-old man in the postanesthesia care unit who underwent a left-carotid endarterectomy earlier in the day. He is having difficulty breathing, and you notice that the left side of his neck appears swollen. As you examine him, he becomes agitated and his oxygen saturation decreases to 92%. You ask for the surgeon be called "stat" and attempt bag mask ventilation. The next step to take is

    A. Wait for the surgeon to arrive
    B. Release the sutures and evacuate the hematoma
    D. Administer naloxone
    E. Apply noninvasive ventilation

12. The most common cause of transient postoperative hypoxemia in the postanesthesia care unit (PACU) is

    A. Microaspiration
    B. Pneumothorax
    C. Alveolar hypoventilation
    D. Pulmonary embolus

13. For every 1-mm Hg increase in arterial Paco₂, minute ventilation increases by

 A. 0.5 L/min
 B. 1 L/min
 C. 2 L/min
 D. 4 L/min

14. Which of the following is not a cause of arterial hypoxemia in the postanesthesia care unit?

 A. Decreased alveolar partial pressure of oxygen
 B. Ventilation-to-perfusion mismatch
 C. Shunt
 D. Decreased venous admixture

15. A healthy 21-year-old college football player is admitted to the postanesthesia care unit with hypoxemia after undergoing an Achilles tendon repair. The patient developed laryngospasm after extubation in the operating room, which resolved after application of positive pressure. What is the likely cause of his pulmonary edema?

 A. Cardiovascular dysfunction
 B. Aspiration
 C. Postobstructive pulmonary edema
 D. Volume overload

16. Administration of 5 L/min of oxygen by nasal cannula results in an Fio₂ delivery of

 A. 0.45
 B. 0.41
 C. 0.34
 D. 0.28

17. Which of the following postoperative hemodynamic abnormalities is the most predictive of unplanned ICU admission and mortality

 A. Tachycardia
 B. Bradycardia
 C. Hypotension
 D. Hypertension

18. The most common cause of systemic hypotension in the postanesthesia care unit (PACU) is

 A. Intravascular volume depletion
 B. Myocardial ischemia
 C. Residual anesthetic effects
 D. Vasodilation

19. A sympathetic block above which level can result in bradycardia and hypotension?

 A. T4
 B. T6
 C. T8
 D. T10

20. Which of the following statements regarding a perioperative anaphylactic reaction is most correct?

 A. Vasopressin is the drug of choice to treat anaphylaxis
 B. The absence of bronchospasm and rash excludes the diagnosis of anaphylaxis
 C. Low serum tryptase concentrations can differentiate between anaphylactic and anaphylactoid reactions
 D. Neuromuscular-blocking drugs are the most common causes of anaphylactic reactions in the perioperative setting

21. You are called to the bedside to evaluate new ST-segment depressions on a routine postoperative EKG of a 42-year-old woman who underwent a partial colectomy. She is asymptomatic. Her heart rate is 80 to 90 bpm, and her blood pressure is 135/60. Your next step in the management includes

    A. Wait and monitor her
    B. Send off one set of troponins
    C. Administer metoprolol for HR control
    D. Call a cardiology consult

22. Which of the following patients warrants a routine postoperative EKG?

    A. An 85-year-old male with hypothyroidism who underwent a cystoscopy and ureteral stent placement
    B. A 72-year-old male with coronary artery disease (CAD) and hypertension who underwent an ankle fusion
    C. A 52-year-old male with hypertension, hyperlipidemia, and diabetes who underwent a radical prostatectomy
    D. A 50-year-old male with rheumatoid arthritis who underwent bilateral knee replacements

23. You are called to evaluate a 68-year-old woman who underwent a right upper lobectomy for lung cancer. She is complaining of chest pain and palpitations and explains to you that she has never had this problem before. Her EKG demonstrates atrial fibrillation with a rate of 152. Her blood pressure is currently 65/40. Which of the following is the most appropriate first step in managing her?

    A. Repeat EKG in 15 minutes
    B. Administer 150 mg IV amiodarone
    C. Administer 5 mg IV metoprolol
    D. Electrical cardioversion

24. Postoperative premature ventricular contractions (PVCs) most commonly are a result of

    A. QT prolongation
    B. Excessive β-blocker administration
    C. Increased sympathetic system stimulation
    D. Residual volatile anesthetics

25. Which of the following could result in bradydysrhythmias in the postoperative period?

    A. Opioid administration
    B. Bowel distention
    C. Increased intraocular pressure
    D. All of the above

26. What percentage of patients over the age of 50 who undergo elective surgery will experience postoperative delirium within the first 5 days following their surgical procedure?

    A. <1%
    B. 5%
    C. 10%
    D. 25%

27. Which of the following intraoperative factors is predictive of postoperative delirium?

    A. Blood loss
    B. Anesthetic technique
    C. Intraoperative hypotension
    D. Intraoperative hypertension

28. Each of the following increases the risk of postoperative delirium, except

    A. Advanced age
    B. Preexisting cognitive impairment
    C. Alcohol abuse
    D. Chronic pain

29. Which of the following statements regarding emergence excitement is most correct?

    A. It is most common in children aged 6 to 8 years
    B. Less than 5% of children experience emergence excitement
    C. It is associated with long-term cognitive sequelae
    D. Preoperative midazolam administration is associated with an increased incidence

30. Oliguria is defined as urine output less than

    A. 0.2 mL/kg/hr
    B. 0.5 mL/kg/hr
    C. 0.7 mL/kg/hr
    D. 1.0 mL/kg/hr

31. Postoperative urinary retention (POUR) is the inability to void despite a bladder volume of

    A. 100 to 200 mL
    B. 300 to 400 mL
    C. 500 to 600 mL
    D. 700 to 800 mL

32. The most common cause of oliguria in the immediate postoperative period is

    A. Low cardiac output
    B. Acute tubular necrosis
    C. Renal vascular obstruction
    D. Hypovolemia

33. An intra-abdominal pressure higher than which of the following is required to impede renal perfusion?

    A. 10 cm H_2O
    B. 15 cm H_2O
    C. 20 cm H_2O
    D. 30 cm H_2O

34. A 42-year-old morbidly obese male undergoes a laparoscopic gastric bypass. The surgical procedure lasts 8 hours. Estimated blood loss is 200 mL, and he receives 4.5 L of crystalloid. In the postanesthesia care unit, his urine output is 5 to 10 mL/hr despite an additional 1 L of crystalloid. The most likely etiology of his oliguria is

    A. Contrast-induced nephropathy
    B. Rhabdomyolysis
    C. Hypovolemia
    D. Surgical injury of ureters

35. All of the following are consequences of moderate hypothermia (33–35°C), except

    A. Inhibition of platelet function
    B. Prolongation of neuromuscular blockade
    C. Inhibition of drug metabolism
    D. Increases coagulation-factor activity

36. The most accurate measurement of core body temperature is obtained via

    A. Axillary
    B. Tympanic membrane
    C. Rectal
    D. Nasopharyngeal

37. The most effective treatment for abolishing postoperative shivering is

    A. Clonidine
    B. Doxapram
    C. Meperidine
    D. Fentanyl

38. A 22-year-old nonsmoking woman with no previous anesthetic history undergoes a laparo-scopic ovarian cystectomy. Her risk of postoperative nausea and vomiting (PONV) is most closely approximated by

    A. 5%
    B. 10%
    C. 20%
    D. 40%

39. A 30-year-old woman who underwent a knee arthroscopy has postoperative nausea and vomiting (PONV) in the postanesthesia care unit (PACU). Per report, she received ondan-setron 4 mg IV 30 minutes prior to the conclusion of her procedure. Which of the following treatments is most appropriate for managing her PONV in the PACU?

    A. Scopolamine patch
    B. Dexamethasone
    C. Ondansetron
    D. Promethazine

40. Which of the following is the most frequent cause of delayed awakening in the postanesthesia care unit (PACU)?

    A. Hypothermia
    B. Hypoglycemia
    C. Residual effects of sedatives
    D. Hypercarbia

41. Which of the following general principles regarding discharge from the postanesthesia care unit (PACU) is correct?

    A. A mandatory minimum stay in the PACU is not required
    B. Patients should not be discharged until they are pain-free
    C. Patients need to void prior to PACU discharge
    D. Patients need to demonstrate the ability to drink and retain clear fluids prior to PACU discharge

42. According to the ASA Standards for Postanesthesia Care, which of the following statements is correct?

    A. A patient is to be transported to the postanesthesia care unit (PACU) by at least one phy-sician
    B. A patient must be monitored by continuous pulse oximetry during transport to the PACU
    C. A patient who solely received regional anesthesia may routinely bypass the PACU
    D. A patient must be discharged from the PACU by a physician

43. An otherwise-healthy adult male breathing room air receives a large dose of opioid that depresses his ventilation to the point that his alveolar $Paco_2$ is 80 mm Hg. What is his predicted alveolar Pao_2?

    A. 40 mm Hg
    B. 50 mm Hg
    C. 70 mm Hg
    D. 90 mm Hg

44. If the patient described in the previous question is administered 2 L of oxygen by nasal cannula, then his alveolar Pao_2 increases to what amount?

    A. 60 mm Hg
    B. 80 mm Hg
    C. 100 mm Hg
    D. 120 mm Hg

45. A 42-year-old woman complains of pain and inability to dorsiflex the first toe. The nerve most likely to be involved is the

    A. Sciatic
    B. Femoral
    C. Tibial
    D. Peroneal

46. Which of the following clinical criteria is associated with transfusion-related acute lung injury (TRALI) as compared to transfusion-associated circulatory overload (TACO)?

    A. Pulmonary edema
    B. Hypoxemia
    C. Leukopenia
    D. Leukocytosis

47. Which of the following statements regarding postoperative shivering is most correct?

    A. Occurs with general anesthesia but not epidural anesthesia
    B. Is always associated with a decrease in body temperature
    C. In normothermic patients is related to a hypothalamic depressant effects of opioids
    D. In normothermic patients results from uninhibited spinal reflexes

48. A 49-year-old woman with nephrolithiasis develops tachycardia, low-grade fever, and hypotension after a ureteral stent placement. Urine output is 5 to 10 mL/hr. All of the following can be used to treat the patient, except

    A. Antibiotics
    B. Fluids
    C. Diuretics
    D. Vasopressors

49. All of the following are advantages of high-flow nasal cannula delivery systems, except

    A. Humidification of the gas
    B. Gas delivery up to 6 L/min
    C. Deliver of gas throughout the respiratory cycle
    D. Ability to deliver warm gas (37°C)

50. Which of the following procedures is most likely to be associated with postoperative hypertension?

    A. Craniotomy
    B. Colectomy
    C. Gastric bypass
    D. Hip arthroplasty

CHAPTER 20 ANSWERS

1. **B.**   Critical respiratory events accounted for more than half of the PACU malpractice claims in the US closed-claims database.

2. **D.**   The ASA has adopted Standards for Postanesthesia Care that delineate the minimum requirements for PACU monitoring and care. All of the statements are contained within the ASA Standards for Postanesthesia Care.

3. **A.**   Airway obstruction is a common and potentially devastating complication in the postoperative period. The most frequent cause of postoperative airway obstruction is the loss of pharyngeal tone due to the residual depressant effects of inhaled and intravenous anesthetics and the persistent effects of neuromuscular-blocking drugs.

4. **D.**   The possibility of residual neuromuscular blockade must be considered as a potential cause of upper airway obstruction in any patient who received neuromuscular-blocking drugs during anesthesia. Residual neuromuscular blockade may not be clinically evident because the diaphragm recovers from neuromuscular blockade before the pharyngeal muscles do. End-tidal carbon dioxide concentrations, oxygen saturation, and tidal volumes may indicate adequate ventilation and oxygenation, while the ability to maintain a patent upper airway and clear upper airway secretions remains compromised.

5. **A.**   Measurement of the TOF ratio is commonly used to assess reversal of neuromuscular blockade. Significant clinical weakness may persist to a ratio of 0.7, and pharyngeal function does not return to baseline until an adductor pollicis TOF ratio is greater than 0.9.

6. **B.**   In awake patients, clinical assessment of reversal of neuromuscular blockade is preferred to the application of painful train-of-four or tetanic stimulation. Clinical evaluation includes grip strength, tongue protrusion, the ability to lift the legs off the bed, and the ability to lift the head off the bed for a full 5 seconds. Of these maneuvers, the 5-second sustained head lift is considered the gold standard because it reflects not only generalized motor strength but, more importantly, the patient's ability to maintain and protect the airway.

7. **A.**   If persistence or return of neuromuscular weakness in the postanesthesia care unit is suspected, prompt review of possible etiologic factors is indicated. Metabolic states that can contribute to prolonged neuromuscular blockade include hypocalcemia, hypermagnesemia, hypothermia, respiratory acidosis, and hepatic and renal failure.

8. **C.**   Laryngospasm refers to a sudden spasm of the vocal cords that completely occludes the laryngeal opening. Although it is most likely to occur in the operating room at the time of tracheal extubation, patients who arrive in the PACU asleep after general anesthesia are also at risk for laryngospasm. Jaw thrust with CPAP is often sufficient stimulation to "break" the laryngospasm. If jaw thrust and CPAP maneuvers fail, then administration of propofol and providing muscle relaxation with succinylcholine are effective treatments.

9. **D.**   Airway edema is a possible complication in patients undergoing prolonged procedures in the prone position and in procedures with large amounts of blood loss, requiring aggressive fluid resuscitation. Although facial and scleral edema are important physical signs that can alert the clinician to the presence of airway edema, significant edema of pharyngeal tissue is often not accompanied by visible external signs. If tracheal extubation is to be attempted in these patients in the postanesthesia care unit, evaluation of airway patency must precede removal of the endotracheal tube (ETT). The patient's ability to breathe around the ETT can be evaluated by a "cuff-leak" test. By deflating the ETT cuff and with occlusion of the proximal end of the ETT, the patient is asked to breathe around the tube. Good air movement suggests that the patent's airway will remain patent after tracheal extubation. Though helpful, the cuff-leak "test" does not fully exclude the presence of airway edema.

10. **A.** Patients with OSA are particularly prone to airway obstruction and, therefore, deserve special consideration in the postanesthesia care unit (PACU). Patients with OSA are exquisitely sensitive to opioids, and when possible, continuous regional anesthesia techniques should be used to provide postoperative analgesia. Benzodiazepines can have a more intense effect on pharyngeal muscle tone than opioids and, therefore, can contribute to airway obstruction in the PACU. When caring for a patient with OSA, plans should be made preoperatively to provide CPAP in the immediate postoperative period. The majority of patients with mild to moderate OSA are undiagnosed at the time of surgery; therefore, care should be taken to identify at-risk patients based on preoperative clinical suspicion, a history of snoring, and daytime sleepiness.

11. **B.** An obstructed upper airway requires immediate attention. It may not be possible to mask-ventilate a patient with severe upper airway obstruction as a result of edema or hematoma. In the case of hematoma after carotid surgery, an attempt should be made to decompress the airway by opening the wound and evacuating the hematoma. This maneuver may not effectively decompress the airway if a significant amount of fluid or blood has infiltrated the tissue planes of the pharyngeal wall. If emergency tracheal intubation is required, it is important to have ready access to difficult airway equipment and surgical backup for performance of an emergency tracheostomy.

12. **C.** Alveolar hypoventilation and atelectasis are the most common causes of transient postoperative hypoxemia in the PACU. Microaspiration, pneumothorax, and pulmonary embolus are less common causes of postoperative hypoxemia.

13. **C.** Under normal conditions, minute ventilation increases by approximately 2 L/min for every 1-mm Hg increase in arterial $Paco_2$. This normal ventilatory response to carbon dioxide can be significantly depressed in the immediate postoperative period by the residual effects of drugs.

14. **D.** Increased venous admixture, decreased alveolar partial pressure of oxygen, ventilation-to-perfusion mismatch, and shunt are causes of arterial hypoxemia in the postoperative period. Increased venous admixture is due to mixing of desaturated venous blood with oxygenated arterial blood. Normally, only 2% to 5% of cardiac output is shunted through the lungs, and this small amount of shunted blood with a normal mixed venous saturation has a minimal effect on Pao_2. In low cardiac output states, or conditions in which the shunt fraction increases (such as pulmonary edema and atelectasis), there is mixing of a greater amount of desaturated shunted blood with saturated arterialized blood, which decreases the Pao_2.

15. **C.** Postobstructive pulmonary edema is a rare, but significant complication resulting from upper airway obstruction produced by the exaggerated negative pressure generated by inspiration against a closed glottis. This exaggerated negative intrathoracic pressure increases venous return, which further promotes the transudation of fluid. Muscular healthy patients are at increased risk because of their ability to generate significant inspiratory force. Laryngospasm is the most common cause of upper airway obstruction leading to postobstructive pulmonary edema, but pulmonary edema may result from any condition that occludes the upper airway. Arterial hypoxemia is usually manifested within 90 minutes after development of postobstructive pulmonary edema and is accompanied by bilateral fluffy infiltrates on the chest radiograph. The diagnosis depends on clinical suspicion once other causes of pulmonary edema are ruled out. Treatment is supportive and includes supplemental oxygen, diuresis, and positive-pressure ventilation.

16. **B.** As a general rule, each L/min of oxygen flow through nasal cannula increases Fio_2 by 0.04, with 5 L/min resulting in approximately 0.41 Fio_2 [$0.04 \times 5 = 0.2 + 0.21$ (room air) $= 0.41$].

17. **D.** Hemodynamic alterations in the postoperative period can have a negative impact on outcome. Surprisingly, postoperative hypertension and tachycardia are more predictive of unplanned admission to the critical care unit and mortality rate than are hypotension and bradycardia.

18. **A.**   Intravascular volume depletion (hypovolemia) is the most common cause of hypotension in the PACU. Common causes of decreased intravascular volume in the immediate postoperative period include ongoing third-space translocation of fluid, inadequate intraoperative fluid replacement, and loss of sympathetic nervous system tone as a result of spinal or epidural blockade. Bleeding should be ruled out as a cause of hypovolemia in patients who have undergone a surgical procedure in which significant blood loss is possible.

19. **A.**   A high sympathetic block (T4) can result in bradycardia and hypotension secondary to blockade of the cardioaccelerator fibers. This should be treated promptly with vasopressors, such as ephedrine, as cardiac arrest secondary to bradycardia and hypotension can ensue. Epinephrine is used when there is severe bradycardia and hypotension.

20. **D.**   Anaphylactic (or anaphylactoid) reactions may be the cause of postoperative hypotension. Anaphylaxis should be considered in cases of sudden refractory hypotension even when not accompanied by the classic signs of bronchospasm and rash. Increased serum tryptase concentrations confirm the occurrence of an allergic reaction, but this change does not differentiate anaphylactic from anaphylactoid reactions. Neuromuscular-blocking drugs are the most common cause of anaphylactic reactions in the operative setting. Epinephrine is the drug of choice to treat anaphylaxis.

21. **A.**   Postoperative ECG changes should be interpreted in light of the patient's cardiac history and risk index. In low-risk patients (<45 years of age, no known cardiac disease, only one risk factor), postoperative ST-segment changes on the ECG do not usually indicate myocardial ischemia. Relatively benign causes of ST-segment changes in these low-risk patients include anxiety, gastroesophageal reflux disease, hyperventilation, and hypokalemia. In general, low-risk patients require only routine postanesthesia care unit observation unless associated signs and symptoms warrant further clinical evaluation.

22. **C.**   A routine postoperative ECG is only recommended for patients with known or suspected CAD who have undergone high- or intermediate-risk surgery. High-risk surgery includes emergency surgery, major vascular surgery, peripheral vascular surgery, and unanticipated prolonged procedures associated with large fluid shifts or blood loss. Intermediate-risk procedures include intra-abdominal and thoracic surgery, carotid endarterectomy, head and neck surgery, orthopedic surgery, and prostate surgery.

23. **D.**   Control of the ventricular response rate is the immediate goal in the treatment of new-onset atrial fibrillation. While most patients can be treated pharmacologically, hemodynamically unstable patients require prompt electrical cardioversion.

24. **C.**   PVCs and ventricular bigeminy are common in the postoperative period. PVCs most often reflect increased sympathetic nervous system stimulation, as many occur with hypoxemia, hypercapnia, and acidemia.

25. **D.**   Bradycardia in the PACU is often iatrogenic. Drug-related causes include administration of α-blockers, opioids, anticholinesterase agents, and treatment with dexmedetomidine. Procedure- and patient-related causes include bowel distention, increased intracranial or intraocular pressure, and spinal anesthesia.

26. **C.**   Approximately 10% of adult patients older than 50 years who undergo elective surgery will develop postoperative delirium within the first five postoperative days.

27. **A.**   Intraoperative factors that are predictive of postoperative delirium include surgical blood loss, the number of intraoperative blood transfusions, and hematocrit less than 30%. Intraoperative hemodynamic derangements and the anesthetic technique do not seem to be predictors of postoperative delirium.

28. **D.**   Many adult patients at risk for postoperative delirium can be identified preoperatively. The most significant preoperative risk factors include (1) advanced age, (2) preoperative cognitive impairment, (3) decreased functional status, (4) alcohol abuse, and (5) a previous history of delirium. Chronic pain is not a risk factor for postoperative delirium.

29. **D.**   Emergence excitement is a transient confusional state that is associated with emergence from general anesthesia. It is common in children, with more than 30% experiencing agitation or delirium at some period during their postanesthesia care unit stay. The peak age of emergence excitement in children is between 2 and 4 years. Unlike delirium, emergence excitement typically resolves quickly and without long-term cognitive sequelae. Preoperative midazolam administration has been associated with an increase in the incidence and duration of emergence delirium in children.

30. **B.**   Postoperative oliguria can result from prerenal, renal, and postrenal causes. Frequently, the cause is multifactorial, with a preexisting renal insufficiency that is exacerbated by an intraoperative insult. Oliguria is defined as urine output less than 0.5 mL/kg/hr.

31. **C.**   POUR is defined as the inability to void despite a bladder volume of more than 500 to 600 mL. Risk factors include male gender, age older than 50 years, intraoperative fluid volume, duration of surgery, and bladder volume on admission. Certain types of surgery are also associated with a higher risk of POUR, including anorectal and joint replacement surgery. Commonly used perioperative medications such as anticholinergics, β-blockers, and narcotics can also contribute to POUR. Diagnosis can be made by clinical examination, bladder catheterization, or ultrasound assessment. Bladder volumes measured by ultrasound imaging correlate well with volumes obtained by urinary catheterization.

32. **D.**   The most common cause of oliguria in the immediate postoperative period is hypovolemia. A fluid challenge is usually effective in restoring urine output. Volume resuscitation to maximize renal perfusion is particularly important in order to prevent the development of acute kidney injury. If an intravascular fluid challenge is contraindicated or oliguria persists, assessment of intravascular volume or cardiac function is indicated to differentiate hypovolemia from low cardiac output states.

33. **D.**   An intra-abdominal pressure higher than 30 cm H_2O can impede renal perfusion, leading to renal ischemia and postoperative renal dysfunction. Bladder pressure should be measured in patients in whom intra-abdominal hypertension is suspected so that abdominal decompression can be performed to relieve intra-abdominal pressure and restore renal perfusion.

34. **B.**   Rhabdomyolysis is a recognized cause of postoperative renal insufficiency in morbidly obese patients, particularly those who have undergone gastric bypass procedures. Risk factors include the body mass index and duration of surgery. Volume loading, diuretics, and alkalinization of urine to flush the renal tubules can prevent ongoing renal tubular damage and subsequent acute renal failure.

35. **D.**   Mild to moderate hypothermia (33–35°C) is a recognized cause of a number of postoperative complications, including inhibition of platelet function, reduced coagulation-factor activity, and decreased drug metabolism. In addition, it exacerbates postoperative bleeding, prolongs neuromuscular blockade, and may delay awakening.

36. **B.**   Core body temperature can most accurately be measured at the tympanic membrane. Axillary, rectal, and nasopharyngeal temperature measurements are less accurate and may underestimate core temperature.

37. **C.**   A number of opioids and clonidine are effective in stopping shivering once it starts, but meperidine is the most effective treatment. Doxapram, a central nervous system stimulant, is somewhat effective in abolishing postoperative shivering.

38. D.   A simple risk score consisting of four factors can be used to identify high-risk patients for PONV. The four risk factors are (1) female gender, (2) history of motion sickness or PONV, (3) nonsmoking, and (4) the use of postoperative opioids. The incidence of PONV correlates with the number of these factors present: zero, one, two, three, or four factors correspond to an incidence of 10%, 21%, 39%, 61%, and 79%, respectively. The patient in the vignette has two risk factors (female, nonsmoker), so her approximate risk of PONV is 40%.

39. D.   When choosing a rescue antiemetic for patients with PONV, both the class of drug and the timing of administration are factors. If an adequate dose of antiemetic given at the appropriate time proves ineffective, simply giving more of the same class of drug in the PACU is unlikely to be of significant benefit. If no prophylactic drug was given, the recommended treatment is a low-dose 5-HT_3 antagonist, ondansetron. Of the choices provided in the vignette, promethazine is likely to be the most effective rescue antiemetic. Since the patient received ondansetron for prophylaxis, additional ondansetron is unlikely to be effective. A scopolamine patch is unlikely to take effect rapidly enough to be beneficial. Dexamethasone, while effective for prophylaxis, is less beneficial for rescue.

40. C.   Even after prolonged surgery and anesthesia, a response to stimulation in 60 to 90 minutes should be expected. The etiology of delayed awakening after anesthesia can be divided into the general categories of pharmacologic, metabolic, and neurologic causes. Of these, residual sedation from drugs used during anesthesia is the most frequent cause of delayed awakening in the PACU.

41. A.   Specific PACU discharge criteria may vary, but certain general principles are universally applicable. These principles include mandatory minimum stay in the PACU is not required, patients must be observed until they are no longer at risk for respiratory depression, and their mental status is clear or has returned to baseline; hemodynamic criteria are based on the patient's baseline hemodynamics without specific systemic blood pressure and heart rate requirements. To facilitate PACU discharge, discharge scoring systems have been developed and modified over time to reflect current anesthesia practice.

42. D.   The Standards for Postanesthesia Care are intended to ensure the quality of postanesthetic patient care. They include the following:

- Standard I: "All patients who have received general anesthesia, regional anesthesia, or monitored anesthesia care shall receive appropriate post anesthesia management"
- Standard II: "A patient transported to the PACU shall be accompanied by a member of the anesthesia care team who is knowledgeable about the patient's condition. The patient shall be continually evaluated and treated during transport with monitoring and support appropriate to the patient's condition"
- Standard III: "Upon arrival to the PACU, the patient shall be reevaluated and a verbal report provided to the responsible PACU nurse by the member of the anesthesia care team who accompanies the patient"
- Standard IV: "The patient's condition shall be evaluated continually in the PACU"
- Standard V: "A physician is responsible for the discharge of the patient from the PACU"

43. B.   At sea level, a normocapnic patient breathing room air will have an alveolar oxygen pressure of 100 mm Hg. Review of the alveolar gas equation demonstrates that hypoventilation alone is sufficient to cause arterial hypoxemia in a patient breathing room air. In this case, a rise in $Paco_2$ from 40 to 80 mm Hg (alveolar hypoventilation) results in an alveolar oxygen pressure (Pao_2) of 50 mm Hg.

$$Pao_2 = Fio_2 \times (Patm - PH_2O) - Paco_2/R$$
$$= 0.21 \times (760 - 47) - 80/0.8$$
$$= 50 \text{ mm Hg}$$

(Patm = atmospheric pressure mm Hg, PH_2O = water vapor pressure mm Hg, R = respiratory quotient—8 CO_2 molecules produced for every oxygen molecule consumed)

44. C.   In the setting of isolated hypoventilation, modest increases in inspired oxygen are remarkably effective at restoring alveolar oxygenation. For this patient, if 2 L of supplemental oxygen is administered by nasal cannula, then the F_{IO_2} increases to approximately 28% and the calculated alveolar Pa_{O_2} is 100 mm Hg.

$$Pa_{O_2} = F_{IO_2} \times (Patm - PH_2O) - Pa_{CO_2}/R$$
$$= 0.28 \times (760 - 47) - 80/0.8$$
$$= 100 \text{ mm Hg}$$

45. D.   An assessment and written documentation of the patient's peripheral nerve function on discharge from the postanesthesia care unit may become useful information should a new peripheral neuropathy develop in the later postoperative period. The peroneal nerve provides the motor innervation for dorsiflexion of the first toe, while the tibial nerve allows plantar flexion of the first toe.

46. C.   TRALI can occur up to 6 hours after transfusion of blood, coagulation factor, or platelet transfusions. Therefore, it should be included in the differential diagnosis of pulmonary edema in the postanesthesia care unit, among patients who received intraoperative transfusions. The resulting noncardiogenic pulmonary edema is often associated with fever, systemic hypotension, and the presence of exudative pulmonary fluid. If a complete blood count is obtained with the onset of symptoms, an acute decrease in the white blood cell count (leukopenia) reflecting the sequestration of granulocytes is seen within the lung. Initially, it may be difficult distinguishing TRALI from TACO caused by volume overload resulting from the blood products transfused. In either case, treatment is supportive and includes supplemental oxygen, dieresis, and mechanical ventilation, if needed.

47. D.   Postoperative shivering commonly occurs after both general and neuraxial anesthesia and is usually, but not always, associated with a decrease in the patient's body temperature. Although thermoregulatory mechanisms can explain shivering in a hypothermic patient, a separate mechanism has been proposed to explain shivering in normothermic patients. The mechanism of normothermic shivering is thought to be a result from uninhibited spinal reflexes, which are manifested as clonic activity.

48. C.   Urinary tract manipulation can result in sepsis in the postanesthesia care unit. In these cases, hypotension is often accompanied by fever and rigor. If sepsis is suspected, fluid resuscitation and vasopressor support should be initiated, blood should be obtained for culture, and antibiotic therapy should be administered. The patient's low urine output should be improved with hemodynamic support. Diuretics are not indicated for a hypovolemic patient with sepsis.

49. B.   Delivery of oxygen by traditional nasal cannula is limited to 6 L/min flow to minimize discomfort and complications that result from inadequate humidification. Alternatively, oxygen can be delivered up to 40 L/min by high-flow nasal cannula systems, which humidify and warm the gas to 99.9% relative humidity and 37°C. Unlike non-rebreather masks, these devices deliver oxygen directly to the nasopharynx throughout the respiratory cycle.

50. A.   A number of patient, procedural, and postoperative factors can contribute to the development of postoperative hypertension. Patients with a history of essential hypertension are at greatest risk for significant systemic hypertension in the postanesthesia care unit. Advanced age, history of cigarette smoking, and preexisting renal disease are other patient-related risk factors for postoperative hypertension. Surgical procedures that predispose the patient to postoperative hypertension include craniotomy and carotid endarterectomy. Other common postoperative causes of hypertension include pain, hypoxemia, hypoventilation and associated hypercapnia, emergence excitement, shivering, bladder distension, drug withdrawal, and hypervolemia.

CHAPTER 21

Miscellaneous Topics

Paul Sikka and Thomas Halaszynski

1. A 90-year-old male is presented to the operating room for surgical repair of a right femoral neck fracture. His medical history is significant for chronic obstructive pulmonary disease (60 pack year smoking history) and is prescribed 4 L/min of continuous home oxygen. A note from his pulmonologist states that this patient is a high-risk candidate for general anesthesia and will prove to be difficult to wean from mechanical ventilation. To properly assess the respiratory risk for this patient, which of the following will provide the least beneficial value?

   A. Stat pulmonary function tests
   B. Baseline chest radiograph
   C. Thorough history and physical examination
   D. Baseline arterial blood gas

2. A 65-year-old female, status post coronary artery bypass grafting (CABG) 2 weeks ago, is scheduled for a fem-fem bypass. The patient has been recovering well since her routine two-vessel cardiac bypass surgery, but continues to experience intermittent claudication symptoms of the left lower extremity. The surgeon informs you that the patient was scheduled for the vascular bypass surgery several weeks ago, but could not undergo the surgery due to her poor cardiac function. Now that cardiac pathology has been resolved, he would like to proceed with the vascular procedure as soon as possible. Your recommendations to the vascular surgeon would be

   A. Provided she is without cardiac symptoms, the vascular surgery can now be performed
   B. The vascular procedure should be delayed for another 2 weeks
   C. The surgeon needs to obtain cardiology clearance prior to the procedure
   D. The vascular surgery should be delayed for at least 6 months following the CABG procedure

3. A 76-year-old female comes to the preadmission clinic for anesthetic evaluation prior to a right total hip replacement (THR) scheduled in 2 weeks. Her medical history is significant for coronary artery disease (status post stent placement 6 months ago) and baseline unstable angina one to two times per month. The patient indicates that her symptoms are relieved by sublingual nitroglycerin. A recent echocardiogram (30 days prior) showed an ejection fraction of 30% along with evidence of inferior-wall-motion abnormality. Examination of the most current EKG shows diffuse T-wave inversions with a heart rate of 60 to 65 bpm (on metoprolol) and a blood pressure of 125/60 mm Hg. In addition, the patient has severe chronic obstructive pulmonary disease, is dependent upon 2 L/min home O_2, and has obstructive sleep apnea (on bi-level positive-airway pressure at night). In order to maximize the preoperative condition of this patient, you will order all of the following diagnostic tests/examinations/consultations, except

   A. Repeat the cardiac catheterization and confirm whether or not the patient requires coronary artery bypass grafting (CABG) surgery prior to THR
   B. Communicate with cardiologist to confirm patient is medically optimized
   C. Would not introduce any more coronary interventions unless new symptoms are present
   D. Maintain hemodynamic stability during THR surgery

4. A 74-year-old patient undergoes a lumbar sympathetic blockade to improve blood flow after sustaining a frostbite injury to the left lower extremity. Clinical findings that would suggest a successful block include

   A. Inability to dorsiflex the foot
   B. Piloerection on the legs
   C. Numbness from the knee to the toes
   D. Temperature increase in the legs

5. The nerve that needs to be blocked to obliterate the gag reflex when applying pressure to the posterior portion of the tongue during an awake fiberoptic intubation is the

   A. Recurrent laryngeal nerve
   B. Glossopharyngeal nerve
   C. Superior laryngeal nerve
   D. Inferior laryngeal nerve

6. A 74-year-old patient undergoes a stellate ganglion block secondary to extreme hot flashes and night awakenings secondary to a long history of breast cancer. Potential complications include all of the following, except

   A. Recurrent laryngeal nerve paralysis
   B. Subarachnoid block
   C. Pneumothorax
   D. All of the above

7. Incorrect statement regarding metabolic equivalent (MET) is

   A. 1 MET = consumption of 3.5 mL O_2/min/kg of body weight
   B. 5 MET = climbing one to two flights of stairs, dancing, or bicycling
   C. 4 MET = equivalent to gardening
   D. 2 MET = equivalent to getting dressed

8. A 35-year-old G2P1 at 30 weeks gestational age is coming to the OR within the next hour for open reduction internal fixation of an ankle fracture. The patient's blood type is O^+ and has hematocrit of 32. All of the following should be arranged, except

   A. Prepare for a perioperative obstetrical (OB) consultation
   B. Type screen and crossmatch for blood
   C. Intraoperative RhoGam injection prior to surgery start
   D. Prepare for perioperative fetal monitoring

9. An E-cylinder of oxygen with a pressure of 1,000 psig and being used at a rate of 2 L/min will run out in

   A. 2 hours
   B. 3 hours
   C. 4 hours
   D. 6 hours

10. A 49-year-old patient is undergoing a craniotomy for tumor resection. Intraoperatively, the patient received drugs including thiopental, vecuronium, isoflurane, and fentanyl. The patient is brought to the postanesthesia care unit with a HR of 58/min, BP of 196/96 mm Hg, and oxygen saturation of 98%. A few moments later the patient has two episodes of vomiting. You would then

   A. Give ondansetron
   B. Give metoclopramide
   C. Give fentanyl
   D. Call the neurosurgeon

11. Parkinsonism is associated with

    A. Loss of dopaminergic neurons alone
    B. Loss of cholinergic neurons alone
    C. Loss of cholinergic and increase in dopaminergic activity
    D. Loss of dopaminergic and increase in cholinergic activity

12. A 36-year-old patient with multiple sclerosis (MS) is to undergo an exploratory laparotomy. The best anesthesia technique to prevent a flare-up of symptoms would be

    A. General anesthesia with endotracheal intubation using a nondepolarizing muscle relaxant
    B. General anesthesia with endotracheal intubation using a depolarizing muscle relaxant
    C. Spinal anesthesia
    D. Combined spinal–epidural anesthesia

13. The primary aim of using succinylcholine for anesthesia for electroconvulsive therapy (ECT) is to

    A. Prevent loss of airway
    B. Control excessive seizure activity
    C. Control cardiovascular sympathetic discharge
    D. Prevent musculoskeletal injuries

14. Cardiovascular response following an electroconvulsive therapy (ECT) is characterized by

    A. An initial parasympathetic discharge followed by a sympathetic discharge
    B. An initial sympathetic discharge followed by a parasympathetic discharge
    C. Sympathetic discharge alone
    D. Parasympathetic discharge alone

15. Nondepolarizing muscle relaxants block which of the following receptors?

    A. Adrenergic
    B. Calcium
    C. Muscarinic
    D. Nicotinic

16. Ipratropium acts to relieve bronchospasm via which of the following receptors?

    A. Nicotinic
    B. Muscarinic
    C. α Receptors
    D. β-Receptors

17. All statements regarding neostigmine are true, except

    A. It inhibits acetylcholinesterase
    B. It inhibits pseudocholinesterase
    C. It shortens the duration of action of succinylcholine
    D. It can cause neuromuscular blockade

18. When using neostigmine to reverse neuromuscular blockade in the presence of severe renal disease, you would use the following dose when compared to a normal patient

    A. Same
    B. Higher
    C. Lower
    D. Titrated

19. Fastest acting neuromuscular reversal agent is

    A. Edrophonium
    B. Neostigmine
    C. Pyridostigmine
    D. Physostigmine

20. Highest plasma concentration of a local anesthetic will occur if infiltrated via which of the following routes?

    A. Tracheal
    B. Caudal
    C. Intercostal
    D. Brachial plexus

21. A 27-year-old 38 weeks pregnant female presents with painless vaginal bleeding. The best step in the management of this patient is

    A. Direct examination with a vaginal speculum and then take the patient to OR for cesarean section
    B. Cesarean section
    C. Bed rest and observation
    D. Epidural after bleeding stops

22. The most frequent cause of delayed emergence in the postanesthesia care unit is

    A. Residual anesthetic agents
    B. Hypoventilation
    C. Hypotension
    D. Hypothermia

23. Emergence from inhalational anesthetics is primarily dependent on

    A. Type of agent used
    B. Cardiac output
    C. Ventilation
    D. Adjunct anesthetic drugs

24. Emergence from intravenous anesthetics is primarily dependent on

    A. Redistribution
    B. Elimination half-life
    C. Type of agent used
    D. Hepatic or renal disease

25. A 35-year-old patient is brought to the postanesthesia care unit (PACU) after undergoing an appendectomy. His anesthetics included propofol 140 mg, isoflurane 2.0 MAC, vecuronium 6 mg, and morphine 6 mg. In the PACU, the patient is shivering. The most likely cause of his shivering is

    A. Use of isoflurane
    B. Presence of infection and dehydration
    C. Use of unwarmed fluids
    D. Use of morphine

26. Best method to prevent shivering is

    A. Use warmed fluids
    B. Warming lights
    C. Meperidine
    D. Forced-air-warming device

27. A 56-year-old patient, with a tracheostomy, is undergoing a radical neck dissection under general anesthesia. The induction is uneventful and you proceed to replace the tracheostomy tube with an endotracheal tube for the procedure. The patient's peak airway inspiratory pressures increase suddenly. The most likely diagnosis is

    A. Bronchospasm
    B. Pneumothorax
    C. Malposition of the endotracheal tube (ETT)
    D. Patient attempting to breath

28. Laryngospasm (LS) is due to stimulation of the

    A. Superior laryngeal nerve
    B. Internal laryngeal nerve
    C. Recurrent laryngeal nerve
    D. External laryngeal nerve

CHAPTER 21 ANSWERS

1. **A.** Pulmonary function test results have not been shown to be beneficial or to guide treatment when planning for intraoperative anesthesia. History and physical exam are the basics and important in anesthesia plan formulation. Baseline chest films along with arterial blood gas results are not indicated in every pulmonary patient, but may be helpful in anesthesia decision-making and intraoperative anesthetic management.

2. **B.** With the exception of emergency surgery, current guidelines suggest waiting at least for a 1-month time interval following a coronary intervention, before proceeding with any elective surgical procedure.

3. **A.** Generally speaking, the indications for cardiovascular investigations are the same in surgical patients as in any other patient. Unless the combined risk of coronary intervention and surgery is less than surgery alone without coronary intervention, preoperative CABG/stent, etc., is not generally suggested.

4. **D.** Indications for a lumbar sympathetic blockade include diagnosis, prognosis, and therapy of circulatory and pain conditions such as inoperable peripheral vascular disease, vasospastic disease (lower), reflexive sympathetic dystrophies and herpes zoster (lower), and the presence of pain (neuropathic, urogenic/pelvic, cancer pain, and phantom limb). Contraindications for a lumbar sympathetic blockade include anticoagulant therapy, hemorrhagic disorder, allergy to injected medications, infection, local neoplasm, and local vascular anomalies. Lumbar sympathetic chain includes L3–L5 ganglia, and is positioned anterior to L2, L3, and L4 vertebral bodies, anterior to the psoas muscle margin and fascia, posterior to the vena cava on the right, and posterior to the aorta on the left. Complications of a lumbar sympathetic blockade include blockade of the L2 somatic nerve root, injection into the subarachnoid/epidural/intravascular (vena cava/aorta/lumbar vessels) spaces, damage by needle or neurolytics to the kidneys/renal pelvis/ureters/intervertebral disks, infection, backache, neuropathic pain, hematoma, sympathalgia, destruction of sympathetic fibers (cramping/burning pain to anterior thigh), sympathectomy-mediated hypotension, intravascular steal (especially arteriosclerotic patient), and failure of ejaculation.

5. **B.** Airway blockade techniques: For anesthesia of nasal mucosa and nasopharynx, and nasal intubation, the sphenopalatine ganglion and ethmoid nerves need to be anesthetized. For anesthesia of the mouth (oropharynx and tongue base), the glossopharyngeal and superior laryngeal nerve blocks need to be performed. For anesthesia of the hypopharynx, larynx, and trachea, the recurrent laryngeal nerve needs to be blocked by performing a transtracheal block.

6. **D.** Complications of stellate ganglion block include hematoma formation (vascular injury to carotid artery, internal jugular vein), nerve injury (vagus, brachial plexus roots), pneumothorax, esophageal perforation, intravascular injection (carotid or vertebral artery, internal jugular vein), epidural or intrathecal injection, hoarseness of voice (recurrent laryngeal nerve), elevated hemidiaphragm (phrenic nerve), infection, and Horner syndrome (ptosis, anhidrosis, miosis).

7. **D.** 1 MET = consumption of 3.5 mL O_2/min/kg of body weight. Typically, 1 MET = dressing or eating; 2 MET = walking downstairs or cooking; 4 MET = gardening; 5 MET = climbing one to two flights of stairs. A patient unable to achieve the level of 4 to 5 MET is at an increasing risk of perioperative complications, typically cardiopulmonary adverse reactions.

8. **C.** The patient is Rh O^+; therefore, there exists no need for RhoGam immunoglobulin injection. OB consultation should be initiated with any pregnant patient, and the obstetrician should decide the need for appropriate perioperative monitoring (continuous monitoring versus pre- and postoperative monitoring) of the mother and the fetus based upon the stage of pregnancy.

9. **B.** An E-cylinder of oxygen at 1,000 psig is approximately half full, that is, it has about 330 L of oxygen. If being consumed at a rate of 2 L/min, it will be exhausted in about 3 hours.

10. **D.** Vomiting in patient who has undergone an intracranial procedure may indicate raised intracranial pressure. Therefore, the patient needs to be evaluated immediately, and the neurosurgeon needs to be notified.

11. **D.** Parkinsonism of Parkinson disease (called when no identifiable cause) is associated with a loss of dopaminergic activity and a reciprocal increase in cholinergic activity in the brain.

12. **A.** General anesthesia is most often used in patients with MS. Regarding muscle relaxants, the use of succinylcholine should be avoided, as demyelination and denervation may increase the risk of succinylcholine-induced hyperkalemia. Nondepolarizing neuromuscular blockers are safe to use, but patients of MS may have altered sensitivity and prolonged duration of action, which may necessitate postoperative ventilation. Therefore, nondepolarizing muscle relaxants should be administered in minimal doses. Regarding regional anesthesia, spinal and epidural anesthesia and peripheral nerve blocks have been successfully used in patients with MS. Although spinal anesthesia has been implicated in postoperative exacerbations of MS symptoms, the finding is not fully confirmed. Furthermore, intraoperatively the patient's temperature should be closely monitored, as even slight increases in body temperature may cause a decline in neurologic function postoperatively.

13. **D.** ECT is performed under general anesthesia. The patient is preoxygenated, and general anesthesia is induced with a hypnotic (methohexital or propofol). Once the patient is asleep, succinylcholine is administered to relax the muscles. Seizures produced by ECT have been known to cause musculoskeletal injuries and joint dislocations. Therefore, succinylcholine is used to relax the muscle and prevent such injuries. Airway is maintained with mask ventilation.

14. **A.** Cardiovascular response following an ECT consists of an initial parasympathetic response followed by a sympathetic response. The parasympathetic response may lead to severe bradycardia in some. Glycopyrrolate administered pre-ECT may attenuate the parasympathetic response and also decrease secretions. The sympathetic response leads to tachycardia and hypertension, which may lead to deleterious effects in patients with coronary artery disease. The sympathetic discharge can be attenuated by using β-blockers (esmolol, metoprolol) or labetalol.

15. **D.** Nondepolarizing muscle relaxants inhibit neuronal transmission to the muscle by blocking the nicotinic acetylcholine receptors. They act as competitive antagonists to acetylcholine (Ach) and prevent the binding of Ach to the receptors.

16. **B.** Ipratropium (atrovent) is a bronchodilator and acts on the muscarinic acetylcholine receptors in the smooth muscles of the bronchi in the lung when inhaled. It is a derivative of atropine, but has a quaternary amine structure and thus it does not cross the blood–brain barrier to cause central effects. Although ipratropium is commonly combined with albuterol as a rescue agent for bronchospasm, it should not be used as a replacement for albuterol.

17. **C.** Neostigmine is a reversible acetylcholinesterase inhibitor, the enzyme that breaks down acetylcholine. This leads to more acetylcholine being available for neuromuscular transmission, which can now competitively displace the nondepolarizing muscle relaxant molecules to cause the return of neuromuscular activity. Since succinylcholine is broken down by a similar enzyme (pseudocholinesterase), neostigmine administration leads to the prolongation of duration of action of succinylcholine. It should be remembered that neostigmine, when given (unintended) without the prior administration of a nondepolarizing muscle relaxant, can directly act as a muscle relaxant when given in sufficient dose.

18. **A.** Renal excretion accounts for about 50% of excretion of neostigmine (about 75% of that of pyridostigmine and edrophonium). It is important to note that the presence of renal failure decreases the plasma clearance of not only neostigmine (and pyridostigmine, edrophonium) but also nondepolarizing muscle relaxants. Therefore, if neostigmine is administered in the usual dosage, and overdoses of muscle relaxants are avoided, renal failure should not be associated with recurarization.

19. **A.** Edrophonium is given in a dose of 0.5 to 1 mg/kg and has an onset of action in 30 to 60 seconds. Peak action occurs in 1 to 5 minutes and duration of action of is about 5 to 20 minutes. Because of its short duration of action, patients should be monitored for the effects of recurarization. Onset of neostigmine's action (0.04–0.07 mg/kg) is in 1 to 3 minutes, peak effect occurs in 5 to 7 minutes, and duration of action is 40 to 60 minutes. Pyridostigmine is not used for neuromuscular reversal, and physostigmine has no role in neuromuscular blockade reversal.

20. **C.** Local anesthetics, when infiltrated into tissues, get absorbed into the circulation to some extent. The amount of local anesthetic absorbed into circulation depends upon the vascularity of the area. Highest blood concentration occurs with intercostal infiltration due to the high vascularity of the area.

21. **B.** Painless vaginal bleeding is most commonly due to placenta previa. A full-term parturient who presents with active painless vaginal bleeding should be taken to the operating room for cesarean section under general anesthesia. Examination with a vaginal speculum may initiate massive hemorrhage and hence should be not performed. Patients should have large-bore IVs (even a central line) for adequate fluid resuscitation, and blood should be available for transfusion. Patients with placenta previa, who are less than 37 weeks of gestation, and with mild bleeding, may be managed with bed rest and observation.

22. **A.** The most common cause of delayed emergence is residual anesthetics. These can be sedatives, analgesics, muscle relaxants, or volatile inhalational agents. Overdose of narcotics can be reversed by naloxone, benzodiazepines can be reversed by flumazenil, muscle relaxants are reversed with an appropriate dose of neostigmine–glycopyrrolate and administered as per the train-of-four twitch monitoring, and volatile agents are washed out by adequate ventilation. Hypoventilation can lead to hypoxia and hypercarbia. Hypothermia potentiates the effects of CNS depressants, and can be prevented by using forced-air-warming devices, using warm intravenous fluids, and raising the ambient room temperature. Other causes of delayed emergence include hypotension and metabolic abnormalities.

23. **C.** Once the administration of volatile agent is stopped at the end of the surgery, the washout or elimination occurs primarily through the lungs. Hence, adequate ventilation is the main route of elimination of volatile inhalational agents. Hypoventilation due to any cause will decrease the washout of volatile anesthetics and delay emergence from anesthesia.

24. **A.** Emergence from intravenous anesthetics depends primarily on redistribution from the brain. However, as the intravenous drugs accumulate, due to repeated administration or infusion, emergence becomes dependent on metabolism and elimination half-life. Presence of hepatic or renal disease, and the pharmacokinetics of the agents, also affects emergence from anesthesia.

25. **A.** Volatile inhalational agents cause peripheral vasodilation and cause redistribution of heat from the body core to the peripheral compartment. Using isoflurane in such a high concentration (2 MAC) is the most likely cause of shivering in the PACU in this patient. Other causes that can cause shivering are cold ambient operating room temperature, using unwarmed intravenous fluids, and an open large wound (exploratory laparotomy). Shivering tries to raise the body's temperature by causing intense vasoconstriction. In addition, shivering can increase

the oxygen demand tremendously, which can be of issue in patients with coronary artery disease. Shivering can be treated with meperidine (12.5–25 mg IV). Hypothermia should be treated by raising the room temperature or by using a forced-air-warming device.

26. **D.** One of the best methods to prevent hypothermia and shivering is using a forced-air-warming device intraoperatively or in the postanesthesia care unit. Meperidine is commonly used to treat shivering, 12.5 to 25 mg IV. Warming lights, raising the room temperature, and using warm intravenous fluids are other methods to prevent or treat hypothermia.

27. **C.** Patients undergoing radical neck dissection for laryngeal cancer often have a tracheostomy tube. After induction, the tracheostomy tube is commonly replaced with an ETT, which is sutured into place by the surgeon. The ETT should be placed carefully, and adequacy of ventilation should be checked by ausculating breath sounds and the presence of end-tidal CO_2. A malposition of the ETT, including placement in a false passage will lead to high peak inspiratory pressures. Other causes listed can also lead to high inspiratory pressures.

28. **A.** LS is a forceful involuntary spasm of laryngeal muscles. It is due to stimulation of the superior laryngeal nerve. LS occurs commonly due to intense stimulation during light anesthesia (during extubation). Also, the presence of oral secretions can lead to LS. Treatment of LS is done by providing positive-pressure breaths (bag and mask) with 100% oxygen. This usually breaks the LS. However, if LS persists, succinylcholine is administered in a small dose (0.25 mg/kg) to relax the laryngeal muscles.

    Side effects of inhaled ipratropium are minimal and include dry mouth, skin flushing, tachycardia, palpitations, and headache. It is contraindicated for use in patients with narrow angle–closure glaucoma. In patients with prostatic hypertrophy, it can lead to urinary retention, and hence should be used with caution in these patients.

    Parkinsonism is characterized by progressive loss of motor function resulting from the degeneration of neurons in substantia nigra region of the brain. The onset of Parkinson disease typically occurs between the ages of 60 and 70 years. Clinical signs include a slight tremor of the thumb and forefinger (pill-rolling tremor), muscular rigidity (arms, legs, neck), bradykinesia (difficulty in initiating movement), postural instability, a shuffling gait, lack of facial expression (masked face), and difficulty in swallowing or speaking. The disease slowly progresses over 10 to 20 years, resulting in paralysis, dementia, and death.